Environmental Health
SOURCEBOOK

Fifth Edition

Fifth Edition

Environmental Health
SOURCEBOOK

*Basic Consumer Health Information about the
Environment and Its Effects on Human Health, Including
Facts about Air, Water, and Soil Contamination, Hazardous
Chemicals, Foodborne Hazards and Illnesses, Household
Hazards Such as Radon, Mold, and Carbon Monoxide,
Consumer Hazards from Toxic Products and Imported
Goods, and Disorders Linked to Environmental Causes,
Including Cancer, Allergies, and Asthma*

*Along with Information about the Impact of
Environmental Hazards on Specific Populations, a
Glossary of Related Terms, and Resources for
Additional Help and Information*

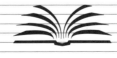

OMNIGRAPHICS

615 Griswold, Ste. 901, Detroit, MI 48226

Bibliographic Note
Because this page cannot legibly accommodate all the copyright notices, the Bibliographic Note portion of the Preface constitutes an extension of the copyright notice.

* * *

OMNIGRAPHICS
Angela L. Williams, *Managing Editor*
***

Copyright © 2018 Omnigraphics
ISBN 978-0-7808-1628-2
E-ISBN 978-0-7808-1629-9

Library of Congress Cataloging-in-Publication Data
Names: Omnigraphics, Inc., issuing body.

Title: Environmental health sourcebook: basic consumer health information about the environment and its effects on human health, including facts about air, water, and soil contamination, hazardous chemicals, foodborne hazards and illnesses, household hazards such as radon, mold, and carbon monoxide, consumer hazards from toxic products and imported goods, and disorders linked to environmental causes, including chemical sensitivity, cancer, allergies, and asthma; along with information about the impact of environmental hazards on specific populations, a glossary of related terms, and resources for additional help and information.

Description: Fifth edition. | Detroit, MI: Omnigraphics, [2018] | Series: Health reference series | Includes bibliographical references and index.

Identifiers: LCCN 2018009596 (print) | LCCN 2018010498 (ebook) | ISBN 9780780816299 (eBook) | ISBN 9780780816282 (hardcover: alk. paper)

Subjects: LCSH: Environmental health. | Environmentally induced diseases. | Environmental toxicology.

Classification: LCC RA565 (ebook) | LCC RA565.E484 2018 (print) | DDC 615.9/02--dc23

LC record available at https://lccn.loc.gov/2018009596

Table of Contents

Part II: Health Concerns and Their Environmental Triggers

Part III: Outdoor Environmental Hazards: Air, Water, and Soil

Part IV: Household and Indoor Hazards

Part V: Foodborne Hazards

Part VI: Consumer Products and Medical Hazards

Part VII: Additional Help and Information

Preface

About This Book

Humans interact with the environment constantly. These interactions affect the quality of life, years of healthy life lived, and health disparities. The World Health Organization (WHO) defines environment, as it relates to health, as "all the physical, chemical, and biological factors external to a person, and all the related behaviors." Environmental health consists of preventing or controlling disease, injury, and disability related to the interactions between people and their environment. Maintaining a healthy environment is central to increasing quality of life and years of healthy life. Globally, 23 percent of all deaths and 26 percent of deaths among children under age 5 are due to preventable environmental factors. Poor environmental quality has its greatest impact on people whose health status is already at risk. Therefore, environmental health must address the societal and environmental factors that increase the likelihood of exposure and disease.

Environmental Health Sourcebook, Fifth Edition offers updated information about the effects of the environment on human health. It discusses specific populations—including pregnant women and their fetuses, children, the elderly, and minorities—in which the effects of environmental exposures are especially harmful and, in some cases, can have a lasting impact that extends to future generations. Airborne, waterborne, foodborne, and chemical hazards are discussed, and facts about cancer, respiratory problems, infertility, autism, and other diseases with suspected environmental triggers are presented. A section on consumer products and medical hazards examines health risks associated with some common household items. The book concludes with a glossary and a directory of resources for additional information.

How to Use This Book

This book is divided into parts and chapters. Parts focus on broad areas of interest. Chapters are devoted to single topics within a part.

Part I: Understanding the Health Effects of Environmental Hazards provides information and risk assessment tools to help readers determine what health threats may be present in the world around them. It offers suggestions for reducing possible exposure to dangers, and it discusses issues of special concern to children, pregnant women, the elderly, and minority populations. It also explains the connection between human health and climatic changes.

Part II: Health Concerns and Their Environmental Triggers provides readers with in-depth details on individual diseases with suspected environmental causes, including cancer, respiratory problems, and certain viruses. It details the effects of the environment on fertility and pregnancy, and it explains how environmental factors might be cause autism.

Part III: Outdoor Environmental Hazards: Air, Water, and Soil explores hazards, both natural and man-made, that are found in the outdoor environment. Readers will learn about pollution in air and water, as well as how chemicals and pesticides have spread through the food chain and how they can be avoided. It also explores hazards—such as noise and light pollution, smog and acid rain, and climate change— caused by the modern urban environment.

Part IV: Household and Indoor Hazards discusses the hazards people face in the environment where they spend up to 90 percent of their time—inside their homes, offices, and schools. These risks include indoor air contaminants, such as carbon monoxide, mold, asbestos, and lead, as well as unsafe indoor activities, such as smoking or inappropriately using chemicals and pesticides. The part concludes with the effects of electric and magnetic field exposure.

Part V: Foodborne Hazards includes facts about food safety regulations, potentially problematic food additives, and chemical contaminants in the food supply. It provides tips for avoiding the most common foodborne illnesses and for safely preparing food at home. Because most Americans rely on the industrial food chain for the majority of their food, it also discusses safety concerns related to food technologies, including genetic engineering, the use of antibiotics and hormones, and nanoparticles.

Part VI: Consumer Products and Medical Hazards tells readers about the health risks they face from consumer products, including everyday objects such as hand soap, insect repellants, and plastics. It discusses the safety of imported goods, now found in virtually every home, and it describes concerns about the use of untested chemicals and additives in personal care products, such as cosmetics and sunscreens.

Part VII: Additional Help and Information includes a glossary of important terms and a directory of organizations providing information and advocacy on environmental health topics.

Bibliographic Note

This volume contains documents and excerpts from publications issued by the following government agencies: Centers for Disease Control and Prevention (CDC); National Cancer Institute (NCI); National Institute of Diabetes and Digestive and Kidney Diseases (NIDDK); National Institute of Environmental Health Sciences (NIEHS); National Institute on Aging (NIA); National Institutes of Health (NIH); *NIH News in Health*; Office of Disease Prevention and Health Promotion (ODPHP); Tox Town; U.S. Department of Education (ED); U.S. Department of Labor (DOL) U.S. Department of Veterans Affairs (VA); U.S. Environmental Protection Agency (EPA); and U.S. Food and Drug Administration (FDA).

About the Health Reference Series

The *Health Reference Series* is designed to provide basic medical information for patients, families, caregivers, and the general public. Each volume takes a particular topic and provides comprehensive coverage. This is especially important for people who may be dealing with a newly diagnosed disease or a chronic disorder in themselves or in a family member. People looking for preventive guidance, information about disease warning signs, medical statistics, and risk factors for health problems will also find answers to their questions in the *Health Reference Series*. The *Series*, however, is not intended to serve as a tool for diagnosing illness, in prescribing treatments, or as a substitute for the physician/patient relationship. All people concerned about medical symptoms or the possibility of disease are encouraged to seek professional care from an appropriate healthcare provider.

A Note about Spelling and Style

Health Reference Series editors use *Stedman's Medical Dictionary* as an authority for questions related to the spelling of medical terms and the *Chicago Manual of Style* for questions related to grammatical structures, punctuation, and other editorial concerns. Consistent adherence is not always possible, however, because the individual volumes within the *Series* include many documents from a wide variety of different producers, and the editor's primary goal is to present material from each source as accurately as is possible. This sometimes means that information in different chapters or sections may follow other guidelines and alternate spelling authorities. For example, occasionally a copyright holder may require that eponymous terms be shown in possessive forms (Crohn's disease vs. Crohn disease) or that British spelling norms be retained (leukaemia vs. leukemia).

Medical Review

Omnigraphics contracts with a team of qualified, senior medical professionals who serve as medical consultants for the *Health Reference Series*. As necessary, medical consultants review reprinted and originally written material for currency and accuracy. Citations including the phrase, "Reviewed (month, year)" indicate material reviewed by this team. Medical consultation services are provided to the *Health Reference Series* editors by:

Dr. Vijayalakshmi, MBBS, DGO, MD
Dr. Senthil Selvan, MBBS, DCH, MD
Dr. K. Sivanandham, MBBS, DCH, MS (Research), PhD

Our Advisory Board

We would like to thank the following board members for providing initial guidance on the development of this series:

- Dr. Lynda Baker, Associate Professor of Library and Information Science, Wayne State University, Detroit, MI

- Nancy Bulgarelli, William Beaumont Hospital Library, Royal Oak, MI

- Karen Imarisio, Bloomfield Township Public Library, Bloomfield Township, MI

- Karen Morgan, Mardigian Library, University of Michigan-Dearborn, Dearborn, MI

- Rosemary Orlando, St. Clair Shores Public Library, St. Clair Shores, MI

Health Reference Series *Update Policy*

The inaugural book in the *Health Reference Series* was the first edition of *Cancer Sourcebook* published in 1989. Since then, the *Series* has been enthusiastically received by librarians and in the medical community. In order to maintain the standard of providing high-quality health information for the layperson the editorial staff at Omnigraphics felt it was necessary to implement a policy of updating volumes when warranted.

Medical researchers have been making tremendous strides, and it is the purpose of the *Health Reference Series* to stay current with the most recent advances. Each decision to update a volume is made on an individual basis. Some of the considerations include how much new information is available and the feedback we receive from people who use the books. If there is a topic you would like to see added to the update list, or an area of medical concern you feel has not been adequately addressed, please write to:

Managing Editor
Health Reference Series
Omnigraphics
615 Griswold, Ste. 901
Detroit, MI 48226

Part One

Understanding the Health Effects of Environmental Hazards

Chapter 1

Environmental Health: Overview

Humans interact with the environment constantly. These interactions affect the quality of life, years of healthy life lived, and health disparities. The World Health Organization (WHO) defines the environment, as it relates to health, as "all the physical, chemical, and biological factors external to a person, and all the related behaviors."

Environmental health consists of preventing or controlling disease, injury, and disability related to the interactions between people and their environment. Creating healthy environments can be complex and relies on continuing research to better understand the effects of exposure to environmental hazards on people's health.

Why Is Environmental Health Important?

Maintaining a healthy environment is central to increasing quality of life and years of healthy life. Globally, 23 percent of all deaths and 26 percent of deaths among children under age 5 are due to preventable environmental factors.

This chapter contains text excerpted from the following sources: Text in this chapter begins with text excerpted from "Environmental Health," Office of Disease Prevention and Health Promotion (ODPHP), U.S. Department of Health and Human Services (HHS), March 26, 2018; Text under the heading "Children's Environmental Health Facts" is excerpted from "Protecting Children's Environmental Health," U.S. Environmental Protection Agency (EPA), March 14, 2018.

Environmental factors are diverse and far-reaching. They include:

- Exposure to hazardous substances in the air, water, soil, and food
- Natural and technological disasters
- Climate change
- Occupational hazards
- The built environment

Poor environmental quality has its greatest impact on people whose health status is already at risk. Therefore, environmental health must address the societal and environmental factors that increase the likelihood of exposure and disease.

Understanding Environmental Health

Outdoor Air Quality

Poor air quality is linked to premature death, cancer, and long-term damage to respiratory and cardiovascular systems. Progress has been made to reduce unhealthy air emissions. Decreasing air pollution is an important step in creating a healthy environment.

Surface and Groundwater

Surface and ground water quality concerns apply to both drinking water and recreational waters. Contamination by infectious agents or chemicals can cause mild to severe illness. Protecting water sources and minimizing exposure to contaminated water sources are important parts of environmental health.

Toxic Substances and Hazardous Wastes

The health effects of toxic substances and hazardous wastes are not yet fully understood. Research to better understand how these exposures may impact health is ongoing. Meanwhile, efforts to reduce exposures continue. Reducing exposure to toxic substances and hazardous wastes is fundamental to environmental health.

Homes and Communities

People spend most of their time at home, work, or school. Some of these environments may expose people to:

- Indoor air pollution

- Inadequate heating and sanitation

- Structural problems

- Electrical and fire hazards

- Lead-based paint hazards

These hazards can impact health and safety. Maintaining healthy homes and communities is essential to environmental health.

Infrastructure and Surveillance

Preventing exposure to environmental hazards relies on many partners, including state and local health departments. Personnel, surveillance systems, and education are important resources for investigating and responding to disease, monitoring for hazards, and educating the public. Additional methods and greater capacity to measure and respond to environmental hazards are needed.

Global Environmental Health

Water quality is an important global challenge. Diseases can be reduced by improving water quality and sanitation and increasing access to adequate water and sanitation facilities.

Emerging Issues in Environmental Health

Environmental health is a dynamic and evolving field. While not all complex environmental issues can be predicted, some known emerging issues in the field include:

Climate Change

Climate change is projected to impact sea level, patterns of infectious disease, air quality, and the severity of natural disasters such as floods, droughts, and storms.

Disaster Preparedness

Preparedness for the environmental impact of natural disasters as well as disasters of human origin includes planning for human health needs and the impact on public infrastructures, such as water and roadways.

Nanotechnology

The potential impact of nanotechnology is significant and offers possible improvements to:

- Disease prevention, detection, and treatment
- Electronics
- Clean energy
- Manufacturing
- Environmental risk assessment

However, nanotechnology may also present unintended health risks or changes to the environment.

The Built Environment

Features of the built environment appear to impact human health-influencing behaviors, physical activity patterns, social networks, and access to resources.

Exposure to Unknown Hazards

Every year, hundreds of new chemicals are introduced to the U.S. market. It is presumed that some of these chemicals may present new, unexpected challenges to human health, and their safety should be evaluated prior to release.

These cross-cutting issues are not yet understood well enough to inform the development of systems for measuring and tracking their impact. Further exploration is warranted. The environmental health landscape will continue to evolve and may present opportunities for additional research, analysis, and monitoring.

Blood Lead Levels (BLLs)

As of 2017, there were approximately 4 million houses or buildings that have children living in them who are potentially being exposed to lead. Nearly half a million U.S. children ages 1–5 have blood lead levels (BLLs) at or above 5 micrograms per deciliter (μg/dL), which is currently the reference level at which the Centers for Disease Control and Prevention (CDC) recommends public health actions be taken. Even blood lead exposure levels as low as 2 μg/dL can affect a child's cognitive function. Since no safe BLL have been identified for children, any exposure should be taken seriously. However, since lead exposure often occurs with no obvious signs or symptoms, it often remains unrecognized.

Children's Environmental Health Facts

Asthma

- Asthma is a common chronic disease among children in the United States.
- Asthma is the third-ranking cause of noninjury related hospital-ization among children less than 15 years of age.

Disparities in Asthma

- Asthma disproportionately affects children from lower income families and children from various racial and ethnic groups.
- African American children have a 500 percent higher mortality rate from asthma as compared with Caucasian children.
- Larger disparities exist within the Hispanic population such that 20 percent of Puerto Rican children were reported to have asthma as compared with 7 percent of Mexican children.
- While national level surveys suggest Asian and Pacific Islander children do not have high rates of asthma, small-scale surveys, however, show a high prevalence of asthma among subgroups of Asian and Pacific Islander children.
- Filipino children have an asthma prevalence of 23.8 percent.
- Pacific Islander children have an asthma prevalence of 21 percent.

Economic Impact of Asthma

- Asthmatic patients and their families pay a higher portion of their medical care costs than patients with other diseases due to heavy reliance on prescription medication combined with lower insurance coverage for prescription drugs

Lead Exposure

- No level of lead in blood has been identified as safe for children. The Centers for Disease Control and Prevention (CDC) recom-mend public health actions be initiated for children with a refer-ence level of 5 micrograms of lead per deciliter of blood.

- Today, elevated blood lead levels in children are due mostly to ingestion of contaminated dust, paint, and soil.

- Other sources of lead exposure include ceramics, drinking water pipes and plumbing fixtures, consumer products, batteries, gasoline, solder, ammunition, imported toys, and cosmetics

- In 2010, an estimated 535,000 children had a blood lead level of 5 μg/dL. The number of children affected by lead poisoning has decreased significantly from 4.7 million in 1978.

- Lead exposure in young children can result in lowered intelligence, reading and learning disabilities (LD), impaired hearing, reduced attention span, hyperactivity, delayed puberty, and reduced postnatal growth.

Disparities in Lead Exposure

- Blood lead levels (BLL) are higher for children ages 1–5 years old from lower-income families and for certain racial and ethnic groups.

- The median BLL in Black non-Hispanic children ages 1–5 years old is higher than the level in White non-Hispanic children, Mexican-American children, and children of "all other races/ethnicities."

- The median BLL for children living in families with incomes below the poverty level is higher than for children living in families at or above the poverty level.

Economic Impact of Lead Exposure

- The cost of reduced cognitive ability is measured by intelligence quotient (IQ) scores and valued in terms of forgone earnings and is estimated to be about $9,600 per IQ point lost.

- The cost of not eliminating lead exposure to children between 2000–2010 is expected to be about $22 billion in forgone earnings.

Childhood Cancer

- Leukemia is the most common cancer in children under 15, accounting for 30 percent of all childhood cancers, followed by brain and other nervous system cancers

- Cancer is the second leading cause of death among children ages 1–14 years of age, with unintentional injuries being the leading cause
- The causes of childhood cancer are poorly understood, though different forms of cancer have different causes. A number of studies suggest that environmental contaminants, including radiation, secondhand smoke, pesticides, and solvents, may play a role in the development of childhood cancers.

Disparities in Childhood Cancer

- Hispanic children were reported to have a higher incidence of acute lymphocytic Leukemia (ALL) than non-Hispanic White children
- Although national studies indicate that Asian Pacific Islander American (APIA) children overall do not have higher rates of cancer compared to non-Hispanic Whites, a smaller scale study conducted in California showed APIA children are at increased risk of developing acute nonlymphocytic Leukemia (ALL) compared with non-Hispanic White infants

Economic Impact of Childhood Cancer

The total cost per case of childhood cancer was estimated to be about $623,000.

Developmental Disabilities

- Between 3–8 percent of the babies born each year will be affected by developmental disorders such as attention deficit hyperactivity disorder (ADHD) or mental retardation

Disparities in Developmental Disabilities

- Mental retardation is more common for children from lower-income families and for certain racial and ethnic groups

Economic Impact of Developmental Disabilities

- The economic costs associated with autism are approximately $35 billion dollars per year
- Expenditures can range from 1.6 times (for students with specific learning disabilities) to 3.1 times (for students with multiple disabilities) higher than expenditures for a regular education student

Chapter 2

Health Risk Assessment: Determining Whether Environmental Substances Pose a Risk to Human Health

Human Health Risk Assessment

A human health risk assessment is the process to estimate the nature and probability of adverse health effects in humans who may be exposed to chemicals in contaminated environmental media, now or in the future.

Human health risk assessment includes 4 basic steps:

- **Planning: Planning and scoping process.** U.S. Environmental Protection Agency (EPA) begins the process of a human health risk assessment with planning and research.

- **Step 1: Hazard identification.** Examines whether a stressor has the potential to cause harm to humans and/or ecological systems and if so, under what circumstances.

- **Step 2: Dose-response assessment.** Examines the numerical relationship between exposure and effects.

This chapter includes text excerpted from "Human Health Risk Assessment," U.S. Environmental Protection Agency (EPA), October 3, 2016.

- **Step 3: The exposure assessment.** Examines what is known about the frequency, timing, and levels of contact with a stressor.

- **Step 4: Risk characterization.** Examines how well the data support conclusions about the nature and extent of the risk from exposure to environmental stressors.

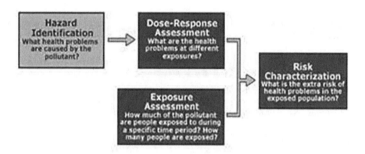

Figure 2.1. *The 4-Step Risk Assessment Process*

A human health risk assessment addresses questions such as:

- What types of health problems may be caused by environmental stressors such as chemicals and radiation?

- What is the chance that people will experience health problems when exposed to different levels of environmental stressors?

- Is there a level below which some chemicals don't pose a human health risk?

- What environmental stressors are people exposed to and at what levels and for how long?

- Are some people more likely to be susceptible to environmental stressors because of factors such as age, genetics, preexisting health conditions, ethnic practices, gender, etc.?

Are some people more likely to be exposed to environmental stressors because of factors such as where they work, where they play, what they like to eat, etc.?

The answers to these types of questions help decision makers, whether they are parents or public officials, understand the possible human health risks from environmental media.

Planning

Even a human health risk assessment starts with a good plan. Before anything though there is a need to make judgments early when planning major risk assessments regarding the purpose, scope, and technical approaches that will be used. To start, risk assessors will typically ask the following questions:

Who / What / Where Is at Risk?

- Individuals

- General population

- Life stages such as children, teenagers, pregnant/nursing women

- Population subgroups—highly susceptible (for example, due to asthma, genetics, etc.) and/or highly exposed (for example, based on geographic area, gender, racial or ethnic group, or economic status)

What Is the Environmental Hazard of Concern?

- Chemicals (single or multiple/cumulative risks)

- Radiation

- Physical (dust, heat)

- Microbiological or biological

- Nutritional (for example, diet, fitness, or metabolic state)

- Socioeconomic (for example, access to healthcare)

Where Do These Environmental Hazards Come From?

- Point sources (for example, smoke or water discharge from a factory; contamination from a superfund site)

- Nonpoint sources (for example, automobile exhaust; agricultural runoff)

- Natural sources

How Does Exposure Occur?

- Pathways (recognizing that one or more may be involved)

- Air

13

- Surface water
- Groundwater
- Soil
- Solid waste
- Food
- Nonfood consumer products, pharmaceuticals
- Routes (and related human activities that lead to exposure)
- Ingestion (both food and water)
- Contact with skin
- Inhalation
- Nondietary ingestion (for example, "hand-to-mouth" behavior)

What Does the Body Do with the Environmental Hazard and How Is This Impacted by Factors Such as Age, Race, Sex, Genetics, Etc.?)

- **Absorption**. Does the body take up the environmental hazard?
- **Distribution**. Does the environmental hazard travel throughout the body or does it stay in one place?
- **Metabolism**. Does the body break down the environmental hazard?
- **Excretion**. How does the body get rid of it?

What Are the Health Effects?

- Example of some health effects includes cancer, heart disease, liver disease, and nerve disease

How Long Does It Take for an Environmental Hazard to Cause a Toxic Effect? Does It Matter When in a Lifetime Exposure Occurs?

- **Acute**. Right away or within a few hours to a day
- **Subchronic**. Weeks or months (for humans generally less than 10% of their lifespan)
- **Chronic**. A significant part of a lifetime or a lifetime (for humans at least seven years)

- Intermittent
- Timing

Step 1. Hazard Identification

The objective of step 1 is to identify the types of adverse health effects that can be caused by exposure to some agent in question and to characterize the quality and weight of evidence supporting this identification.

Hazard identification is the process of determining whether exposure to a stressor can cause an increase in the incidence of specific adverse health effects (e.g., cancer, birth defects). It is also whether the adverse health effect is likely to occur in humans.

In the case of chemical stressors, the process examines the available scientific data for a given chemical (or group of chemicals) and develops a weight of evidence to characterize the link between the negative effects and the chemical agent.

Exposure to a stressor may generate many different adverse effects in a human: diseases, the formation of tumors, reproductive defects, death, or other effects.

Sources of Data

Statistically controlled clinical studies on humans provide the best evidence linking a stressor, often a chemical, to a resulting effect. However, such studies are frequently not available since there are significant ethical concerns associated with human testing of environmental hazards.

Epidemiological studies involve a statistical evaluation of human populations to examine whether there is an association between exposure to a stressor and a human health effect. The advantage of these studies is that they involve humans while their weakness results from generally not having accurate exposure information and the difficulty of teasing out the effects of multiple stressors.

When data from human studies are unavailable, data from animal studies (rats, mice, rabbits, monkeys, dogs, etc.) are relied on to draw inference about the potential hazard to humans. Animal studies can be designed, controlled, and conducted to address specific gaps in knowledge, but there are uncertainties associated with extrapolating results from animal subjects to humans.

Key Components of Hazard Identification

A wide variety of studies and analysis are used to support a hazard identification analysis.

- **Toxicokinetics** considers how the body absorbs, distributes, metabolizes, and eliminates specific chemicals

- **Toxicodynamics** focus on the effects that chemicals have on the human body. Models based on these studies can describe mechanisms by which a chemical may impact human health, thus providing insights into the possible effects of a chemical.

When assessing a chemical for potential carcinogenic behavior, the EPA current practice is to focus on the analysis of a mode of action. Mode of action is a sequence of key events and processes, starting with interaction of an agent and a cell, proceeding through operational and anatomical changes, and resulting in cancer formation. A given agent may work by more than one mode of action, both at different tumor sites as well as at the same site.

Analysis of mode of action is based on physical, chemical, and biological information that helps to explain key events in an agent's influence on tumor development.

A key component of hazard characterization involves evaluating the weight of evidence regarding a chemical's potential to cause adverse human health effects. The weight of evidence narrative may include some standard 'descriptors' that signify certain qualitative threshold levels of evidence or confidence have been met, such as 'carcinogenic to humans' or 'suggestive evidence of carcinogenic potential'.

Step 2. Dose Response

The objective of step 2 is to document the relationship between dose and toxic effect.

A dose-response relationship describes how the likelihood and severity of adverse health effects (the responses) are related to the amount and condition of exposure to an agent (the dose provided). Although this chapter refers to the "dose-response" relationship, the same principles generally apply for studies where the exposure is to a concentration of the agent (e.g., airborne concentrations applied in inhalation exposure studies), and the resulting information is referred to as the "concentration-response" relationship.

The term "exposure-response" relationship may be used to describe either a dose-response or a concentration response, or other specific exposure conditions.

Typically, as the dose increases, the measured response also increases. At low doses, there may be no response. At some level of dose, the responses begin to occur in a small fraction of the study population or at a low probability rate. Both the dose at which response begin to appear and the rate at which it increases given increasing dose can be variable between different pollutants, individuals, exposure routes, etc.

The shape of the dose-response relationship depends on the agent, the kind of response (tumor, the incidence of disease, death, etc.), and the experimental subject (human, animal) in question. For example, there may be one relationship for a response such as 'weight loss' and a different relationship for another response such as 'death'. Since it is impractical to study all possible relationships for all possible responses, toxicity research typically focuses on testing for a limited number of adverse effects.

Upon considering all available studies, the response (adverse effect), or a measure of response that leads to an adverse effect (known as a 'precursor' to the effect), that occurs at the lowest dose is selected as the critical effect for risk assessment. The underlying assumption is that if the critical effect is prevented from occurring, then no other effects of concern will occur.

Step 3. Exposure Assessment

The objective of step 3 is to calculate a numerical estimate of exposure or dose.

Exposure assessment is the process of measuring or estimating the magnitude, frequency, and duration of human exposure to an agent in the environment or estimating future exposures for an agent that has not yet been released. An exposure assessment includes some discussion of the size, nature, and types of human populations exposed to the agent, as well as discussion of the uncertainties in the above information.

Exposure can be measured directly, but more commonly is estimated indirectly through consideration of measured concentrations in the environment, consideration of models of chemical transport and fate in the environment, and estimates of human intake over time.

Different Kinds of Doses

Exposure assessment considers both the exposure pathway (the course an agent takes from its source to the person(s) being contacted) as well as the exposure route (means of entry of the agent into the body). The exposure route is generally further described as intake (taken in through a body opening, e.g., as eating, drinking, or inhaling) or uptake (absorption through tissues, e.g., through the skin or eye).

The applied dose is the amount of agent at the absorption barrier that is available for absorption. The potential dose is the amount of agent that is ingested, inhaled, or applied to the skin. The applied dose may be less than the potential dose if the agent is only partly bioavailable.

The internal dose or absorbed dose is the amount of an agent that has been absorbed and is available for interaction with biologically significant receptors within the human body. Finally, the delivered dose is the amount of agent available for interaction with any specific organ or cell.

Range of Exposure

For any specific agent or site, there is a range of exposures actually experienced by individuals. Some individuals may have a high degree of contact for an extended period (e.g., factory workers exposed to an agent on the job). Other individuals may have a lower degree of contact for a shorter period (e.g., individuals using a recreational site downwind of the factory). EPA policy for exposure assessment requires consideration of a range of possible exposure levels.

Two common scenarios for possible exposure are "central tendency" and "high end." "Central tendency" exposure is an estimate of the average experienced by the affected population, based on the amount of agent present in the environment and the frequency and duration of exposure.

"High end" exposure is the highest dose estimated to be experienced by some individuals, commonly stated as approximately equal to the 90th percentile exposure category for individuals.

Quantifying Exposure

There are three basic approaches for quantifying exposure. Each approach is based on different data, and has different strengths and weaknesses; using the approaches in combination can greatly strengthen the credibility of an exposure risk assessment.

- **Point of contact measurement.** The exposure can be measured at the point of contact (the outer boundary of the body) while it is taking place, measuring both exposure concentration and time of contact, then integrating them;

- **Scenario evaluation.** The exposure can be estimated by separately evaluating the exposure concentration and the time of contact, then combining this information;

- **Reconstruction.** The exposure can be estimated from dose, which in turn can be reconstructed through internal indicators (biomarkers, body burden, excretion levels, etc.) after the exposure has taken place (reconstruction).

Step 4. Risk Characterization

The objective of step 4 is to summarize and integrate information from the proceeding steps of the risk assessment to synthesize an overall conclusion about risk.

A risk characterization conveys the risk assessor's judgment as to the nature and presence or absence of risks, along with information about how the risk was assessed, where assumptions and uncertainties still exist, and where policy choices will need to be made. Risk characterization takes place in both human health risk assessments and ecological risk assessments.

In practice, each component of the risk assessment (e.g., hazard assessment, dose-response assessment, exposure assessment) has an individual risk characterization written to carry forward the key findings, assumptions, limitations, and uncertainties. The set of these individual risk characterizations provide the information basis to write an integrative risk characterization analysis.

The final, overall risk characterization thus consists of the individual risk characterizations plus an integrative analysis.

Principles of Conducting Risk Characterizations

A good risk characterization will restate the scope of the assessment, express results clearly, articulate major assumptions and uncertainties, identify reasonable alternative interpretations, and separate scientific conclusions from policy judgments.

The EPA's Risk Characterization Policy calls for conducting risk characterizations in a manner that is consistent with the following principles:

- **Transparency**. The characterization should fully and explicitly disclose the risk assessment methods, default assumptions, logic, rationale, extrapolations, uncertainties, and overall strength of each step in the assessment.

- **Clarity**. The products from the risk assessment should be readily understood by readers inside and outside of the risk assessment process. Documents should be concise, free of jargon, and should use understandable tables, graphs, and equations as needed.

- **Consistency**. The risk assessment should be conducted and presented in a manner which is consistent with the FDA policy, and consistent with other risk characterizations of similar scope prepared across programs within the EPA.

- **Reasonableness**. The risk assessment should be based on sound judgment, with methods and assumptions consistent with the current state-of-the-science and conveyed in a manner that is complete and balanced, informative.

These four principles are referred to collectively as transparent, clear, consistent, and reasonable (TCCR) principles. In order to achieve TCCR in a risk characterization, the same principles need to have been applied in all of the prior steps in the risk assessment which lead up to the risk characterization.

Chapter 3

Environmental Hazards for Children

Children's Health

Children are often more vulnerable to pollutants than adults due to differences in behavior and biology, that can lead to greater exposure and/or unique windows of susceptibility during development.

Children Are Not Little Adults

Children are often more likely to be at risk from environmental hazards than adults because of:

- Unique activity patterns and behavior
- Physiological differences
- Windows of susceptibility during early life stages including fetal development and puberty

Children are also dependent upon adults to ensure that their environment is safe.

This chapter includes text excerpted from "Protecting Children's Environmental Health," U.S. Environmental Protection Agency (EPA), March 14, 2018.

Unique Activity Patterns Plus Behavior

- Children crawl and play close to the ground making them more likely to come into contact with dirt and dust, which can include toxicants

- Children often put their hands, toys, and other items into their mouths

Physiology

- Children eat, breathe, and drink more relative to their body mass than adults do

- Children's natural defenses are less developed

- More permeable blood-brain barrier

- Less effective filtration in nasal passages

- Highly permeable skin

- Lower levels of circulation of plasma proteins

- Digestive system, metabolic pathways, renal clearances, and vital organs are still developing

Windows of Susceptibility

The timing of exposure to chemicals or other insults is critical in determining the consequences to children's health. Because of the different windows of susceptibility, the same dose of a chemical during different periods of development can have very different consequences. For example, fetal loss or birth defects are most likely to occur as a result of exposures to chemicals during the embryonic period, when organs are beginning to differentiate.

Even after the basic structure of an organ has been established, disruption of processes such as growth and cell migration can have lifelong consequences on the function of key organ systems. Due to the complexity and speed of development during the prenatal period, organ system development is particularly susceptible to adverse effects resulting from environmental exposures (Figure 3.1).

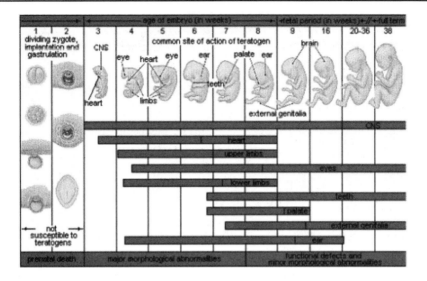

Figure 3.1. *Development of Child during Prenatal Period*

What You Can Do to Protect Children from Environmental Risks

Keep Pesticides and Other Toxic Chemicals Away from Children

- Store food and trash in closed containers to keep pests from coming into your home.

- Use baits and traps when you can; place baits and traps where kids can't get them.

- Read product labels and follow directions.

- Store pesticides and toxic chemicals where kids can't reach them—never put them in other containers that kids can mistake for food or drink.

- Keep children, toys, and pets away when pesticides are applied; don't let them play in fields, orchards, and gardens after pesticides have been used for at least the time recommended on the pesticide label.

- Wash fruits and vegetables under running water before eating— peel them before eating, when possible.

Protect Children from Chemical Poisoning

If a child has swallowed or inhaled a toxic product such as a household cleaner or pesticide or gotten it in their eye or on their skin

- Call 911 if the child is unconscious, having trouble breathing, or having convulsions.
- Check the label for directions on how to give first aid.
- Call the Poison Control Center (PCC) at 800-222-1222 for help with first aid information.

Help Children Breathe Easier

- Don't smoke and don't let others smoke in your home or car.
- Keep your home as clean as possible. Dust, mold, certain household pests, secondhand smoke, and pet dander can trigger asthma attacks and allergies.
- Limit outdoor activity on ozone alert days when air pollution is especially harmful.
- Walk, use bicycles, join or form carpools, and take public transportation.
- Limit motor vehicle idling.
- Avoid open burning.
- Limit outdoor activity on poor air quality days.

Protect Children from Lead Poisoning

- Get kids tested for lead by their doctor or healthcare provider.
- Test your home for lead paint hazards if it was built before 1978.
- Wash children's hands before they eat; wash bottles, pacifiers, and toys often.
- Wash floors and window sills to protect kids from dust and peeling paint contaminated with lead—especially in older homes.
- Run cold water until it becomes as cold as it can get. Use only cold water for drinking, cooking, and making baby formula.

Protect Children from Carbon Monoxide (CO) Poisoning

- Have fuel-burning appliances, furnace flues, and chimneys checked once a year.

- Never use gas ovens or burners for heat; never use barbecues or grills indoors or in the garage.

- Never sleep in rooms with unvented gas or kerosene space heaters.

- Don't run cars or lawnmowers in the garage.

- Install in sleeping areas a carbon monoxide (CO) alarm that meets underwriters laboratories (UL), International Accounting Standards (IAS), or Canadian standards.

Protect Children from Contaminated Fish and Polluted Water

- Be alert for local fish advisories and beach closings. Contact your local health department.

- Take used motor oil to a recycling center; properly dispose of toxic household chemicals.

- Learn what's in your drinking water—call your local public water supplier for annual drinking water quality reports; for private drinking water wells, have them tested annually by a certified laboratory. Call 800-426-4791 for help.

Safeguard Children from High Levels of Radon

- Test your home for radon with a home test kit.

- Fix your home if your radon level is 4 picocuries (pCi)/L or higher. For help, call your state radon office or 800-SOS-RADON (800-767-7236).

Protect Children from Too Much Sun

- Wear hats, sunglasses, and protective clothing.

- Use sunscreen with sun protection factor (SPF) 15+ on kids over six months; keep infants out of direct sunlight.

- Limit time in the mid-day sun—the sun is most intense between 10–4.

Keep Children and Mercury Apart

- Eat a balanced diet but avoid fish with high levels of mercury.
- Replace mercury thermometers with digital thermometers.
- Don't let kids handle or play with mercury.
- Never heat or burn mercury.
- Contact your state or local health or environment department if mercury is spilled—never vacuum a spill.

Promote Healthier Communities

- Walk, use bicycles, join or form carpools, and take public transportation to reduce air pollution, including greenhouse gases.
- Spearhead a clean school bus campaign in your community. Clean School Bus U.S.A emphasizes three ways to reduce public school bus emissions:

  - **Anti-idling strategies.** Unnecessary idling pollutes the air, wastes fuel, and causes excess engine wear. It also wastes money and results in the wear and tear of the vehicle's engine.

  - **Engine retrofit and clean fuels.** Retrofitted engines run cleaner because they have been fitted with devices designed to reduce pollution and/or use cleaner fuel.

  - **Bus replacement.** Older buses are not equipped with today's pollution control or safety features.

- Develop safe routes so that children can walk to and from school, limiting vehicle use and increasing physical activity. Conduct walkability audits in your community to understand where you can and cannot walk. Children can help with a fun and educational activity.

- Promote green building. Green building considerations include:

  - Careful site selection to minimize impacts on the surrounding environment and increase alternative transportation options

  - Energy and water conservation to help ensure efficient use of natural resources and lower utility bills

  - Responsible stormwater management to help limit disruption of natural watershed functions and reduce the environmental impacts of stormwater runoff

- Improved indoor air quality through the use of low volatile organic compound products and careful ventilation practices during construction and renovation

- Use indoor air quality design tools to create healthy school environments. Indoor air quality (IAQ) is a critically important aspect of creating and maintaining school facilities. IAQ Design Tools for Schools provides detailed guidance and links to other resources to help design new schools and repair, renovate and maintain existing facilities. IAQ Design Tools for Schools is web-based guidance to assist school districts, architects, and facility planners design and construct the next generation of schools.

- Support local smart growth activities. Smart growth is a development that serves the economy, the community, and the environment. The U.S. Environmental Protection Agency (EPA) helps states and communities realize the economic, community, and environmental benefits of smart growth by:

  - Providing information, model programs, and analytical tools to inform communities about growth and development

  - Working to remove federal barriers that may hinder smarter community growth

  - Creating new resources and incentives for states and communities pursuing smart growth

- Protect children's environmental health. Children may be more vulnerable to environmental exposures than adults because:

  - Their bodily systems are still developing

  - They eat more, drink more, and breathe more in proportion to their body size

  - Their behavior can expose them more to chemicals and organisms.

- Contact your local health department and ask about cooling centers, disaster preparedness, and other issues of concern to you.

- Sign up for weather, air quality, water quality, and pollen count alert systems through your local government.

- Plant trees, walk instead of driving, teach your children to ride bikes, support neighborhood gardens, recycle paper, compost kitchen waste, and conserve water—taking simple steps to improve the environment really does help!

Storms and Floods

- Have a battery-powered weather radio and a basic emergency supply kit.

- Make an evacuation and communication plan in place for the family during floods and storms.

- If children are exposed to flood waters, watch for diarrhea.

- Check for local drinking water advisories.

- Drink bottled water or boil tap water to disinfect it.

- Check local advisories about recreational activities, such as beach closures.

- After a major storm, check your child's mental health, school performance, sleeping and eating patterns for signs of change, and seek treatment if needed.

Too Much Heat

- If you are pregnant, try to stay cool, stretch your legs, and sip water more often than usual to prevent dehydration.

- Infants and young children overheat quickly and are less able to adapt to extreme heat. Offer sips of water often.

- Dress infants and children loose, lightweight, and light color clothing.

- Children may not ask for water and may not be aware that they need to cool down.

- Never leave infants in a parked car.

- Help children find places to cool off when they are overheated.

- Ensure that children drink plenty of water before and after athletic events.

- Monitor children, and even teenagers, for signs of heat-related illness, provide water and have a plan to combat heat illness.

- Communities can work together to create cooling centers for children, to issue heat warnings and alerts, and to air condition schools.

- Seek medical care right away if your child has signs of heat-related illness.

Avoiding Ticks

- Keep the ticks away from your child to prevent Lyme disease

- Have children wear protective clothing, such as socks, shoes, and long pants if possible

- Reduce tick habitats by keeping the grass short and removing brush from play areas

- Parents should apply insect repellent rated for ticks on children. Always follow label instructions and avoid applying to hands or near eyes and mouth.

- Check children for ticks after they have been outdoors, especially in wooded areas and meadows, and especially from April–October

- Teach children how to check themselves for ticks, and what to do if they find one

- Have children bathe or shower after playing in woods or grassy fields

- Remove ticks promptly

- Call your child's health professional if you suspect Lyme disease—some early signs can include a red expanding "bullseye" rash around the spot a tick attached, fatigue, chills, fever, headache, muscle and joint aches, and swollen lymph nodes (particularly of note when other children or members of the family aren't sick)

Stopping Mosquito Bites

- Use insect repellents when your children play outdoors. Always follow the label directions.

- Wear long sleeves and pants from dusk through dawn when mosquitoes are most active.

- Install or repair screens on windows and doors. If you can, use your air conditioning.

- Help reduce the number of mosquitoes around your home by emptying standing water from containers, flower pots, gutters, buckets, pool covers, pet dishes, tires, and birdbaths.

Protecting Children's Health during and after Natural Disasters

Children's Health in the Aftermath of Floods

Children are different from adults. They may be more vulnerable to chemicals and organisms they are exposed to in the environment because:

- Children's nervous, immune response, digestive and other bodily systems are still developing and are more easily harmed;

- Children eat more food, drink more fluids, and breathe more air than adults in proportion to their body size—so it is important to take extra care to ensure the safety of their food, drink, and air;

- The way children behave—such as crawling and placing objects in their mouths—can increase their risk of exposure to chemicals and organisms in the environment.

Mold

After homes have been flooded, moisture can remain in drywall, wood furniture, cloth, carpet, and other household items and surfaces and can lead to mold growth. Exposure to mold can cause hay-fever-like reactions (such as stuffy nose, red, watery or itchy eyes, sneezing) to asthma attacks. It is important to dry water damaged areas and items within 24–48 hours to prevent mold growth. Buildings wet for more than 48 hours will generally contain visible and extensive mold growth.

Some children are more susceptible than others to mold, especially those with allergies, asthma and other respiratory conditions. To protect your child from mold exposure, you can clean smooth, hard surfaces such as metal and plastics with soap and water and dry thoroughly. Flood water damaged items made of more absorbent materials cannot be cleaned and should be discarded. These items include paper, cloth, wood, upholstery, carpets, padding, curtains, clothes, stuffed animals, etc.

If there is a large amount of mold, you may want to hire professional help to clean up the mold. If you decide to do the cleanup yourself, please remember:

- Clean and dry hard surfaces such as showers, tubs, and kitchen countertops.

- If something is moldy, and can't be cleaned and dried, throw it away.

- Use a detergent or use a cleaner that kills germs.

- Do not mix cleaning products together or add bleach to other chemicals.

- Wear an N-95 respirator, goggles, gloves so that you don't touch mold with your bare hands, long pants, a long-sleeved shirt, and boots or work shoes.

Homes or apartments that have sustained heavy water damage will be extremely difficult to clean and will require extensive repair or complete remodeling. It's strongly advised that children not stay in these buildings.

Carbon Monoxide (CO)

NEVER use portable generators indoors! Place generators outside and as far away from buildings as possible. Do not put portable generators on balconies or near doors, vents, or windows and do not use them near where you or your children are sleeping. Due to loss of electricity, gasoline or diesel-powered generators may be used in the aftermath of floods. These devices release CO, a colorless, odorless, and deadly gas. Simply opening doors and windows or using fans will not prevent CO buildup in the home or in partially enclosed areas such as a garage.

If your children or anyone else in your family starts to feel sick, dizzy or weak or experiences a headache, chest pain or confusion, get to fresh air immediately and seek medical care as soon as possible. Your child's skin under the fingernails may also turn cherry red if he/ she has been exposed to high levels of CO. Fetuses and infants are especially vulnerable to the life-threatening effects of CO.

Install a CO detector that is Nationally Recognized Testing Laboratory (NRTL) approved (such as UL). These are generally available at local hardware stores. CO is lighter than air, so detectors should be placed closer to the ceiling. Detectors should be placed close enough to sleeping areas to be heard by sleeping household members.

Contaminated Water

While all people need safe drinking water, it is especially important for children because they are more vulnerable to harm from contaminated water. If a water source may be contaminated with flood waters, children, pregnant women, and nursing mothers should drink only bottled water, which should also be used to mix baby formula and for cooking. It's also recommended that sponge bathe your children with warm bottled water until you are certain your tap water is safe to drink.

Your child may or may not show symptoms or become ill from swallowing small amounts of contaminated water. Symptoms can vary by a contaminant. If your child drinks water contaminated with disease-causing organisms, he/she may come down with symptoms similar to the "stomach flu." These include stomach ache, nausea, vomiting, and diarrhea, and may cause dehydration.

Some contaminants, such as pesticides and gasoline, may cause the water to smell and taste strange, and others such as lead and disease-causing organisms may not be detectable. Drinking water contaminated with chemicals such as lead or gasoline may not cause immediate symptoms or cause your child to become ill but could still potentially harm your child's developing brain or immune system.

Because you cannot be sure if the water is safe until private wells are professionally tested or city water is certified as safe by local officials, parents are urged to take every precaution to make sure their child's drinking water is safe.

If you have a flooded well, do NOT turn on the pump, and do NOT flush the well with water. Contact your local or state health department or agriculture extension agent for specific advice on disinfecting your well.

Your public water system or local health agency will inform you if you need to boil water prior to using it for drinking and cooking. View additional information about emergency disinfection of drinking water.

Tap water that has been brought to a rolling boil for at least 1 minute will kill disease-causing organisms. Boiling will not remove many potentially harmful chemicals, and may actually increase concentrations of heavy metals (including lead), which can be harmful to a child's developing immune system. Chemically treating tap water with either chlorine or iodine will kill many disease-causing organisms, but will not remove harmful chemicals or heavy metals.

Household Items Contaminated by Floodwaters

Drinking water containers. Clean thoroughly with soap and water, then rinse. For gallon-sized containers, add approximately 1 teaspoon of bleach to a gallon of water to make a bleach solution. Cover the container and agitate the bleach solution thoroughly, allowing it to contact all inside surfaces. Cover and let stand for 30 minutes, then rinse with potable water.

Kitchenware and utensils. In general, metal and glazed ceramic that are thoroughly washed and dried can be sanitized and kept. Follow local public health guidance on effective and safe sanitation procedures. Wood items must be thrown away, as these items can absorb contaminants or grow mold from the exposure to flood water and they cannot be properly sanitized.

Children's toys and baby items. Throw away ALL soft or absorbent toys because it is impossible to clean them and they could harm your child. Throw away ALL baby bottles, nipples, and pacifiers that have come in contact with flood waters or debris.

Other Flood Topics

Teenagers. Teens are still growing and developing especially their reproductive, nervous and immune systems. Teens are less likely to understand dangers and may underestimate the dangers of certain situations, or they may be reluctant to voice their concerns about potential dangers. Whenever possible, teens should not participate in the post-flood cleanup that would expose them to contaminated water, mold, and hazardous chemicals. Older teens may help adults with minor cleanups if they wear protective gear including goggles, heavy work gloves, long pants, shirts, socks, boots, and a properly fitting N-95 respirator.

Older adults and people living with chronic diseases: Flooding often leads to the development of microorganisms and the release of dangerous chemicals into the air and water. Older adults and people living with chronic diseases are especially vulnerable to these contaminants.

Bleach. Household bleach contains chlorine, a very corrosive chemical which can be harmful if swallowed or inhaled. It is one of the most common cleaners accidentally swallowed by children. Children—especially those with asthma—should not be in the room while using these products. Call Poison Control at 800-222-1212 immediately in case of poisoning.

Formerly flooded or debris-filled areas. Children in these areas may be at risk of exposure to dirt and debris that may have been contaminated with hazardous chemicals like lead, asbestos, oil, and gasoline. Children can be exposed by direct contact with their skin, by breathing in dust particles or fumes, or by putting their hands in their mouths.

Mosquitoes and disease-causing pests. Flood water may increase the number of mosquitoes and other disease-causing pests. To protect your child, ensure that they use insect repellents containing up to 30 percent N,N-diethyl-meta-toluamide (DEET), picaridin, or oil of lemon eucalyptus. The American Academy of Pediatrics (AAP) recommends that DEET not be used on infants less than 2 months of age and that oil of lemon eucalyptus not be used on children under 3 years of age. Other ways to protect children include staying indoors while the sun is down, wearing light-colored, long-sleeved shirts and pants, covering baby carriages and playpens with mosquito netting, and clear standing water or empty flower pots, etc. of water.

Extreme Heat: Effects on Children and Pregnant Women

Heat-related illnesses are common, yet preventable on hot days. Children and pregnant women need to take extra precautions to avoid overheating on days of extreme heat. Dehydration, heat stroke, and other heat illnesses may affect a child or pregnant woman more severely than the average adult.

Why Are Children More Susceptible to Extreme Heat?

- **Physical characteristics.** Children have a smaller body mass to surface area ratio than adults, making them more vulnerable to heat-related morbidity and mortality. Children are more likely to become dehydrated than adults because they can lose more fluid quickly.

- **Behaviors.** Children play outside more than adults, and they may be at greater risk of heat stroke and exhaustion because they may lack the judgment to limit exertion during hot weather and to rehydrate themselves after long periods of time in the heat. There are also regular reports of infants dying when left in unattended vehicles, which suggests a low awareness of the dangers of heat events.

How Do I Know If My Child Is Dehydrated?

- Decreased physical activity
- Lack of tears when crying

- Dry mouth
- Irritability and fussiness

What Should I Do If My Child Has Become Dehydrated?

- Have the child or infant drink fluid replacement products.
- Allow for rehydration to take a few hours, over which children should stay in a cool, shaded area and sip fluids periodically.
- Call your doctor if symptoms do not improve or if they worsen.

How Do I Know If My Child Has Suffered a Heat Stroke?

Heat stroke, a condition in which the body becomes overheated in a relatively short span of time, can be life-threatening and requires immediate medical attention.

- Skin is flushed, red, and dry
- Little or no sweating
- Deep breathing
- Dizziness, headache, and/or fatigue
- Less urine is produced, of a dark yellowish color
- Loss of consciousness

What Should I Do If My Child Has Suffered a Heat Stroke?

- Immediately remove the child from heat and place in a cool environment.
- Place the child in a bath of cool water and massage skin to increase circulation (do not use water colder than 60°F—this may restrict blood vessels).
- Take the child to hospital or doctor as soon as possible.

How Can Children Be Protected from the Effects of Extreme Heat?

- **Hydration.** Make sure children are drinking plenty of fluids while playing outside, especially if they are participating in sports or rigorous physical activity. Fluids should be drunk before, during, and after periods of time in extreme heat.

- **Staying indoors**. Ideally, children should avoid spending time outdoors during periods of extreme heat. Playing outside in the morning or evenings can protect children from dehydration or heat exhaustion. Never leave a child in a parked car, even if the windows are open.

- **Light clothing.** Children should be dressed in light, loose-fitting clothes on extremely hot days. Breathable fabrics such as cotton are ideal because sweat can evaporate and cool down the child's body.

How Do I Care for My Infant during Hot Weather?

- Check your baby's diaper for concentrated urine, which can be a sign of dehydration.

- If your infant is sweating, he or she is too warm. Remove him or her from the sun immediately and find a place for the baby to cool down.

- Avoid using a fan on or near your baby; it dehydrates them faster.

- A hat traps an infant's body heat and should only be worn in the sun to avoid sunburn.

- Never leave an infant in a parked car, even if the windows are open.

Why Are Pregnant Women Especially at Risk during Periods of Extreme Heat?

An increase in the core body temperature of a pregnant woman may affect the fetus, especially during the first trimester.

How Can Pregnant Women Protect Themselves from the Effects of Extreme Heat?

- Wear light loose fitting clothing

- Stay hydrated by drinking six to eight glasses of water a day

- Avoid caffeine, salt, and alcohol

- Balance fluids by drinking beverages with sodium and other electrolytes

- Limit midday excursions when temperatures are at their highest

- Call a doctor or go to emergency room if a woman feels dizzy, short of breath, or lightheaded

Children's Health and Volcanic Ash

Wildfires expose children to a number of environmental hazards, e.g., fire, smoke, psychological conditions, and the by-products of combustion. After a wildfire, children may be exposed to a different set of environmental hazards involving not only their homes, but also nearby structures, land, and recovery activities.

What Does Volcanic Ash Consist of?

Volcanic ash consists of tiny pieces of rock and glass that are spread over large areas by the wind.

Risks of Volcanic Ash Exposure

During volcanic ash fall, people should take measures to avoid unnecessary exposure to airborne ash and gases. Short-term exposure to ash usually does not cause significant health problems for the general public, but special precautions should be taken to protect susceptible people such as infants and children. Most volcanic gases such as carbon dioxide (CO_2) and hydrogen sulfide (H_2S) blow away quickly. Sulfur dioxide (SO_2) is an irritant volcanic gas that can cause the airways to narrow, especially in people with asthma. Precaution should be taken to ensure that children living close to the volcano or in low-lying areas (where gases may accumulate) are protected from respiratory and eye irritation.

While children face the same health problems from volcanic ash particles suspended in the air as adults (namely respiratory and irritation of the nose, throat, and eyes), they may be more vulnerable to exposure due to their smaller physical size, developing respiratory systems, and decreased the ability to avoid unnecessary exposure. Small volcanic ash particles—those less than 10 micrometers in diameter—pose the greatest health concern because they can pass through the nose and throat and get deep into the lungs. This size range includes fine particles, with diameters less than 2.5 micrometers, and coarse particles, which range in size from 2.5–10 micrometers in diameter. Particles larger than 10 micrometers do not usually reach the lungs, but they can irritate your eyes, nose, and throat. The volcanic ash may exacerbate the symptoms of children suffering from existing respiratory illnesses such as asthma, cystic fibrosis (CF), or tuberculosis (TB).

37

Precautions for Children If Ash Is Present

- Always pay attention to warnings and obey instructions from local authorities

- Check the Air Quality Index (AQI) forecast for your area

- Stay alert to news reports about volcanic ash warnings

- Keep children indoors

  - Children should avoid running or strenuous activity during ash fall. Exertion leads to heavier breathing which can draw ash particles deeper into the lungs.

  - Parents may want to plan indoor games and activities that minimize activity when ash is present.

  - If your family must be outdoors when there is ash in the air, they should wear a disposable mask. If no disposable masks are available, makeshift masks can be made by moistening fabric such as handkerchiefs to help to block out large ash particles.

  - Volcanic ash can irritate the skin; long-sleeved shirts and long pants should be worn if children must go outdoors.

- Children should not play in areas where ash is deep or piled up, especially if they are likely to roll or lie in the ash piles.

- Children should wear glasses instead of a contact lens to avoid eye irritation.

- Create a "clean room" where children sleep and play to help to minimize exposure to ash in the indoor air.

  - Keep windows and doors closed. Close any vents or air ducts (such as chimneys) that may allow ash to enter the house.

  - Run central air conditioners on the "recirculate" option (instead of "outdoor air intake"). Clean the air filter to allow good air flow indoors.

  - Avoid vacuuming as it will stir up ash and dust into the air.

  - Do not smoke or burn anything (tobacco, candles, incense) inside the home. This will create more indoor pollutants.

  - If it is too warm or difficult to breathe inside with the windows closed, seek shelter elsewhere.

- A portable room air filter may be effective to remove particles from the air.

- Choosing to buy an air cleaner is ideally a decision that should be made before a smoke/ash emergency occurs. Going outside to locate an appropriate device during an emergency may be hazardous, and the devices may be in short supply.

- An air cleaner with a high-efficiency particulate air (HEPA) filter, an electrostatic precipitator (ESP), or an ionizing air cleaner may be effective at removing air particles provided it is sized to filter two or three times the room air volume per hour

- Avoid ozone generators, personal air purifiers, "pure air" generators, and "super oxygen" purifiers as these devices emit ozone gas into the air at levels that can irritate airways and exacerbate existing respiratory conditions. These devices are also not effective at removing particles from the air.

Chapter 4

Environmental Hazards for Pregnant Women

More than three million healthy babies are born annually in the United States. While most women have a normal term pregnancy and deliver a normal infant, a safe and healthy pregnancy is not experienced by all women. Certain genetic, behavioral, social, and environmental factors can affect the parents' ability to conceive, carry, and deliver a healthy, full-term baby.

Reproductive and Birth Outcomes and the Environment

Our understanding of risk factors for reproductive problems such as infertility, low birth weight, prematurity, fetal and infant death has increased over the past decades. Certain health conditions, social and economic factors, and behaviors can increase the risk of adverse reproductive and birth outcomes. It's also learned that environmental exposures can play a role in reproductive and birth outcomes. However, there is still much not known.

Exposure and Risk

The following are some of the possible environmental exposure and risk factors that are associated with reproductive and birth outcomes:

- **Environmental tobacco smoke.** Exposure of nonsmoking pregnant women to environmental tobacco smoke (also known as

This chapter includes text excerpted from "Reproductive and Birth Outcomes," Centers for Disease Control and Prevention (CDC), January 10, 2017.

secondhand smoke) may be a risk factor for preterm birth, low birth weight, and possibly fetal death or miscarriage.

- **Air pollution.** Exposure to air pollution may be related to both low birth weight and preterm birth, even at low levels.

- **Lead.** A pregnant woman's exposure to lead may cause preterm birth, low birth weight, and spontaneous fetal death or miscarriage.

- **Pesticides.** Exposure to pesticides has been associated with fetal death (miscarriage) and babies being born too small, but more research is needed in this area.

- **Environmental contaminants.** Although age and certain health conditions are more commonly associated with infertility, it is believed that environmental contaminants may cause infertility by creating other health conditions. For example, some research suggests that environmental contaminants can affect a woman's menstruation and ovulation. Low-level exposures to compounds such as lead and pesticides are suspected risk factors for women. Exposure to compounds such as lead and polychlorinated biphenyls (PCBs) have been linked to decreased sperm quality among men. Much more research needs to be done to find out how environmental contaminants may be affecting human fertility.

- **Endocrine Disruptors.** Some scientists have suggested that environmental hazards can affect how many males are born. Parents and the fetus can be exposed to different hazards referred to as endocrine disruptors. Fewer males are conceived when exposure to endocrine disruptors causes a decrease in testosterone. Diethylstilbestrol (DES), a synthetic estrogen widely prescribed to pregnant women during the mid-1900s, is a strong endocrine disruptor. Previous studies have suggested an association between endocrine disrupting compounds and the secondary sex ratio (the sex ratio of the grandchildren of the exposed women). Several studies show that declines in the sex ratio of males to females at birth may be associated with occupational exposure or exposure to air pollution.

Prevention

Women who are pregnant or may become pregnant should follow their doctor's advice on how they can have a healthy baby. Doctors can also answer questions on fertility and give advice on conceiving. Early and regular prenatal care helps identify conditions and behaviors that can result in adverse reproductive and birth outcomes.

Here are some ways to prevent environmental exposures:

- Stop smoking and avoid secondhand smoke.

- Limit outdoor activity when the air quality index (AQI) shows unhealthy levels of air pollutants.

- Cut out or reduce any indoor sources of particulate matter, like wood burning stoves and fireplaces, and try to reduce the amount of time spent outdoors near areas with higher levels of air pollution, such as areas with a lot of traffic.

- Stay away from lead.

- Stay away from mercury. Some fish, especially albacore tuna, may have been contaminated with mercury. State health departments send out public fish consumption guidelines that pregnant women can follow.

- Do not use pesticides if you are pregnant. Stay away from rooms that have been recently sprayed with insecticides and from other areas with potential pesticide exposure.

Chapter 5

Environmental Hazards for the Elderly

Chapter Contents

Section 5.1

The Elderly and Hazards of Falling and Fractures

This section includes text excerpted from "Prevent Falls and Fractures," National Institute on Aging (NIA), National Institutes of Health (NIH), March 15, 2017.

A simple thing can change your life—like tripping on a rug or slipping on a wet floor. If you fall, you could break a bone, like thousands of older men and women, do each year. For older people, a break can be the start of more serious problems, such as a trip to the hospital, injury, or even disability.

If you or an older person you know has fallen, you're not alone. More than one in three people age 65 years or older fall each year. The risk of falling—and fall-related problems—rises with age.

Many Older Adults Fear Falling

The fear of falling becomes more common as people age, even among those who haven't fallen. It may lead older people to avoid activities such as walking, shopping, or taking part in social activities.

But don't let a fear of falling keep you from being active. Overcoming this fear can help you stay active, maintain your physical health, and prevent future falls. Doing things like getting together with friends, gardening, walking, or going to the local senior center helps you stay healthy. The good news is, there are simple ways to prevent most falls.

Causes and Risk Factors for Falls

Many things can cause a fall. Your eyesight, hearing, and reflexes might not be as sharp as they were when you were younger. Diabetes, heart disease, or problems with your thyroid, nerves, feet, or blood vessels can affect your balance. Some medicines can cause you to feel dizzy or sleepy, making you more likely to fall. Other causes include safety hazards in the home or community environment.

Scientists have linked several personal risk factors to falling, including muscle weakness, problems with balance and gait, and blood pressure that drops too much when you get up from lying down or sitting (called postural hypotension). Foot problems that cause pain and unsafe footwear, like backless shoes or high heels, can also increase your risk of falling.

Confusion can sometimes lead to falls. For example, if you wake up in an unfamiliar environment, you might feel unsure of where you are. If you feel confused, wait for your mind to clear or until someone comes to help you before trying to get up and walk around.

Some medications can increase a person's risk of falling because they cause side effects like dizziness or confusion. The more medications you take, the more likely you are to fall.

Take the Right Steps to Prevent Falls

If you take care of your overall health, you may be able to lower your chances of falling. Most of the time falls and accidents don't "just happen." Here are a few tips to help you avoid falls and broken bones:

- **Stay physically active.** Plan an exercise program that is right for you. Regular exercise improves muscles and makes you stronger. It also helps keep your joints, tendons, and ligaments flexible. Mild weight-bearing activities, such as walking or climbing stairs, may slow bone loss from osteoporosis.

- **Have your eyes and hearing tested?** Even small changes in sight and hearing may cause you to fall. When you get new eyeglasses or contact lenses, take time to get used to them. Always wear your glasses or contacts when you need them. If you have a hearing aid, be sure it fits well and wear it.

- **Find out about the side effects of any medicine you take.** If a drug makes you sleepy or dizzy, tell your doctor or pharmacist.

- **Get enough sleep.** If you are sleepy, you are more likely to fall.

- **Limit the amount of alcohol you drink.** Even a small amount of alcohol can affect your balance and reflexes. Studies show that the rate of hip fractures in older adults increases with alcohol use.

- **Stand up slowly.** Getting up too quickly can cause your blood pressure to drop. That can make you feel wobbly. Get your blood pressure checked when lying and standing.

- **Use an assistive device if you need help feeling steady when you walk.** Appropriate use of canes and walkers can prevent falls. If your doctor tells you to use a cane or walker, make sure it is the right size for you and the wheels roll smoothly. This is important when you're walking in areas you don't know well or where the walkways are uneven. A physical or occupational therapist can help you decide which devices might be helpful and teach you how to use them safely.

- **Be very careful when walking on wet or icy surfaces.** They can be very slippery! Try to have sand or salt spread on icy areas by your front or back door.

- **Wear nonskid, rubber soled, low-heeled shoes, or lace-up shoes with nonskid soles that fully support your feet.** It is important that the soles are not too thin or too thick. Don't walk on stairs or floors in socks or in shoes and slippers with smooth soles.

- **Always tell your doctor if you have fallen since your last checkup, even if you aren't hurt when you fall.** A fall can alert your doctor to a new medical problem or problems with your medications or eyesight that can be corrected. Your doctor may suggest physical therapy, a walking aid, or other steps to help prevent future falls.

What to Do If You Fall

Whether you are at home or somewhere else, a sudden fall can be startling and upsetting. If you do fall, stay as calm as possible.

Take several deep breaths to try to relax. Remain still on the floor or ground for a few moments. This will help you get over the shock of falling.

Decide if you are hurt before getting up. Getting up too quickly or in the wrong way could make an injury worse.

If you think you can get up safely without help, roll over onto your side. Rest again while your body and blood pressure adjust. Slowly get up on your hands and knees, and crawl to a sturdy chair.

Put your hands on the chair seat and slide one foot forward so that it is flat on the floor. Keep the other leg bent so the knee is on the floor. From this kneeling position, slowly rise and turn your body to sit in the chair.

If you are hurt or cannot get up on your own, ask someone for help or call 911. If you are alone, try to get into a comfortable position and wait for help to arrive.

Carrying a mobile or portable phone with you as you move about your house could make it easier to call someone if you need assistance. An emergency response system, which lets you push a button on a special necklace or bracelet to call for help, is another option.

Keep Your Bones Strong to Prevent Falls

Falls are a common reason for trips to the emergency room and for hospital stays among older adults. Many of these hospital visits are for fall-related fractures. You can help prevent fractures by keeping your bones strong.

Having healthy bones won't prevent a fall, but if you fall, it might prevent breaking a hip or other bone, which may lead to a hospital or nursing home stay, disability, or even death. Getting enough calcium and vitamin D can help keep your bones strong. So can physical activity. Try to get at least 150 minutes per week of physical activity.

Other ways to maintain bone health include quitting smoking and limiting alcohol use, which can decrease bone mass and increase the chance of fractures. Also, try to maintain a healthy weight. Being underweight increases the risk of bone loss and broken bones.

Osteoporosis is a disease that makes bones weak and more likely to break. For people with osteoporosis, even a minor fall may be dangerous. Talk to your doctor about osteoporosis.

Section 5.2

Hot Weather Safety for Older Adults

This section includes text excerpted from "Hot Weather Safety for Older Adults," National Institute on Aging (NIA), National Institutes of Health (NIH), June 15, 2016.

Too much heat is not safe for anyone. It is even riskier if you are older or have health problems. It is important to get relief from the heat quickly. If not, you might begin to feel confused or faint. Your heart could become stressed and stop beating.

Being hot for too long can be a problem. It can cause several illnesses, all grouped under the name hyperthermia.

- **Heat syncope** is a sudden dizziness that can happen when you are active in hot weather. If you take a heart medication called a beta blocker or are not used to hot weather, you are even more likely to feel faint. Rest in a cool place, put your legs up, and drink water to make the dizzy feeling go away.

- **Heat cramps** are the painful tightening of muscles in your stomach, arms, or legs. Cramps can result from hard work or exercise. Though your body temperature and pulse usually stay normal during heat cramps, your skin may feel moist and cool. Find a way to cool your body down. Rest in the shade or in a cool building. Drink plenty of fluids, but not those with alcohol or caffeine.

- **Heat edema** is a swelling in your ankles and feet when you get hot. Put your legs up to help reduce swelling. If that doesn't work fairly quickly, check with your doctor.

- **Heat exhaustion** is a warning that your body can no longer keep itself cool. You might feel thirsty, dizzy, weak, uncoordinated, and nauseated. You may sweat a lot. Your body temperature may stay normal, but your skin may feel cold and clammy. Some people with heat exhaustion have a rapid pulse. Rest in a cool place and get plenty of fluids. If you don't feel better soon, get medical care. Be careful—heat exhaustion can progress to heat stroke.

Heat Stroke—A Medical Emergency

If you have heat stroke, you need to get medical help right away. Older people living in homes or apartments without air conditioning or fans are at most risk. People who become dehydrated or those with chronic diseases or alcoholism are also at most risk. Signs of heat stroke are:

- Fainting (possibly the first sign) or becoming unconscious

- A change in behavior—confusion, agitation, staggering, being grouchy, or acting strangely

- Body temperature over 104°F (40°C)

- Dry, flushed skin and a strong, rapid pulse or a slow, weak pulse

- Not sweating, even if it is hot

Who Is at Risk?

Each year, most people who die from hyperthermia are over 50 years old. Health problems that put you at greater risk include:

- Heart or blood vessel problems

- Poorly working sweat glands or changes in your skin caused by normal aging

- Heart, lung, or kidney disease, as well as any illness that makes you feel weak all over or results in a fever

- Conditions treated by drugs, such as diuretics, sedatives, tranquilizers, and some heart and high blood pressure medicines; they may make it harder for your body to cool itself

- Taking several prescription drugs; ask your doctor if any of your medications make you more likely to become overheated

- Being very overweight or underweight

- Drinking alcoholic beverages

How Can I Lower My Risk?

Things you can do to lower your risk of heat-related illness:

- Drink plenty of liquids, such as water or fruit or vegetable juices. Stay away from drinks containing alcohol or caffeine. If your doctor has told you to limit your liquids, ask what you should do when it is very hot.

- If you live in a home or apartment without fans or air conditioning, try to keep your house as cool as possible. Limit your use of the oven. Keep your shades, blinds, or curtains closed during the hottest part of the day. Open your windows at night.

- If your house is hot, try to spend time during mid-day someplace that has air conditioning—for example, go to the shopping mall, movies, library, senior center, or a friend's house

- If you need help getting to a cool place, ask a friend or relative. Some religious groups, senior centers, and Area Agencies on Aging (AAA) provide this service. If necessary, take a taxi or call for senior transportation. Don't stand outside in the heat waiting for a bus.

- Dress for the weather. Some people find natural fabrics, such as cotton, to be cooler than synthetic fibers.

- Don't try to exercise or do a lot of activities outdoors when it's hot.

- Avoid crowded places when it's hot outside. Plan trips during non-rush-hour times.

What Should I Remember?

Older people can have a tough time dealing with heat and humidity. The temperature inside or outside does not have to reach 100°F (38°C) to put them at risk for a heat-related illness.

A headache, confusion, dizziness, or nausea could be a sign of a heat-related illness. Go to the doctor or an emergency room to find out if you need treatment.

To keep heat-related illnesses from becoming a dangerous heat stroke, remember to:

- Get out of the sun and into a cool place—air conditioning is best.

- Drink fluids, but avoid alcohol and caffeine. Water and fruit or vegetable juices are good choices.

- Shower, bathe, or sponge off with cool water.

- Lie down and rest in a cool place.

- Visit your doctor or go to an emergency room if you don't cool down quickly.

Section 5.3

Cold Weather Safety for Older Adults

This section includes text excerpted from "Cold Weather Safety for Older Adults," National Institute on Aging (NIA), National Institutes of Health (NIH), January 1, 2018.

If you are like most people, you feel cold every now and then during the winter. What you may not know is that just being really cold can make you very sick.

Older adults can lose body heat fast—faster than when they were young. Changes in your body that come with aging can make it harder for you to be aware of getting cold. A big chill can turn into a dangerous problem before an older person even knows what's happening. Doctors call this serious problem hypothermia.

What Is Hypothermia?

Hypothermia is what happens when your body temperature gets very low. For an older person, a body temperature of 95°F or lower can cause many health problems, such as a heart attack, kidney problems, liver damage, or worse.

Being outside in the cold, or even being in a very cold house, can lead to hypothermia. Try to stay away from cold places, and pay attention to how cold it is where you are. You can take steps to lower your chance of getting hypothermia.

Keep Warm Inside

Living in a cold house, apartment, or other building can cause hypothermia. In fact, hypothermia can happen to someone in a nursing home or group facility if the rooms are not kept warm enough. If someone you know is in a group facility, pay attention to the inside temperature and to whether that person is dressed warmly enough.

People who are sick may have special problems keeping warm. Do not let it get too cold inside and dress warmly. Even if you keep your temperature between 60–65°F, your home or apartment may not be warm enough to keep you safe. This is a special problem if you live alone because there is no one else to feel the chilliness of the house or notice if you are having symptoms of hypothermia.

Here are some tips for keeping warm while you're inside:

- Set your heat to at least 68–70°F. To save on heating bills, close off rooms you are not using. Close the vents and shut the doors in these rooms, and keep the basement door closed. Place a rolled towel in front of all doors to keep out drafts.

- Make sure your house isn't losing heat through windows. Keep your blinds and curtains closed. If you have gaps around the windows, try using weather stripping or caulk to keep the cold air out.

- Dress warmly on cold days even if you are staying in the house. Throw a blanket over your legs. Wear socks and slippers.

- When you go to sleep, wear long underwear under your pajamas, and use extra covers. Wear a cap or hat.

- Make sure you eat enough food to keep up your weight. If you don't eat well, you might have less fat under your skin. Body fat helps you to stay warm.

- Drink alcohol moderately, if at all. Alcoholic drinks can make you lose body heat.

- Ask family or friends to check on you during cold weather. If a power outage leaves you without heat, try to stay with a relative or friend.

You may be tempted to warm your room with a space heater. But, some space heaters are fire hazards, and others can cause carbon monoxide (CO) poisoning.

Bundle Up on Windy, Cold Days

A heavy wind can quickly lower your body temperature. Check the weather forecast for windy and cold days. On those days, try to stay inside or in a warm place. If you have to go out, wear warm clothes, and don't stay out in the cold and wind for a long time.

Here are some other tips:

- Dress for the weather if you have to go out on chilly, cold, or damp days

- Wear loose layers of clothing. The air between the layers helps to keep you warm.

- Put on a hat and scarf. You lose a lot of body heat when your head and neck are uncovered.

- Wear a waterproof coat or jacket if it's snowy

- Change your clothes right away if they get damp or wet

Illness, Medicines, and Cold Weather

Some illnesses may make it harder for your body to stay warm.

- Thyroid problems can make it hard to maintain a normal body temperature.

- Diabetes can keep blood from flowing normally to provide warmth.

- Parkinson disease (PD) and arthritis can make it hard to put on more clothes, use a blanket, or get out of the cold.

- Memory loss can cause a person to go outside without the right clothing.

Talk with your doctor about your health problems and how to prevent hypothermia.

Taking some medicines and not being active also can affect body heat. These include medicines you get from your doctor and those you buy over-the-counter (OTC), such as some cold medicines. Ask your doctor if the medicines you take may affect body heat. Always talk with your doctor before you stop taking any medication.

Here are some topics to talk about with your doctor to stay safe in cold weather:

- Ask your doctor about signs of hypothermia

- Talk to your doctor about any health problems and medicines that can make hypothermia a special problem for you. Your doctor can help you find ways to prevent hypothermia.

- Ask about safe ways to stay active even when it's cold outside

What Are the Warning Signs of Hypothermia?

Sometimes it is hard to tell if a person has hypothermia. Look for clues. Is the house very cold? Is the person not dressed for cold weather? Is the person speaking slower than normal and having trouble keeping his or her balance?

Watch for the signs of hypothermia in yourself, too. You might become confused if your body temperature gets very low. Talk to your family and friends about the warning signs so they can look out for you.

Early signs of hypothermia:

- Cold feet and hands

- Puffy or swollen face

- Pale skin

- Shivering (in some cases the person with hypothermia does not shiver)

- Slower than normal speech or slurring words

- Acting sleepy

- Being angry or confused

Later signs of hypothermia:

- Moving slowly, trouble walking, or being clumsy

- Stiff and jerky arm or leg movements

- Slow heartbeat

- Slow, shallow breathing

- Blacking out or losing consciousness

Call 911 right away if you think someone has warning signs of hypothermia.

What to do after you call 911:

- Try to move the person to a warmer place.

- Wrap the person in a warm blanket, towels, or coats—whatever is handy. Even your own body warmth will help. Lie close, but be gentle.

- Give the person something warm to drink, but avoid drinks with alcohol or caffeine, such as regular coffee.

- Do not rub the person's legs or arms.

- Do not try to warm the person in a bath.

- Do not use a heating pad.

Chapter 6

Climate Change and Human Health

Climate change is a significant threat to the health of the American people. It is the result of the buildup of greenhouse gases in the atmosphere, primarily from the burning of fossil fuels, such as oil and gasoline, for energy and other human activities. These gases, such as carbon dioxide (CO_2) and methane (CH_4), warm and alter the global climate. Temperatures and the frequency of heavy rain and snow have been increasing in the United States. The changes in temperature and precipitation, as well as other changes, such as more intense severe weather and rising sea levels, all have effects on people's environments that can, in turn, harm their health and well-being. Climate change is anticipated to worsen all of the major climate trends in the United States.

How Does Climate Change Affect Human Health?

While climate change is a global process, it has both local and regional impacts that profoundly affect communities. Some of these effects are relatively direct, as when heat waves or intense hurricanes cause injury and illness, and even death. Some health effects of climate change are less direct and involve changes in our environment that in turn can affect human health and diseases. For example, changes in

This chapter includes text excerpted from "Climate Change and Human Health," National Institute of Environmental Health Sciences (NIEHS), April 1, 2016.

temperatures and rainfall can have a strong effect on the life cycles of insects and other species that transmit disease, such as Lyme disease and West Nile virus, leading to new outbreaks or shifts in places where these diseases occur. Rising sea levels can worsen the flooding from hurricanes in coastal areas, leading to human exposures to water and areas contaminated by industrial pollutants and hazardous wastes. In all cases, the effects of climate change occur in combination with other well-known health stressors, such as poverty, social disadvantage, impaired language ability, and others. Often referred to as the social determinants of health, these factors lead to certain people being more vulnerable, by making it more likely they may be exposed to climate change-related risks or less able to cope with such exposures and their health impacts. Examples of the varied ways that climate change can affect people's health are shown in the following table.

Table 6.1. Examples of Climate Change Impacts on Health

	Climate Driver	Exposure	Health Outcome	Impact
Extreme Heat	More frequent, severe, prolonged heat events	Elevated temperatures	Heat-related death and illness	Rising temperatures will lead to an increase in heat-related deaths and illnesses.
Outdoor Air Quality	Increasing temperatures and changing precipitation patterns	Worsened air quality (ozone, particulate matter, and higher pollen counts)	Premature death, acute and chronic cardiovascular and respiratory illnesses	Rising temperatures and wildfires and decreasing precipitation will lead to increases in ozone and particulate matter, elevating the risks of cardiovascular and respiratory illnesses and death.

Table 6.1. Continued

	Climate Driver	Exposure	Health Outcome	Impact
Flooding	Rising sea level and more frequent or intense extreme precipitation, hurricanes, and storm surge events	Contaminated water, debris, and disruptions to essential infrastructure	Drowning, injuries, mental health consequences, gastrointestinal and other illness	Increased coastal and inland flooding exposes populations to a range of negative health impacts before, during, and after events.
Vector-borne Infection (Lyme disease)	Changes in temperature extremes and seasonal weather patterns	Earlier and geographically expanded tick activity	Lyme disease	Ticks will show earlier seasonal activity and a generally northward range expansion, increasing risk of human exposure to Lyme disease-causing bacteria.
Water-related Infection (Vibrio vulnificus)	Rising sea surface temperature, changes in precipitation, and runoff affecting coastal salinity	Recreational water or shellfish contaminated with Vibrio vulnificus	Vibrio vulnificus induced diarrhea and intestinal illness, wound and bloodstream infections, death	Increases in water temperatures will alter timing and location of Vibrio vulnificus growth, increasing exposure and risk of waterborne illness.

Table 6.1. Continued

	Climate Driver	Exposure	Health Outcome	Impact
Food-related Infection (Salmonella)	Increases in temperature, humidity, and season length	Increased growth of pathogens, seasonal shifts in incidence of *Salmonella* exposure	*Salmonella* infection, gastrointestinal outbreaks	Rising temperatures increase *Salmonella* prevalence in food; longer seasons and warming winters increase risk of exposure and infection.
Mental Health and Well-being	Climate change impacts especially extreme weather	Level of exposure to traumatic events, like disasters	Distress, grief, behavioral health disorders, social impacts, resilience	Changes in exposure to climate- or weather-related disasters cause or exacerbate stress and mental health consequences, and with greater risk for certain populations.

Who Is Most at Risk from Climate Change?

Although the U.S. has a well developed public health and medical system, every American is vulnerable to the impacts of climate change at some point in their lives, no matter where they live. Globally, the effects of climate change will have even more severe consequences for human health. Certain U.S. populations are more vulnerable to climate change health threats as a result of specific physical, environmental, and socio-demographic factors, as well as age and life stage. Some of these groups and the challenges they face from climate change include the following.

Low Income Groups

People with low incomes live with many factors that increase their vulnerability to health impacts of climate change. They are more likely to live in risk-prone areas, such as urban heat islands, isolated rural areas, or coastal and other flood-prone areas, or where there is older or poorly maintained infrastructure. Low-income group softens face an increased burden of air or other toxic pollution that may be increased or mobilized by climate change impacts like severe storms. They experience relatively greater incidence of chronic medical conditions, such as cardiovascular and kidney disease, diabetes, asthma, and chronic obstructive pulmonary disease (COPD), all of which may be worsened by climate change impacts. Also, limited transportation and access to health education can impede their ability to prepare for, respond to, and cope with climate-related health risks.

Indigenous Peoples

A number of health risks are higher among indigenous populations, such as poor mental health-related to historical or personal trauma, environmental exposures from pollutants or toxic substances, and diabetes. Because of existing vulnerabilities, indigenous people, especially those who are dependent on the environment for sustenance or who live in geographically isolated or impoverished communities, are likely to experience greater exposure and lower resilience to climate-related health effects. Indigenous communities already face threats to their homes, food sources, and cultural traditions from climate impacts on the environment, such as reductions in sea ice, increases in flooding and landslides, damage to wildlife habitats, loss of medicinal plants, and effects on abundance and nutrition of certain traditional foods.

Children and Pregnant Women

Children have a proportionately higher intake of air, food, and water relative to their body weight compared to adults. They also share unique behaviors and interactions with their environment, such as more time spent outdoor sand placing hands in their mouth. These factors, combined with climate changes, may increase their exposure to environmental contaminants. Extreme heat threatens student-athletes who practice outdoors, as well as children in homes or schools without air conditioning. Children may be vulnerable to injury during extreme weather events as they depend on adults to escape harm, and can suffer emotional trauma from displacement, loss of home or school, and exposure to the event itself. Climate-related exposures may lead to adverse pregnancy outcomes, including spontaneous abortion, low birth weight, preterm birth, and risks to newborns, and infants, including increased neonatal death, dehydration, malnutrition, diarrhea, and respiratory diseases.

Older Adults

The number of older adults, age 65 and older, is growing substantially in the United States, and they make up a population of concern for climate impacts from extreme heat and weather events, degrade air quality, vector-borne diseases, and others. Older adults may be further challenged by climate change impacts due to factors such as social isolation and living in older structures that make them vulnerable to heat and extreme events, such as hurricanes and floods; preexisting health conditions, such as respiratory conditions that may be worsened by climate changes; and mental health challenges, such as depression, dementia, and other cognitive impairments. Older adults are also more likely to be taking medications to treat chronic medical conditions that make them more vulnerable to complications from heat exposure, including antidepressant and antipsychotic drugs and diuretics.

Occupational Groups

Outdoor workers are often among the first to be exposed to the effects of climate change. Climate change is expected to affect the health of outdoor workers through increases in ambient temperature, degraded air quality, extreme weather, vector-borne diseases, industrial exposures, and changes in the built environment. Workers affected by climate change include farmers, ranchers, and other agricultural workers; commercial fishermen; construction workers; paramedics, firefighters and other first responders; and transportation workers. Also, laborers exposed to hot indoor work environments, such as steel mills, dry cleaners, manufacturing facilities, warehouses, and other areas that lack air conditioning, are at risk for extreme heat exposure. Military personnel who train and conduct operations in hot field environments are at risk for heat-related illness, and may also be at increased risk for certain vector-borne diseases.

Persons with Disabilities or Chronic Medical Conditions

The term disability covers a wide variety of functional limitations-related to hearing, speech, vision, cognition, and mobility. An increase in extreme weather can be expected to disproportionately affect populations with disabilities. Preexisting medical conditions present risk factors for increased illness and death associated with climate-related stressors, especially exposure to extreme heat. The prevalence of common chronic medical conditions, including cardiovascular disease, respiratory disease, diabetes, asthma, and obesity, is anticipated to increase over the coming decades, resulting in larger populations at risk of medical complications from climate change-related exposures. Communities that are both medically underserved and have a high prevalence of chronic medical conditions can be especially at risk.

What Are the Co-Benefits of Mitigating and Adapting to Climate Change?

In addition to investigating how climate change can affect human health, NIEHS is also working to understand how responses to climate change can also affect health. Some responses to climate change may lead to substantial reductions in harmful exposures to people, so-called co-benefits, or additional benefits to people's health beyond the benefits of reducing the severity of climate change itself. For example, measures to reduce emissions of carbon dioxide (CO_2) from burning fossil fuels can also greatly reduce toxic air pollution that causes tens of thousands of deaths in the United States each year. Increases in physical activity from policies that lead people to walk, bicycle, or use public transportation, rather than drive, can improve health even as they reduce the combustion of gasoline or other fossil fuels used for transportation. Other examples of co-benefits include healthy changes in food production and consumption that reduce methane emissions from agricultural sources and improved housing insulation that helps people use less energy while adapting to more extreme temperatures.

Impacts of Climate Change on Human Health in the United States

Every person in the United States is vulnerable to the health impacts of climate change at some point in their lives, no matter where they live. This finding is part of a report by the U.S. Global Change Research Program (UCRP), *The Impacts of Climate Change on Human Health in the United States: A Scientific Assessment*. The report, which estimates the current and future impacts of climate change on public health, finds that climate change is exacerbating existing health threats and creating new ones. Nearly all of the health threats, from increases in heat; more frequent or severe extreme events, such as floods or hurricanes; degraded air quality; diseases transmitted through food, water, and vectors, such as ticks and mosquitoes; and stresses to mental health, are expected to worsen with climate change. Certain populations, including low-income groups; some communities of color; limited English proficiency; and immigrant groups; as well as indigenous peoples, children, pregnant women, older adults, certain workers, persons with disabilities, and people with preexisting medical conditions, are more vulnerable to climate change health impacts.

Part Two

Health Concerns and Their Environmental Triggers

Chapter 7

Human Health Problems with Environmental Causes

The air, the water, the sun, the dust, plants and animals, and the chemicals and metals of our world... They support life. They make it beautiful and fun. But, as wonderful as they are... They can also make some people sick. Here are some diseases that are related to your environment from A to Z and some ideas for preventing or caring for them.

Allergies and Asthma

Slightly more than half of the 300 million people living in the United States are sensitive to one or more allergens. They sneeze, their noses run, and their eyes itch from pollen, dust, and other substances. Some suffer sudden attacks that leave them breathless and gasping for air. This is allergic asthma. Asthma attacks often occur after periods of heavy exercise or during sudden changes in the weather. Some can be triggered by pollutants and other chemicals in the air and in the home. Doctors can test to find out which substances are causing reactions. They can also prescribe drugs to relieve the symptoms.

This chapter includes text excerpted from "Environmental Diseases from A to Z," National Institute of Environmental Health Sciences (NIEHS), June 2007. Reviewed April 2018.

Birth Defects

Sometimes, when pregnant women are exposed to chemicals or drink a lot of alcohol, harmful substances reach the fetus. Some of these babies are born with an organ, tissue, or body part that has not developed in a normal way. Aspirin and cigarette smoking can also cause birth problems. Birth defects are the leading cause of death for infants during the first year of life. Many of these could be prevented.

Cancer

Cancer occurs when a cell or group of cells begin to multiply more rapidly than normal. As the cancer cells spread, they affect nearby organs and tissues in the body. Eventually, the organs are not able to perform their normal functions. Cancer is the second leading cause of death in the United States, causing more than 500,000 deaths each year. Some cancers are caused by substances in the environment: cigarette smoke, asbestos, radiation, natural and artificial chemicals, alcohol, and sunlight. People can reduce their risk of getting cancer by limiting their exposure to these harmful agents.

Dermatitis

Dermatitis is a fancy name for inflamed, irritated skin. Many of us have experienced the oozing bumps and itching caused by poison ivy, oak, and sumac. Some chemicals found in paints, dyes, cosmetics, and detergents can also cause rashes and blisters. Too much wind and sun make the skin dry and chapped. Fabrics, foods, and certain medications can cause unusual reactions in some individuals. People can protect themselves from poison ivy by following a simple rule: "Leaves of three, leave them be." Smart folks know their poisons.

Emphysema

Air pollution and cigarette smoke can break down sensitive tissue in the lungs. Once this happens, the lungs cannot expand and contract properly. This condition is emphysema. About two million Americans have this disease. For these people, each breath is hard work.

Even moderate exercise is difficult. Some emphysema patients must breathe from tanks of oxygen.

Fertility Problems

Fertility is the ability to produce children. However, one in eight couples has a problem. However, more than 10 percent of couples cannot conceive after one year of trying to become pregnant. Infertility can be caused by infections that come from sexual diseases or from exposure to chemicals on the job or elsewhere in the environment. Researchers at the National Institute of Environmental Health Sciences (NIEHS) have shown that too much caffeine in the diet can temporarily reduce a woman's fertility.

Goiter

Sometimes people don't get enough iodine from the foods they eat. This can cause a small gland called the thyroid to grow larger. The thyroid can become so large that it looks like a baseball sticking out of the front of your neck. This is called goiter. Since the thyroid controls basic functions like growth and energy, goiter can produce a wide range of effects. Some goiter patients are unusually restless and nervous. Others tend to be sluggish and lethargic. Goiter became rare after public health officials decided that iodine should be added to salt.

Heart Disease

Heart disease is the leading cause of death in the United States and is a major cause of disability. Almost 700,000 Americans die of heart disease each year. While these may be due in part to poor eating habits and/or lack of exercise, environmental chemicals also play a role. While most chemicals that enter the body are broken down into harmless substances by the liver, some are converted into particles called free radicals that can react with proteins in the blood to form fatty deposits called plaques, which can clog blood vessels. A blockage can cut off the flow of blood to the heart, causing a heart attack.

Immune Deficiency Diseases

The immune system fights germs, viruses, and poisons that attack the body. It is composed of white blood cells and other warrior cells.

When a foreign particle enters the body, these cells surround and destroy this "enemy." We have all heard of AIDS [acquired immunodeficiency syndrome] and the harm it does to the immune system. Some chemicals and drugs can also weaken the immune system by damaging its specialized cells. When this occurs, the body is more vulnerable to diseases and infections.

Job-Related Illnesses

Every job has certain hazards. Even a writer can get a paper cut. But did you know that about 137 workers die from job-related diseases every day? This is more than eight times the number people of who die from job-related accidents. Many of these illnesses are caused by chemicals and other agents present in the workplace.

Factories and scientific laboratories can contain poisonous chemicals, dyes, and metals. Doctors and other health workers have to work with radiation. People who work in airports or play in rock concerts can suffer hearing loss from loud noise. Some jobs involve extreme heat or cold. Workers can protect themselves from hazards by wearing special suits and using goggles, gloves, ear plugs, and other equipment.

Kidney Diseases

About 7.5 million adults have some evidence of chronic kidney disease. These diseases range from simple infections to total kidney failure. People with kidney failure cannot remove wastes and poisons from their blood. They depend on expensive kidney machines in order to stay alive. Some chemicals found in the environment can produce kidney damage. Some nonprescription drugs, when taken too often, can also cause kidney problems. Be sure to read the label and use drugs as directed.

Lead Poisoning

Sometimes, infants and children will pick up and eat paint chips and other objects that contain lead. Lead dust, fumes, and lead-contaminated water can also introduce lead into the body. Lead can damage the brain, kidneys, liver, and other organs. Severe lead poisoning can produce headaches, cramps, convulsions, and even death.

Even small amounts can cause learning problems and changes in behavior. Doctors can test for lead in the blood and recommend ways to reduce further exposure.

Mercury Poisoning

Mercury is a silvery metal that is extremely poisonous. Very small amounts can damage the kidneys, liver, and brain. Years ago, workers in hat factories were poisoned by breathing the fumes from mercury used to shape the hats. Remember the "Mad Hatter" in Alice in Wonderland? Today, mercury exposure usually results from eating contaminated fish and other foods that contain small amounts of mercury compounds. Since the body cannot get rid of mercury, it gradually builds up inside the tissues. If it is not treated, mercury poisoning can eventually cause pain, numbness, weak muscles, loss of vision, paralysis, and even death.

Nervous System Disorders

The nervous system, which includes the brain, spinal cord, and nerves, commands and controls our thoughts, feelings, movements, and behavior. The nervous system consists of billions of nerve cells. They carry messages and instructions from the brain and spinal cord to other parts of the body. When these cells are damaged by toxic chemicals, injury, or disease, this information system breaks down.

This can result in disorders ranging from mood changes and memory loss to blindness, paralysis, and death. Proper use of safety devices such as seat belts, child restraints, and bike helmets can prevent injuries and save lives.

Osteoporosis

Over 10 million Americans have osteoporosis, while 18 million others have lost bone mass and are likely to develop osteoporosis in the future. About 25 million Americans suffer from some kind of bone thinning. As people get older, back problems become more common, and bones in the spine, hip, and wrists break more easily. Young people can lower their chances of getting osteoporosis in later years by exercising and eating calcium-rich foods like milk and yogurt.

Pneumoconiosis

Ordinary house and yard dust do not pose a serious health hazard. But some airborne particles can be very dangerous. These include fibers from asbestos, cotton, and hemp, and dust from such compounds as silica, graphite, coal, iron, and clay. These particles can damage sensitive areas of the lung, turning healthy tissue into scar tissue. This condition is called pneumoconiosis, or black lung. Chest pains and shortness of breath often progress to bronchitis, emphysema, and/or early death. Proper ventilation and the use of protective masks can greatly reduce the risk of lung disease.

Queensland Fever

People do not usually get diseases from farm animals. However, those who work with hides and animal products can get sick from breathing the infected dust around them. This illness is called Queensland fever because it was first discovered among cattle ranchers and dairy farmers in Queensland, Australia. It is caused by a tiny organism that infects livestock and then spreads to the milk and feces. Symptoms include fever, chills, and muscle aches and pains. Researchers have developed vaccines to protect livestock workers from this illness.

Reproductive Disorders

Beginning in the late 1940s, many women who were in danger of losing their unborn babies have prescribed a synthetic female hormone called DES (diethylstilbestrol). In 1971, scientists discovered that some of the daughters of these women were developing a very rare cancer of the reproductive organs. Since then, the use of DES and other synthetic hormones during pregnancy has been discontinued. NIEHS and other agencies are studying the possibility that some natural chemicals and artificial pesticides may cause similar problems. They are finding that some of these chemicals are so similar to female estrogen that they may actually "mimic" this important hormone. As a result, they may interfere with the development of male and female reproductive organs. This can lead to an increased risk of early puberty, low sperm counts, ovarian cysts, and cancer of the breast or testicles.

Sunburn and Skin Cancer

Almost everyone has stayed in the sun too long and been burned.

Too much sunlight can also produce the most common type of cancer—skin cancer. Some skin cancers are easy to treat because they do not spread beyond the surrounding tissue. Others, like melanoma, are much more dangerous because they spread to other parts of the body.

Deaths due to melanoma are increasing by 4 percent each year. More than 7,800 people died from melanomas of the skin in 2003.

Tooth Decay

In the 1930s, health experts noticed that people who lived in areas where the water contained natural chemicals called fluorides had fewer cavities.

At present, all U.S. residents are exposed to fluoride to some degree, and its use has resulted in a significant decline in tooth decay. National surveys report that the incidence of tooth decay among children 12–17 years of age has declined from 90 percent in 1971 to 67 percent in 1988. Dentists can also protect young teeth by applying special coatings called sealants.

Uranium Poisoning

Uranium is a dangerous element because it is radioactive. This means it gives off high-energy particles that can go through the body and damage living tissue. A single high dose of radiation can kill. Small doses over a long period can also be harmful. For example, miners who are exposed to uranium dust are more likely to get lung cancer. Uranium poisoning can also damage the kidneys and interfere with the body's ability to fight infection. While most people will never come in contact with uranium, those who work with medical X-rays or radioactive compounds are also at risk. They should wear lead shields and follow recommended safety guidelines to protect themselves from unnecessary exposure.

Vision Problems

Our eyes are especially sensitive to the environment. Gases found in polluted air can irritate the eyes and produce a burning sensation.
Tiny particles of smoke and soot can also cause redness and itching of the eyes. Airborne organisms like molds and fungus can cause infections of the eyes and eyelids. Too much exposure to the sun's rays can eventually produce a clouding of the lens called a cataract.

Waterborne Diseases

Even our clearest streams, rivers, and lakes can contain chemical pollutants. Heavy metals like lead and mercury can produce severe organ damage. Some chemicals can interfere with the development of organs and tissues, causing birth defects. Others can cause normal cells to become cancerous. Some of our waterways also contain human and animal wastes. The bacteria in the wastes can cause high fever, cramps, vomiting, and diarrhea.

Xeroderma Pigmentosa

Xeroderma is a rare condition that people inherit from their parents. When these people are exposed to direct sunlight, their skin breaks out into tiny dark spots that look like freckles. If this condition is not treated, the spots can become cancerous. These areas must then be removed by a surgeon.

Yusho Poisoning

In 1968, more than 1,000 people in western Japan became seriously ill. They suffered from fatigue, headache, cough, numbness in the arms and legs, and unusual skin sores. Pregnant women later delivered babies with birth defects. These people had eaten food that was cooked in contaminated rice oil. Toxic chemicals called PCBs (polychlorinated biphenyls) had accidentally leaked into the oil during the manufacturing process. Health experts now refer to this illness as "Yusho," which means "oil disease."

For years, PCBs were widely used in the manufacturing of paints, plastics, and electrical equipment. When scientists discovered that low levels of PCBs could kill fish and other wildlife, their use was dramatically reduced. By this time, PCBs were already leaking into the environment from waste disposal sites and other sources. Today, small amounts of these compounds can still be found in our air, water, soil, and some of the foods we eat.

Zinc Deficiency/Poisoning

Zinc is a mineral that the body needs to function properly. In rare cases, people can be poisoned if there is too much zinc in their food or water. However, most people can take in large quantities without any harmful effects. In areas where nutrition is a problem, people may not get enough zinc from their diet. This can lead to retarded growth, hair loss, delayed sexual maturation, eye and skin lesions, and loss of appetite.

Chapter 8

Cancer and Environmental Concerns

Chapter Contents

Section 8.1

Environmental Causes of Cancer

This section includes text excerpted from
"Cancer-Causing Substances in the Environment,"
National Cancer Institute (NCI), May 18, 2015.

Cancer is caused by changes in certain genes that alter the way our cells function. Some of these genetic changes occur naturally when deoxyribonucleic acid (DNA) is replicated during the process of cell division. But others are the result of environmental exposures that damage DNA. These exposures may include substances, such as the chemicals in tobacco smoke, or radiation, such as ultraviolet (UV) rays from the sun. People can avoid some cancer-causing exposures, such as tobacco smoke and the sun's rays. But others are harder to avoid, especially if they are in the air we breathe, the water we drink, the food we eat, or the materials we use to do our jobs. Scientists are studying which exposures may cause or contribute to the development of cancer. Understanding which exposures are harmful, and where they are found, may help people to avoid them.

The substances listed below are among the most likely carcinogens to affect human health. Simply because a substance has been designated as a carcinogen, however, does not mean that the substance will necessarily cause cancer. Many factors influence whether a person exposed to a carcinogen will develop cancer, including the amount and duration of the exposure and the individual's genetic background.

Cancer-Causing Substances in the Environment

Cancer-causing substances in the environment include:

Aflatoxins

What Are Aflatoxins?

Aflatoxins are a family of toxins produced by certain fungi that are found on agricultural crops such as maize (corn), peanuts, cottonseed, and tree nuts. The main fungi that produce aflatoxins are *Aspergillus flavus* and *Aspergillus parasiticus*, which are abundant in warm and humid regions of the world. Aflatoxin-producing fungi can contaminate crops in the field, at harvest, and during storage.

How Are People Exposed to Aflatoxins?

People can be exposed to aflatoxins by eating contaminated plant products (such as peanuts) or by consuming meat or dairy products from animals that ate contaminated feed. Farmers and other agricultural workers may be exposed by inhaling dust generated during the handling and processing of contaminated crops and feeds.

Which Cancers Are Associated with Exposure to Aflatoxins?

Exposure to aflatoxins is associated with an increased risk of liver cancer.

How Can Aflatoxin Exposure Be Reduced?

You can reduce your aflatoxin exposure by buying only major commercial brands of nuts and nut butter and by discarding nuts that look moldy, discolored, or shriveled. To help minimize risk, the U.S. Food and Drug Administration (FDA) tests foods that may contain aflatoxins, such as peanuts and peanut butter. To date, no outbreak of human illness caused by aflatoxins has been reported in the United States, but such outbreaks have occurred in some developing countries.

Aristolochic Acids (AAs)

What Are AAs?

Aristolochic acids (AA) are a group of acids found naturally in many types of plants known as Aristolochia (birthworts or pipelines) and some types of plants known as Asarum (wild ginger), which grow worldwide.

How Are AAs Used?

Plants containing AAs are used in some herbal products intended to treat a variety of symptoms and diseases, such as arthritis, gout, and inflammation. These products have not been approved by the FDA and are often marketed as dietary supplements or "traditional medicines."

How Are People Exposed to AAs?

Exposure may occur through intentionally or unknowingly eating or drinking herbal or food products that contain AAs.

Which Cancers Are Associated with Exposure to AAs?

Cancers of the upper urinary tract (renal pelvis and ureter) and bladder have been reported among individuals who had kidney damage caused by the consumption of herbal products containing AAs.

How Can Exposures Be Reduced?

To reduce your risk, do not use herbal products that contain AAs.

Arsenic

What Is Arsenic?

Arsenic is a naturally occurring substance that can be found in air, water, and soil. It can also be released into the environment by certain agricultural and industrial processes, such as mining and metal smelting. Arsenic comes in two forms (organic and inorganic); the inorganic form is more toxic than the organic form.

How Are People Exposed to Arsenic?

People in the general population may be exposed to arsenic by smoking tobacco, being around tobacco smoke, drinking contaminated water, or eating food from plants that were irrigated with contaminated water. Inorganic arsenic is naturally present at high levels in the groundwater of certain countries, including the United States. Exposure to arsenic in contaminated drinking water is generally thought to be more harmful to human health than exposure to arsenic in contaminated foods.

In the past, people were exposed to arsenic during certain medical treatments and through contact with pesticides. Research showed that an arsenic compound, arsenic trioxide (As_2O_3), was effective in the treatment of acute promyelocytic leukemia (APL).

Which Cancers Are Associated with Exposure to Arsenic?

Prolonged ingestion of arsenic-containing drinking water is associated with an increased risk of bladder cancer. In addition, cancers of the skin, lung, digestive tract, liver, kidney, and lymphatic and hematopoietic systems have been linked to arsenic exposure.

How Can Exposures Be Reduced?

Access to a safe water supply for drinking, food preparation, and irrigation of food crops is the most important way to prevent exposures to arsenic.

Asbestos

What Is Asbestos?

Asbestos is the name given to a group of naturally occurring fibrous minerals that are resistant to heat and corrosion. Because of these properties, asbestos has been used in commercial products such as insulation and fireproofing materials, automotive brakes, and wall-board materials.

How Are People Exposed to Asbestos?

If products containing asbestos are disturbed, tiny asbestos fibers are released into the air. When asbestos fibers are breathed in, they may get trapped in the lungs and remain there for a long time. Over time, accumulated asbestos fibers can cause tissue inflammation and scarring, which can affect breathing and lead to serious health problems.

Low levels of asbestos fibers are present in the air, water, and soil. Most people, however, do not become ill from this type of exposure. People who become ill from asbestos usually have been exposed to it on a regular basis, most often in a job where they have worked directly with the material or through substantial environmental contact.

Most heavy exposures to asbestos occurred in the past. The heaviest exposures today tend to occur in the construction industry and in ship repair, particularly during the removal of asbestos-containing materials due to renovation, repairs, or demolition. Workers may also be exposed during the manufacture of asbestos-containing products, such as textiles, friction products, insulation, and other building materials.

Which Cancers Are Associated with Exposure to Asbestos?

Exposure to asbestos is associated with an increased risk of lung cancer and mesothelioma, which is a cancer of the thin membranes that line the chest and abdomen. Mesothelioma is the most common form of cancer associated with asbestos exposure, although the disease is relatively rare.

What Can Be Done to Reduce the Hazards of Asbestos?

The use of asbestos is now highly regulated in the United States. The Occupational Safety and Health Administration (OSHA) has issued standards for the construction industry, general industry, and shipyard employment sectors.

How Does Smoking Tobacco Affect the Risk of Asbestos-Associated Cancers?

Many studies have shown that the combination of tobacco smoking and asbestos exposure is particularly hazardous. However, there is also evidence that quitting smoking reduces the risk of lung cancer among asbestos-exposed workers.

Benzene

What Is Benzene?

Benzene is a colorless or light-yellow liquid chemical at room temperature. It is used primarily as a solvent in the chemical and pharmaceutical industries, as a starting material and an intermediate in the synthesis of numerous chemicals, and in gasoline. Benzene is produced by both natural and artificial processes. It is a natural component of crude oil, which is the main source of benzene produced today. Other natural sources include gas emissions from volcanoes and forest fires.

How Are People Exposed to Benzene?

People are exposed to benzene primarily by breathing air that contains the chemical. Workers in industries that produce or use benzene may be exposed to the highest levels of the chemical, although federal and state regulations have reduced these exposures in recent decades. Similarly, limits on the amount of benzene allowed in gasoline have contributed to reduced exposures.

Mainstream cigarette smoke is another source of benzene exposure, accounting for about half of the total U.S. population exposure to this chemical. Among smokers, 90 percent of benzene exposures come from smoking. Benzene may also be found in glues, adhesives, cleaning products, and paint strippers. Outdoor air contains low levels of benzene from secondhand tobacco smoke, gasoline fumes, motor vehicle exhaust, and industrial emissions.

Which Cancers Are Associated with Exposure to Benzene?

Exposure to benzene may increase the risk of developing leukemia and other blood disorders.

How Can Exposure Be Reduced?

Don't smoke and avoid exposure to secondhand tobacco smoke. Try to limit exposure to gasoline fumes.

Benzidine

What Is Benzidine?

Benzidine is a manufactured chemical that does not occur in nature. In the past, large amounts of benzidine were used to produce dyes for cloth, paper, and leather. It was also used in clinical laboratories for detecting blood, as a rubber-compounding agent, and in the manufacture of plastic films. It is no longer used in medical laboratories or in the rubber and plastics industries.

How Are People Exposed to Benzidine?

Inhalation and accidental ingestion are the main ways people can be exposed to benzidine-based dyes in the United States. As benzidine-based dyes were removed from both industrial and consumer markets and replaced with other types of dyes, the potential for exposure has declined.

Which Cancers Are Associated with Exposure to Benzidine?

Occupational exposure to benzidine results in an increased risk of bladder cancer, according to studies of workers in different geographic locations.

Beryllium

What Is Beryllium?

Beryllium is a metal that is found in nature, especially in beryl and bertrandite rock. It is extremely lightweight and hard, is a good conductor of electricity and heat, and is nonmagnetic. Because of these properties, beryllium is used in high-technology consumer and commercial products, including aerospace components, transistors, nuclear reactors, and golf clubs.

How Are People Exposed to Beryllium?

Most exposures to beryllium that cause disease are related to beryllium processing. The major route of human exposure is through airborne particles of beryllium metal, alloys, oxides, and ceramics. Beryllium particles are inhaled into the lungs and upper respiratory tract. Hand-to-mouth exposures and skin contact with ultrafine particles can also occur.

Although beryllium occurs in nature, the major source of its emission into the environment is through the combustion of fossil fuels (primarily coal), which releases beryllium-containing particulates and fly ash into the atmosphere.

Which Cancers Are Associated with Exposure to Beryllium?

An increased risk of lung cancer has been observed in workers exposed to beryllium or beryllium compounds.

1,3-Butadiene

What Is 1,3-Butadiene?

1,3-Butadiene is a colorless gas at room temperature with a gasoline-like odor. It is used to produce synthetic rubber products, such as tires, resins, and plastics, and other chemicals.

How Are People Exposed to 1,3-Butadiene?

Exposure to 1,3-butadiene mainly occurs among workers who breath contaminated air on the job. Other sources of exposure include automobile exhaust; tobacco smoke; and polluted air and water near chemical, plastic, or rubber facilities.

Which Cancers Are Associated with Exposure to 1,3-Butadiene?

Studies have consistently shown an association between occupational exposure to 1,3-butadiene and an increased incidence of leukemia.

How Can Exposures Be Reduced?

People can also reduce their exposure to 1,3-butadiene by avoiding tobacco smoke.

Cadmium (Cd)

What Is Cadmium (Cd)?

Cadmium (Cd) is a natural element found in tiny amounts in air, water, soil, and food. All soils and rocks, including coal and mineral fertilizers, contain some cadmium. Most cadmium used in the United States is extracted during the production of other metals such as zinc, lead, and copper. Cd does not corrode easily and has been used to manufacture batteries, pigments, metal coatings, and plastics.

How Are People Exposed to Cd?

Exposure to Cd occurs mostly in workplaces where Cd products are made. The major routes of occupational exposure are inhalation of dust and fumes and incidental ingestion of dust from contaminated hands, cigarettes, or food.

The general population is exposed to cadmium by breathing tobacco smoke or eating Cd-contaminated foods, which is the major source of Cd exposure for nonsmokers. The expanding nickel–cadmium (NiCd) battery recycling industry is also a potential source of exposure.

Which Cancers Are Associated with Exposure to Cd?

Occupational exposure to various Cd compounds is associated with an increased risk of lung cancer.

How Can Exposures Be Reduced?

Dispose of NiCd batteries properly, and do not allow children to play with these batteries. Avoid tobacco smoke. If you work with Cd, use all recommended safety precautions to avoid carrying Cd-containing dust home from work on your clothing, skin, hair, or tools.

Coal Tar and Coal-Tar Pitch

What Is Coal Tar?

Coal tar is derived from coal. It is a by-product of the production of coke, a solid fuel that contains mostly carbon, and coal gas. Coal tar is used primarily for the production of refined chemicals and coal-tar products, such as creosote and coal-tar pitch. Certain preparations of coal tar have long been used to treat various skin conditions, such as eczema, psoriasis, and dandruff.

What Is Coal-Tar Pitch?

Coal-tar pitch is a thick black liquid that remains after the distillation of coal tar. It is used as a base for coatings and paint, in roofing and paving, and as a binder in asphalt products. Both coal tar and coal-tar pitch contain many chemical compounds, including carcinogens such as benzene.

How Are People Exposed to Coal Tar and Coal-Tar Pitch?

The primary routes of human exposure to coal tars and coal-tar products are inhalation, ingestion, and absorption through the skin. Exposure to coal tars and coal-tar pitches may occur at foundries and during coke production, coal gasification, and aluminum production. Other workers who may be exposed to coal-tar pitches include those who produce or use pavement tar, roofing tar, coal-tar paints, coal-tar enamels, other coal-tar coatings, or refractory bricks.

The general population may be exposed to coal tars in environmental contaminants and through the use of coal tar preparations to treat skin disorders such as eczema, psoriasis, and dandruff.

Which Cancers Are Associated with Exposure to Coal Tar and Coal-Tar Pitch?

Occupational exposure to coal tar or coal-tar pitch is associated with an increased risk of skin cancer. Other types of cancer, including lung, bladder, kidney, and digestive tract cancer, have also been linked to occupational exposure to coal tar and coal-tar pitch.

How Can Exposures Be Reduced?

Exposures to coal tar and coal-tar pitch are regulated under OSHA air contaminants standard for general industry, shipyard employment, and the construction industry.

Coke Oven Emissions

What Are Coke Oven Emissions?

Coke oven emissions come from large ovens that are used to heat coal to produce coke, which is used to manufacture iron and steel. The emissions are complex mixtures of dust, vapors, and gases that typically include carcinogens such as Cd and arsenic. Chemicals recovered from coke oven emissions are used as raw materials for producing items such as plastics, solvents, dyes, paints, and insulation.

How Are People Exposed to Coke Oven Emissions?

Workers at coking plants and coal-tar production plants may be exposed to coke oven emissions. Occupational exposures can also occur among workers in the aluminum, steel, graphite, electrical, and construction industries. The primary routes of potential human exposure to coke oven emissions are inhalation and absorption through the skin.

Which Cancers Are Associated with Exposure to Coke Oven Emissions?

Exposure to coke oven emissions is associated with an increased risk of lung cancer.

Crystalline Silica

What Is Crystalline Silica?

An abundant natural material, crystalline silica is found in stone, soil, and sand. It is also found in concrete, brick, mortar, and other construction materials. Crystalline silica comes in several forms, with quartz being the most common. Quartz dust is respirable crystalline silica, which means it can be taken in by breathing.

How Are People Exposed to Crystalline Silica?

Exposure to tiny particles of airborne silica, primarily quartz dust, occurs mainly in industrial and occupational settings. For example, workers who use handheld masonry saws to cut materials such as concrete and brick may be exposed to airborne silica. When inhaled, these particles can penetrate deep into the lungs.

The primary route of exposure for the general population is inhaling airborne silica while using commercial products containing quartz. These products include cleansers, cosmetics, art clays and glazes, pet litter, talcum powder, caulk, and paint.

Which Cancers Are Associated with Exposure to Crystalline Silica?

Exposure of workers to respirable crystalline silica is associated with elevated rates of lung cancer. The strongest link between human lung cancer and exposure to respirable crystalline silica has been seen in studies of quarry and granite workers and workers involved in ceramic, pottery, refractory brick, and certain earth industries.

How Can Exposures Be Reduced?

The Mine Safety and Health Administration (MSHA) and OSHA have regulations related to silica.

Erionite

What Is Erionite?

Erionite is a naturally occurring fibrous mineral that belongs to a group of minerals called zeolites. It forms fibrous masses in the hollows of rock formations. Some of the mineral's properties are similar to those of asbestos; for example, the fibers pose a hazard only if they are disturbed and become airborne.

How Are People Exposed to Erionite?

In the past, occupational exposure occurred during erionite mining and production operations, but erionite is no longer mined or marketed for commercial purposes. The erionite-related disease has been reported most often among road construction and maintenance workers who may have been exposed to erionite-containing gravel used in road surfacing.

Little is known about current exposures experienced by workers in the United States. However, erionite is found in some other commercial zeolite products. Therefore, the use of other zeolites may result in exposure to erionite among workers and members of the general population who use the zeolites in various processes and products. The commercial uses of other natural zeolites include pet litter, soil conditioners, animal feed, wastewater treatment, and gas absorbents.

Which Cancers Are Associated with Exposure to Erionite?

Exposure to erionite is associated with increased risks of lung cancer and mesothelioma.

How Can Exposures Be Reduced?

There are no regulatory or consensus standards or occupational exposure limits for airborne erionite fibers. OSHA's guidance for working with asbestos could serve as a model for limiting the generation and inhalation of dust known or thought to be contaminated with erionite.

Ethylene Oxide (EtO)

What Is Ethylene Oxide (EtO)?

At room temperature, EtO is a flammable colorless gas with a sweet odor. It is used primarily to produce other chemicals, including antifreeze. In smaller amounts, EtO is used as a pesticide and a sterilizing agent. The ability of ethylene oxide to damage DNA makes it an effective sterilizing agent but also accounts for its cancer-causing activity.

How Are People Exposed to EtO?

The primary routes of human exposure to EtO are inhalation and ingestion, which may occur through occupational, consumer, or environmental exposure. Because EtO is highly explosive and reactive, the equipment used for its processing generally consists of tightly closed and highly automated systems, which decreases the risk of occupational exposure.

Despite these precautions, workers and people who live near industrial facilities that produce or use EtO may be exposed to EtO through uncontrolled industrial emissions. The general population may also be exposed to tobacco smoke and the use of products that have been sterilized with EtO, such as medical products, cosmetics, and beekeeping equipment.

Which Cancers Are Associated with Exposure to EtO?

Lymphoma and leukemia are the cancers most frequently reported to be associated with occupational exposure to EtO.

Formaldehyde (FA)

What Is Formaldehyde (FA)?

Formaldehyde (FA) is a colorless, strong-smelling, flammable chemical that is produced industrially and used in building materials such as particle-board, plywood, and other pressed-wood products. In addition, it is commonly used as a fungicide, germicide, and disinfectant, and as a preservative in mortuaries and medical laboratories. FA also occurs naturally in the environment. It is produced during the decay of plant material in the soil and during normal chemical processes in most living organisms. It is also a combustion product found in tobacco smoke.

How Are People Exposed to FA?

People are exposed primarily by inhaling FA gas or vapor from the air or by absorbing liquids containing FA through the skin. Workers who produce FA or products that contain FA—as well as laboratory technicians, certain healthcare professionals, and mortuary employees—may be exposed to higher levels of FA than the general public.

The general public may be exposed to FA by breathing contaminated air from sources such as pressed-wood products, tobacco smoke, and automobile tailpipe emissions. Another potential source of exposure to FA is the use of unvented fuel-burning appliances, such as gas stoves, wood-burning stoves, and kerosene heaters.

Which Cancers Are Associated with Exposure to FA?

Studies of workers exposed to high levels of formaldehyde, such as industrial workers and embalmers, have found that FA causes myeloid leukemia and rare cancers, including cancers of the paranasal sinuses, nasal cavity, and nasopharynx.

How Can Exposures Be Reduced?

The U.S. Environmental Protection Agency (EPA) recommends the use of "exterior-grade" pressed-wood products to limit FA exposure in the home. FA levels in homes and work settings can also be reduced by ensuring adequate ventilation, moderate temperatures, and reduced humidity levels through the use of air conditioners and dehumidifiers.

Hexavalent Chromium (Cr) Compounds

What Is Chromium (Cr) and What Are Hexavalent Chromium Cr(VI) Compounds?

Chromium (Cr) is an odorless and tasteless metallic element that is found in the earth's crust. It is also found in air, water, soil, and food.

Hexavalent Cr compounds are a group of chemicals that have useful properties, such as corrosion resistance, durability, and hardness. These compounds have been used widely as corrosion inhibitors and in the manufacture of pigments, metal finishing and chrome plating, stainless steel production, leather tanning, and wood preservatives.

They have also been used in textile-dyeing processes, printing inks, drilling muds, fireworks, water treatment, and chemical synthesis.

How Are People Exposed to Cr(VI) Compounds?

Occupational exposure to Cr(VI) can occur from inhalation of dust, mists, or fumes containing Cr(VI), or from eye or skin contact. Industries with the largest number of workers exposed to high concentrations of airborne Cr(VI) compounds include electroplating, welding, and chromate paint.

Which Cancers Are Associated with Exposure to Cr(VI) Compounds?

Occupational exposure to these compounds is associated with increased risks of lung cancer and cancer of the paranasal sinuses and nasal cavity.

Indoor Emissions from the Household Combustion of Coal

What Are Indoor Emissions from the Household Combustion of Coal?

Burning coal inside the home for the purposes of heating or cooking produces particulate and gas emissions that may contain a number of harmful chemicals, such as benzene, carbon monoxide (CO), FA, and polycyclic aromatic hydrocarbons (PAHs).

How Are People Exposed to Indoor Emissions from the Household Combustion of Coal?

People in some parts of the world, particularly in certain regions of China, have been exposed to indoor emissions from coal combustion through the use of unvented stoves and fire pits.

Which Cancers Are Associated with Exposure to Indoor Coal Combustion Emissions?

Lung cancer is associated with exposure to indoor coal combustion emissions.

How Can Exposures Be Reduced?

Installing indoor stoves with chimneys can reduce the level of indoor air pollution.

Mineral Oils: Untreated and Mildly Treated

What Are Mineral Oils?

The name mineral oil has been used to describe many colorless, odorless liquids. Most often, the term refers to a liquid by-product of the distillation of petroleum to produce gasoline and other petroleum-based products from crude oil. These oils, including lubricant base oils and products derived from them, are used in manufacturing, mining, construction, and other industries.

A complete description of mineral oils should include how the oils are refined. Oils used in cosmetic products are typically highly refined, whereas those used in automotive oils and fluids tend to be unrefined or only mildly treated.

How Are People Exposed to Mineral Oils?

Occupational exposure to mineral oils may occur among workers in various industries, including the manufacture of automobiles, airplanes, steel products, screws, pipes, and transformers. Workers in brass and aluminum production, engine repair, copper mining, and newspaper and commercial printing may also be exposed to mineral oils. The general population may be exposed to mineral oils that occur naturally or are present as environmental contaminants.

Which Cancers Are Associated with Exposure to Mineral Oils?

Exposure to mineral oils is strongly associated with an increased risk of nonmelanoma skin cancer, particularly of the scrotum.

Nickel (Ni) Compounds

What Are Ni and Ni Compounds?

Nickel (Ni) is a silvery-white metallic element found in the earth's crust. It can be combined with other elements to form Ni compounds. Because of its unique properties, Ni has many industrial uses. Most Ni is used in metal alloys because it imparts useful properties, such as corrosion resistance, heat resistance, hardness, and strength.

How Are People Exposed to Ni and Ni Compounds?

Occupational exposure is common in workplaces where Ni and Ni compounds are produced or used, including mining, smelting, welding, casting, and grinding. Occupational exposure to Ni occurs mainly through inhalation of dust particles and fumes or through skin contact. The general population is exposed to low levels of nickel in the air, water, food, and tobacco smoke. Ni and its compounds get into the atmosphere through natural processes, such as the spread of dust and volcanic eruptions by the wind, as well as through industrial activities. The general public may also be exposed to Ni-plated materials, such as coins, jewelry, and stainless steel cooking and eating utensils.

Which Cancers Are Associated with Exposure to Ni and Ni Compounds?

Exposure to various Ni compounds is associated with increased risks of lung cancer and nasal cancer.

How Can Exposures Be Reduced?

Exposures of the general population to nickel compounds are almost always too low to be of concern. To protect workers, OSHA has issued exposure limits for Ni compounds.

Radon

What Is Radon?

Radon is a radioactive gas that is released from the normal decay of the elements uranium, thorium, and radium in rocks and soil. The invisible, odorless gas seeps up through the ground and diffuses into the air. In a few areas, depending on local geology, radon dissolves into groundwater and can be released into the air when the water is used. Radon gas usually exists at very low levels outdoors, but the gas can accumulate in areas without adequate ventilation, such as underground mines.

How Are People Exposed to Radon?

Radon is present in nearly all air, so everyone breathes in radon every day, usually at very low levels. Radon can enter homes through cracks in floors, walls, or foundations, and collect indoors. It can also be released from building materials, or from water obtained from wells that contain radon. Radon levels may be higher in homes that are well insulated, tightly sealed, and/or built on soil rich in the elements uranium, thorium, and radium. Basements and first floors typically have the highest radon levels because of their closeness to the ground.

Workers employed in uranium, hard rock and phosphate mining potentially are exposed to radon at high concentrations. Uranium miners generally are believed to have the highest exposures.

Which Cancers Are Associated with Exposure to Radon?

Radon was identified as a health problem when scientists noted that underground uranium miners who were exposed to it died of lung cancer at high rates. Experimental studies in animals confirmed the results of the miner studies by showing higher rates of lung tumors among rodents exposed to high levels of radon. There has been a suggestion of an increased risk of leukemia associated with radon exposure in adults and children; the evidence, however, is not conclusive.

How Can Exposures Be Reduced?

Check the radon levels in your home regularly. The U.S. Environmental Protection Agency (EPA) has more information about residential radon exposure and what people can do about it in its *Consumer's Guide to Radon Reduction.*

Secondhand Tobacco Smoke (Environmental Tobacco Smoke)

What Is Secondhand Tobacco Smoke?

Secondhand tobacco smoke is the combination of the smoke given off by a burning tobacco product and the smoke exhaled by a smoker. It is also called environmental tobacco smoke, involuntary smoke, and passive smoke.

More than 7,000 chemicals have been identified in secondhand tobacco smoke. At least 69 of these chemicals are carcinogens, including arsenic, benzene, beryllium, chromium, and formaldehyde.

How Are People Exposed to Secondhand Smoke?

People can be exposed to secondhand smoke in homes, cars, the workplace, and public places. In the United States, the source of most secondhand smoke is from cigarettes, followed by pipes, cigars, and other tobacco products.

Which Cancers Are Associated with Secondhand Smoke?

Inhaling secondhand smoke causes lung cancer in nonsmokers. Some research also suggests that secondhand smoke may increase the risk of some other cancers as well, though more research is needed on this subject.

How Can Exposures Be Reduced?

There is no safe level of exposure to secondhand smoke; even low levels of secondhand smoke can be harmful. In the United States, legislation has helped to reduce exposures. Federal law bans smoking on all domestic airline flights, nearly all flights between the United States and foreign destinations, interstate buses, and most trains. Smoking is also banned in most federally owned buildings. Many state and local governments have also passed laws prohibiting smoking in public facilities, such as schools, hospitals, and airports, as well as private workplaces, including restaurants and bars.

Internationally, a growing number of nations require all workplaces, including bars and restaurants, to be smoke-free.

Soot

What Is Soot?

Soot is a by-product of the incomplete burning of organics (carbon-containing) materials, such as wood, fuel oil, plastics, and household refuse. The fine black or brown powder that makes up soot may contain a number of carcinogens, including arsenic, cadmium, and chromium.

How Are People Exposed to Soot?

People may be exposed to soot by inhalation, ingestion, or absorption through the skin. Chimney sweeps likely to have the highest occupational exposure to soot. Heating-unit service personnel, brick masons, building demolition personnel, horticulturists, and anyone who works where organic materials are burned may also be exposed through their work. The general public may be exposed through fireplaces, furnaces, engine exhaust, and particulate emissions from any combustion source.

Which Cancers Are Associated with Exposure to Soot?

Exposure to soot was first associated with skin cancer of the scrotum among British chimney sweeps in 1775. Since then, many studies have found that chimney sweeps have an increased risk of scrotal and other skin cancers. Studies of chimney sweeps in several European countries have also found associations with other cancers, including lung, esophageal, and bladder cancers.

How Can Exposures Be Reduced?

In the United States, professional organizations for chimney sweeps keep members up to date on changing technology and safety issues.

Strong Inorganic Acid Mists Containing Sulfuric Acid

What Are Strong Inorganic Acid Mists Containing Sulfuric Acid?

At room temperature, sulfuric acid is a clear, colorless, oily, corrosive liquid. Strong inorganic acid mists containing sulfuric acid may be generated during various manufacturing processes.

How Are People Exposed to Strong Inorganic Acid Mists Containing Sulfuric Acid?

The major routes of occupational exposure are inhalation, ingestion, or absorption through the skin. Workers with potential exposure include those involved in manufacturing phosphate fertilizer, isopropanol, sulfuric acid, nitric acid, and lead batteries. Exposure may also occur during copper smelting, pickling (removing scale and oxides from metal surfaces), and other acid treatment of metals.

Which Cancers Are Associated with Exposure to Strong Inorganic Acid Mists Containing Sulfuric Acid?

Occupational exposure to strong inorganic acid mists containing sulfuric acid is associated with increased risks of laryngeal and lung cancer.

Thorium

What Is Thorium?

Thorium is a naturally occurring radioactive metal that is found in soil, rock, and water. It is formed by the radioactive decay of uranium.

Minerals such as monazite, thorite, and thorianite are rich in thorium and may be mined for the metal. Thorium has coloring properties that have made it useful in ceramic glazes. Thorium also has been widely used in lantern mantles for the brightness it imparts (though alternatives are replacing it), and in welding rods, which burn better with small amounts of added thorium.

How Are People Exposed to Thorium?

The primary ways people are exposed to thorium are inhalation, intravenous injection, ingestion, and absorption through the skin. Once injected, Thorotrast remains in the body, resulting in lifelong exposure to thorium.

Although thorium is widespread in the environment, most people are not exposed to dangerous levels of the metal. However, people who live near thorium-mining areas or facilities that manufacture products with thorium may have increased exposure, especially if their water comes from a private well. Analytical laboratories can test water for thorium content.

Which Cancers Are Associated with Exposure to Thorium?

Studies of patients who received intravascular injections of Thorotrast found an increased risk of liver tumors among these individuals. And there is research evidence that inhaling thorium dust increases the risk of lung and pancreatic cancer. Individuals exposed to thorium also have an increased risk of bone cancer because thorium may be stored in bone.

How Can Exposures Be Reduced?

Occasionally, household items may be found to contain thorium, such as some older ceramic wares in which uranium was used in the glaze, or gas lantern mantles. Although these exposures generally do not pose serious health risks, such household items should be retired from use to avoid unnecessary exposures. A radiation counter is required to confirm if ceramics contain thorium.

Vinyl Chloride

What Is Vinyl Chloride?

Vinyl chloride is a colorless gas that burns easily. It does not occur naturally and must be produced industrially for its commercial uses.

Vinyl chloride is used primarily to make polyvinyl chloride (PVC); PVC is used to make a variety of plastic products, including pipes, wire and cable coatings, and packaging materials. Vinyl chloride is also produced as a combustion product in tobacco smoke.

How Are People Exposed to Vinyl Chloride?

Workers at facilities where vinyl chloride is produced or used may be exposed primarily through inhalation. The general population may be exposed by inhaling contaminated air or tobacco smoke. In the environment, the highest levels of vinyl chloride are found in the air around factories that produce vinyl products. If a water supply is contaminated, vinyl chloride can enter the household air when the water is used for showering, cooking, or laundry.

Which Cancers Are Associated with Exposure to Vinyl Chloride?

Vinyl chloride exposure is associated with an increased risk of a rare form of liver cancer (hepatic angiosarcoma), as well as brain and lung cancers, lymphoma, and leukemia.

Wood Dust

What Is Wood Dust?

Wood dust is created when machines or tools are used to cut or shape wood. High amounts of wood dust are produced in sawmills, and in the furniture-making, cabinet-making, and carpentry industries.

How Are People Exposed to Wood Dust?

Individuals who use machinery or tools to cut or shape wood are exposed to wood dust. When the dust is inhaled, it is deposited in the nose, throat, and other airways. Occupations with high exposure to wood dust include sander operators in the transportation equipment industry, press operators in the wood products industry, lathe operators in the furniture industry, and sander operators in the wood cabinet industry.

Which Cancers Are Associated with Exposure to Wood Dust?

Strong and consistent associations with cancers of the paranasal sinuses and nasal cavity have been observed both in studies of people whose occupations were associated with wood-dust exposure and in studies that directly estimated wood-dust exposure.

How Can Exposures Be Reduced?

Exposures can be reduced through design and engineering modifications, such as installing an exhaust ventilation system with collectors placed at points where dust is produced. Personal protective equipment, such as respirators, is another short-term solution for reducing exposure.

Section 8.2

Carcinogens

This section includes text excerpted from
"Environmental Carcinogens and Cancer Risk,"
National Cancer Institute (NCI), March 20, 2015.

Environmental Carcinogens and Cancer Risk

Does Any Exposure to a Known Carcinogen Always Result in Cancer?

Any substance that causes cancer is known as a carcinogen. But simply because a substance has been designated as a carcinogen does not mean that the substance will necessarily cause cancer. Many factors influence whether a person exposed to a carcinogen will develop cancer, including the amount and duration of the exposure and the individual's genetic background. Cancers caused by involuntary exposures to environmental carcinogens are most likely to occur in subgroups of the population, such as workers in certain industries who may be exposed to carcinogens on the job.

How Can Exposures to Carcinogens Be Limited?

In the United States, regulations have been put in place to reduce exposures to known carcinogens in the workplace. Outside

97

of the workplace, people can also take steps to limit their exposure to known carcinogens, such as testing their basement for radon, quitting smoking, limiting sun exposure, or maintaining a healthy weight.

How Many Cancers Are Caused by Involuntary Exposure to Carcinogens in the Environment?

This question cannot be answered with certainty because the precise causes of most cancers are not known. Some researchers have suggested that, in most populations, environmental exposures are responsible for a relatively small proportion of total cancers (less than 4 percent), whereas other researchers attribute a higher proportion (19 percent) to environmental exposures.

Who Decides Which Environmental Exposures Cause Cancer in Humans?

Two organizations—the National Toxicology Program (NTP), an interagency program of the U.S. Department of Health and Human Services (HHS), and the International Agency for Research on Cancer (IARC), the cancer agency of the World Health Organization (WHO)— have developed lists of substances that, based on the available scientific evidence, are known or are reasonably anticipated to be human carcinogens.

Specifically, the NTP publishes the *Report on Carcinogens* every few years. This congressionally mandated publication identifies agents, substances, mixtures, or exposures (collectively called "substances") in the environment that may cause cancer in humans. The 2014 edition lists 56 known human carcinogens and includes descriptions of the process for preparing the science-based report and the criteria used to list a substance as a carcinogen.

IARC also produces science-based reports on substances that can increase the risk of cancer in humans. Since 1971, the agency has evaluated more than 900 agents, including chemicals, complex mixtures, occupational exposures, physical agents, biological agents, and lifestyle factors. Of these, more than 400 have been identified as carcinogenic, probably carcinogenic, or possibly carcinogenic to humans.

IARC convenes expert scientists to evaluate the evidence that an agent can increase the risk of cancer. The agency describes the principles, procedures, and scientific criteria that guide the evaluations. For instance, agents are selected for review based on two main criteria: (a) there is evidence of human exposure and (b) there is some evidence or suspicion of carcinogenicity.

How Does the NTP Decide Whether to Include a Substance on Its List of Known Human Carcinogens?

As new potential carcinogens are identified, they are evaluated scientifically by the NTP's Board of Scientific Counselors and the NTP Director. Next, a draft report on carcinogens monograph is prepared, which is reviewed by other scientific experts as needed, the public, and other federal agencies. The draft monograph is then revised as necessary and released for additional public comment and peer review by a dedicated panel of experts. Lastly, a finalized monograph and recommendation for listing is sent to the HHS Secretary for approval.

Section 8.3

Cancer Clusters

This section includes text excerpted from "Cancer Clusters," National Cancer Institute (NCI), March 18, 2014. Reviewed April 2018.

What Is a Cancer Cluster?

A cancer cluster is the occurrence of a greater than expected number of cancer cases among a group of people in a defined geographic area over a specific time period. A cancer cluster may be suspected when people report that several family members, friends, neighbors, or co-workers have been diagnosed with the same or related types of cancer.

Cancer clusters can help scientists identify cancer-causing substances in the environment. For example, in the early 1970s, a cluster of cases of angiosarcoma of the liver, rare cancer, was detected among workers in a chemical plant. Further investigation showed that the workers were all exposed to vinyl chloride and that workers in other plants that used vinyl chloride also had an increased rate of angiosarcoma of the liver. Exposure to vinyl chloride is now known to be a major risk factor for angiosarcoma of the liver.

However, most suspected cancer clusters turn out, on detailed investigation, not to be true cancer clusters. That is, no cause can be identified, and the clustering of cases turns out to be a random occurrence.

Where to Report a Suspected Cancer Cluster or Find out If One Is Being Investigated?

Concerned individuals can contact their local or state health department to report a suspected cancer cluster or to find out if one is being investigated. Health departments provide the first response to questions about cancer clusters because they, together with state cancer registries, will have the most up-to-date data on cancer incidence in the area. If additional resources are needed to investigate a suspected cancer cluster, the state health department may request assistance from federal agencies, including the Centers for Disease Control and Prevention (CDC) and the Agency for Toxic Substances and Disease Registry (ATSDR), which is part of the CDC.

Although National Cancer Institute (NCI) does not lead investigations of individual cancer clusters, NCI researchers and staff may provide assistance to other investigative agencies as needed. In addition, scientists at NCI and researchers who are funded by NCI analyze variations in cancer trends, including the frequency, distribution, and patterns of cancer in groups of people. These analyses can detect patterns of cancer in specific populations. For example, NCI's Cancer Mortality Maps website uses data on deaths from the National Center for Health Statistics (NCHS), which is part of the CDC, and population estimates from the U.S. Census Bureau to provide dynamically generated maps that show geographic patterns of cancer death rates throughout the United States.

How Are Suspected Cancer Clusters Investigated?

Health departments use established criteria to investigate reports of cancer clusters. CDC and the Council of State and Territorial Epidemiologists (CSTE) have released updated guidelines for investigating suspected cancer clusters and responding to community concerns.

As a first step, the investigating agency gathers information from the person who reported the suspected cancer cluster. The investigators ask for details about the suspected cluster, such as the types of cancer and number of cases of each type, the age of the people with cancer, and the area and time period over which the cancers were diagnosed. They also ask about specific environmental hazards or concerns in the affected area.

If the review of the findings from this initial investigation suggests the need for further evaluation, investigators then compare information about cases in the suspected cluster with records in the state cancer registry and census data.

If the second step reveals a statistically significant excess of cancer cases, the third step is to determine whether an epidemiologic study can be carried out to investigate whether the cluster is associated with risk factors in the local environment. Sometimes, even if there is a clear excess of cancer cases, it is not feasible to carry out the further study—for example, if the total number of cases is very small.

Finally, if an epidemiologic study is feasible, the fourth step is to determine whether the cluster of cancer cases is associated with a suspect contaminant in the environment. Even if a possible association with an environmental contaminant is found, however, further studies would be needed to confirm that the environmental contaminant did cause the cluster.

What Are the Challenges in Investigating Suspected Cancer Clusters?

Investigators face several challenges when determining whether a greater than expected number of cancer cases represents a cancer cluster.

Understanding the Kind of Cancers Involved

To assess a suspected cancer cluster accurately, investigators must determine whether the type of cancer involved is primary cancer (cancer that is located in the original organ or tissue where cancer started) or cancer that has metastasized (spread) to another site in the body from the original tissue or organ where cancer began (also called secondary cancer). Investigators consider only primary cancer when they investigate a suspected cancer cluster. A confirmed cancer cluster is more likely if it involves one type of cancer than if it involves multiple different cancer types. This is because most carcinogens in the environment cause only a specific cancer type rather than causing cancer in general.

Ascertaining the Number of Cancer Cases in the Suspected Cluster

Many reported clusters include too few cancer cases for investigators to determine whether the number of cancer cases is statistically significantly greater than the expected number.

Determining Statistical Significance

To confirm the existence of a cluster, investigators must show that the number of cancer cases in the cluster is statistically significantly greater than the number of cancer cases expected given the age, sex, and racial distribution of the group of people who developed the disease. If the difference between the actual and expected number of cancer cases is statistically significant, the finding is unlikely to be the result of chance alone. However, it is important to keep in mind that even a statistically significant difference between actual and expected numbers of cases can arise by chance.

Determining the Relevant Population and Geographic Area

An important challenge in confirming a cancer cluster is accurately defining the group of people who should be considered potentially at risk of developing specific cancer (typically the total number of people who live in a specific geographic area). When defining a cancer cluster, there can be a tendency to expand the geographic borders as additional cases of the suspected disease are discovered. However, if investigators define the borders of a cluster based on where they find cancer cases, they may alarm people about cancers that are not related to the suspected cluster. Instead, investigators first define the population and geographic area that is "at risk" and then identify cancer cases within those parameters.

Identifying a Cause for a Cluster

A confirmed cancer cluster—that is, a finding of a statistically significant excess of cancers—may not be the result of any single external cause or hazard (also called an exposure). A cancer cluster could be the result of chance, an error in the calculation of the expected number of cancer cases, differences in how cancer cases were classified, or a known cause of cancer, such as smoking. Even if a cluster is confirmed, it can be very difficult to identify the cause. People move in and out of a geographic area over time, which can make it difficult for investigators

102

to identify hazards or potential carcinogens to which they may have been exposed and to obtain medical records to confirm the diagnosis of cancer. Also, it typically takes a long time for cancer to develop, and any relevant exposure may have occurred in the past or in a different geographic area from where the cancer was diagnosed.

Section 8.4

Lung Cancer and the Environment

This section includes text excerpted from "Cancer—
Lung Cancer and the Environment," Centers for Disease
Control and Prevention (CDC), January 10, 2017.

Lung cancer is the leading cause of cancer deaths in the United States. Lung cancer forms in the tissue of the lung, usually in the cells lining the air passages. Cigarette smoking is the single most crucial risk factor for, and the leading cause of, lung cancer. Exposure to radon is the second leading cause of lung cancer.

The International Agency for Research on Cancer (IARC) has identified the following substances as lung cancer-causing agents:

- Arsenic

- Asbestos

- Bischloromethyl ether

- Chromium (Cr)

- Nickel

- Polycyclic aromatic compounds

- Radon

- Vinyl chloride

A history of certain lung diseases also increases the risk for lung cancer. Diets low in fruits and vegetables might increase the risk of lung cancer in persons who smoke.

103

Environmental tobacco smoke (also called secondhand smoke) is a well-established cause of lung cancer. Air pollution and diesel exhaust have also been shown to have a slight increase in lung cancer morbidity and/or mortality. However, the impact of outdoor air pollution on lung cancer needs further study.

Exposure and Risk

Cigarette smoking is the most common cause of lung cancer. It remains the leading preventable cause of death in the United States. Even for nonsmokers, exposure to environmental tobacco smoke increases the risk for lung cancer. The Surgeon General's report says the evidence suggests that secondhand smoke exposure can cause lung cancer in lifetime nonsmokers, regardless of where the exposure occurs (e.g., home, work, restaurants). Every year, about 3,000 nonsmokers in the United States die from lung cancer caused by secondhand smoke. There is no risk-free level of secondhand smoke exposure.

Studies also indicate that exposure to certain chemicals may increase the risk for lung cancer, especially among smokers. These chemicals include:

• Arsenic

• Chromium (Cr)

• Silica

• Substances used or produced in foundries and substances produced by processing coal

Radon exposure is the second leading cause of lung cancer after tobacco smoke. Radon is a naturally occurring, colorless, odorless, tasteless, radioactive gas that can be found throughout the United States. It can infiltrate homes, offices, and schools, and cause high indoor radon levels. The greatest exposure likely occurs in homes where most personal time is spent.

Prevention

Not smoking is the most effective way to reduce the risk for lung cancer. Limiting exposure to environmental tobacco smoke and testing homes for radon also reduce the risk for lung cancer. Eating fresh fruits and vegetables may also decrease risk, as well as help, prevent other diseases. Also, workers in high-risk jobs should follow appropriate health and safety rules, like wearing protective equipment.

Chapter 9

Respiratory Problems with Environmental Triggers

Chapter Contents

Section 9.1

Asthma and Air Pollution

This section includes text excerpted from "Asthma,"
Centers for Disease Control and Prevention (CDC),
January 10, 2017.

Asthma is a chronic disease that affects the airways that carry oxygen in and out of the lungs. If a person has asthma, the inside of these airways is irritated and swollen. Asthma can cause shortness of breath, wheezing, coughing, and tightness in the chest. For some people, asthma symptoms only appear when they are exposed to something that irritates their breathing. Others have a kind of asthma that makes breathing difficult all of the time.

A person can get asthma at any age. Asthma affects all races, ages, and genders. Although asthma affects people of all ages, it often starts in childhood and is more common in children than in adults.

Asthma has no cure, but it can be controlled. The majority of problems associated with asthma, including staying in the hospital, can be prevented if asthma is managed properly.

Asthma and the Environment

Asthma attacks have been linked to exercise, respiratory infections, and exposure to environmental factors such as allergens, tobacco smoke, and indoor and outdoor air pollution. Asthma attacks can be reduced by taking medication and avoiding exposure to known triggers.

A number of studies have reported associations between air pollution exposures and asthma. For example, researchers have found an association between increased hospital admissions for asthma and particulate matter, an outdoor air pollutant.

Air pollution, such as ozone and particle pollution, can make asthma symptoms worse and trigger attacks. Adults and children with asthma are more likely to have symptoms when ozone and particle pollution are in the air. Ozone is often found in smog and particle pollution is often found in haze, smoke, and dust.

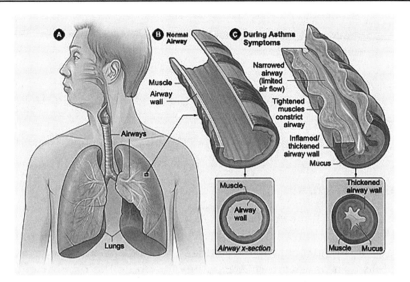

Figure 9.1. *Asthma* (Source: "Asthma," National Heart, Lung, and Blood Institute (NHLBI).)

Figure A shows the location of the lungs and airways in the body. Figure B shows a cross-section of a normal airway. Figure C shows a cross-section of an airway during asthma symptoms.

Ozone is often worst on hot summer days, especially in the afternoons and early evenings. Particle pollution can be bad any time of year, even in winter. It can be especially bad:

- when the weather is calm, and air pollution can build up
- near busy roads, during rush hour, and around factories that produce air pollution
- when smoke is in the air from wood stoves, fireplaces, or burning vegetation

Important asthma triggers are:

- environmental tobacco smoke, also known as secondhand smoke
- dust mites
- outdoor air pollution
- cockroach allergen
- pets

107

- mold

- strenuous physical exercise

- some medicines

- bad weather, such as thunderstorms, high humidity, or freezing temperatures

- some foods and food additives; and strong emotional states that can lead to hyperventilation and an asthma attack

Tracking Asthma

Tracking asthma involves collecting data about people diagnosed and living with asthma and collecting data about people who experience asthma attacks. This includes tracking the number of people ever told by a physician that they have asthma, the number of asthma-related physician visits, the number of clinics or emergency room visits, and the number of deaths due to asthma. Public health officials rely on many sources of data including:

- surveys of self-reported symptoms or diagnoses

- medical encounters of people receiving care for asthma

- death certificates

While the survey data can be used to estimate the number of people suffering from asthma attacks, data on exactly when, where, and how often individuals have asthma attacks are not available.

The National Environmental Public Health Tracking Network (Tracking Network) includes data on asthma hospital stays, emergency department visits for asthma, and asthma prevalence which is the number of people diagnosed with and living with asthma. These data are useful in providing estimates on the geographic distribution and effects of asthma among different populations. These estimates can be used to plan and evaluate asthma interventions.

The emergency department visits for asthma data available on the Tracking Network can be used to identify trends and patterns of emergency department visits over time and in different geographic areas. These data are obtained from state emergency department records and the U.S. Census Bureau.

The asthma prevalence data used on the Tracking Network are obtained from Centers for Disease Control and Prevention's (CDC) Behavioral Risk Factor Surveillance Survey (BRFSS). The BRFSS is a state-based system of health surveys established in 1984.

Asthma Indicators

Asthma Prevalence among Adults and Children

This indicator uses data collected from the Behavior Risk Factor Surveillance Survey (BRFSS). The BRFSS is a state-based system of health surveys established in 1984 by the CDC. Prevalence estimates are organized by different variables to estimate the number of people with asthma in different time periods and geographic areas, such as states and counties. Self-reported data have some limitations because respondents may have difficulty recalling events and understanding questions. Furthermore, cultural and language barriers and limited health knowledge can affect the quality of self-reported data.

Emergency Department Visits for Asthma

This indicator uses data from state emergency department records and the U.S. Census Bureau. It estimates the number and rate of emergency department visits for asthma. These data can be used to identify trends and patterns of emergency department visits over time and in different geographic areas, such as states and counties.

Hospitalizations for Asthma

This indicator uses data collected by hospitals. It can be used to identify trends and patterns in the occurrence of asthma hospital-izations across time and space. The data are organized by different variables to help estimate the number of asthma hospital admissions in different time periods, age groups, and geographic areas, such as states and counties. Asthma hospital admissions tend to be more severe asthma attacks and do not include asthma among individuals who do not receive medical care, who are not hospitalized, or who are treated in outpatient settings. Differences between geographic areas may be the result of differences in the underlying population or in the diagnostic or coding techniques used by the reporting hospital.

109

Section 9.2

Airborne Allergies

This section includes text excerpted from "Seeking Allergy
Relief—When Breathing Becomes Bothersome," NIH News in
Health, National Institutes of Health (NIH), June 2016.

A change in season can brighten your days with vibrant new colors. But blooming flowers and falling leaves can usher in more than beautiful backdrops. Airborne substances that irritate your nose can blow in with the weather. When sneezing, itchy eyes, or a runny nose suddenly appears, allergies may be to blame.

Allergies arise when the body's immune system overreacts to substances, called allergens, that are normally harmless. When a person with allergies breathes in allergens—such as pollen, mold, pet dander, or dust mites—the resulting allergic reactions in the nose are called allergic rhinitis, or hay fever.

Allergy is one of the most common long-term health conditions. "Over the past several decades, the prevalence of allergies has been increasing," says Dr. Paivi Salo, an allergy expert at the National Institutes of Health (NIH). "Currently, airborne allergies affect approximately 10–30 percent of adults and 40 percent of children."

Avoiding your allergy triggers is the best way to control your symptoms. But triggers aren't always easy to identify. Notice when and where your symptoms occur. This can help you figure out the cause.

"Most people with allergies are sensitive to more than one allergen," Salo explains. "Grass, weed and tree pollens are the most common causes of outdoor allergies." Pollen is often the source if your symptoms are seasonal. Indoor allergens usually trigger symptoms that last all year.

If your symptoms become persistent and bothersome, visit your family physician or an allergist. They can test for allergy sensitivities by using a skin or blood test. The test results, along with a medical exam and information about when and where your symptoms occur, will help your doctor determine the cause.

Even when you know your triggers, avoiding allergens can be difficult. When pollen counts are high, stay inside with the windows closed and use the air conditioning. Avoid bringing pollen indoors. "If you go outside, wash your hair and clothing," Salo says. Pets can also bring in pollen, so clean them too.

For indoor allergens, keep humidity levels low in the home to keep dust mites and mold under control. Avoid upholstered furniture and carpets because they harbor allergens. Wash your bedding in hot water, and vacuum the floors once a week.

Allergies run in families. Your children's chances of developing allergies are higher if you have them. While there's no "magic bullet" to prevent allergies, experts recommend breastfeeding early in life. "Breast milk is the least likely to trigger allergic reactions, it's easy to digest, and it strengthens an infant's immune system," Salo says.

Sometimes, avoiding allergens isn't possible or isn't enough. Untreated allergies are associated with chronic conditions like sinus infections and asthma. Over-the-counter (OTC) antihistamines, nasal sprays, and decongestants can often ease mild symptoms. Prescription medications and allergy shots are sometimes needed for more severe allergies. Talk with your doctor about treatment options.

Allergy relief can help clear up more than just itchy, watery eyes. It can allow you to breathe easy again and brighten your outlook on seasonal changes.

Section 9.3

Chronic Obstructive Pulmonary Disease (COPD)

This section includes text excerpted from "Chronic Obstructive Pulmonary Disease (COPD)," Centers for Disease Control and Prevention (CDC), August 4, 2017.

What Is COPD?

Chronic Obstructive Pulmonary Disease, or COPD, refers to a group of diseases that cause airflow blockage and breathing-related problems. It includes emphysema, chronic bronchitis, and in some cases asthma.

111

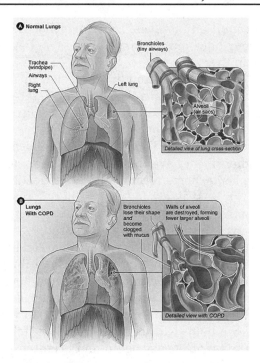

Figure 9.2. *Normal Lungs and Lungs with COPD* (Source: "COPD," National Heart, Lung, and Blood Institute (NHLBI).)

Figure A shows the location of the lungs and airways in the body. The inset image shows a detailed cross-section of the bronchioles and alveoli. Figure B shows lungs damaged by COPD. The inset image shows a detailed cross-section of the damaged bronchioles and alveolar walls.

What Causes COPD?

In the United States, tobacco smoke is a key factor in the development and progression of COPD, although exposure to air pollutants in the home and workplace, genetic factors, and respiratory infections also play a role. In the developing world, indoor air quality is thought to play a larger role in the development and progression of COPD than it does in the United States.

Who Has COPD?

Chronic lower respiratory disease, primarily COPD, was the third leading cause of death in the United States in 2014. Almost 15.7 million Americans (6.4%) reported that they have been diagnosed with COPD. More than 50 percent of adults with low pulmonary function were not aware that they had COPD, so the actual number may be higher. The following groups were more likely to report COPD in 2013.

- People aged 65–74 years and ≥ 75 years
- American Indian/Alaska Natives and multiracial non-Hispanics
- Women
- Individuals who were unemployed, retired, or unable to work
- Individuals with less than a high school education
- Individuals who were divorced, widowed, or separated
- Current or former smokers
- People with a history of asthma

What Are the Complications or Effects of COPD?

Compared to adults without COPD, adults with COPD are more likely to:

- Have activity limitations such as difficulty walking or climbing stairs
- Be unable to work
- Need special equipment such as portable oxygen tanks
- Not engage in social activities such as eating out, going to places of worship, going to group events, or getting together with friends or neighbors
- Have increased confusion or memory loss
- Have more emergency room visits or overnight hospital stays
- Have other chronic diseases such as arthritis, congestive heart failure (CHF), diabetes, coronary heart disease (CHD), stroke, or asthma
- Have depression or other mental or emotional conditions
  Report a fair or poor health status

How Can COPD Be Prevented?

Avoid inhaling tobacco smoke, home, and workplace air pollutants, and respiratory infections to prevent developing COPD. Early detection of COPD might change its course and progress. A simple test,

113

called spirometry, can be used to measure pulmonary—or lung—function and detect COPD in anyone with breathing problems.

How Is COPD Treated?

Treatment of COPD requires a careful and thorough evaluation by a physician. COPD treatment can alleviate symptoms, decrease the frequency and severity of exacerbations, and increase exercise tolerance. For those who smoke, the most important aspect of treatment is smoking cessation. Avoiding tobacco smoke and removing other air pollutants from the patient's home or workplace is also important. Symptoms such as coughing or wheezing can be treated with medication. Pulmonary rehabilitation is an individualized treatment program that teaches COPD management strategies to increase the quality of life. Plans may include breathing strategies, energy conserving techniques, exercise training, and nutritional counseling. Lung infections can cause serious problems in people with COPD. Certain vaccines, such as flu and pneumococcal vaccines, are especially important for people with COPD. Respiratory infections should be treated with antibiotics, if appropriate. Patients who have low blood oxygen levels are often given supplemental oxygen.

Chapter 10

Viruses Spread through Hazards in the Environment

Chapter Contents

Section 10.1

Avian Influenza (Bird Flu)

This section includes text excerpted from "Influenza (Flu)—Avian
Influenza A Virus Infections in Humans," Centers for Disease
Control and Prevention (CDC), April 18, 2017.

Avian Influenza A Virus Infections in Humans

Although avian influenza A viruses usually do not infect people,
rare cases of human infection with these viruses have been reported.
Infected birds shed avian influenza virus in their saliva, mucus, and
feces. Human infections with bird flu viruses can happen when enough
virus gets into a person's eyes, nose or mouth, or is inhaled. This can
happen when the virus is in the air (in droplets or possibly dust) and
a person breathes it in, or when a person touches something that has
a virus on it then touches their mouth, eyes or nose. Rare human
infections with some avian viruses have occurred most often after
unprotected contact with infected birds or surfaces contaminated with
avian influenza viruses. However, some infections have been identified
where direct contact was not known to have occurred. Illness in people
has ranged from mild to severe.

The spread of avian influenza A viruses from one ill person to
another has been reported very rarely, and when it has been reported
it has been limited, inefficient and not sustained. However, because of
the possibility that avian influenza A viruses could change and gain the
ability to spread easily between people, monitoring for human infection
and person-to-person spread is extremely important for public health.

Signs and Symptoms of Avian Influenza a Virus Infections in Humans

The reported signs and symptoms of avian influenza A virus infections in humans have ranged from mild to severe and included con-
junctivitis, influenza-like illness (e.g., fever, cough, sore throat, muscle
aches) sometimes accompanied by nausea, abdominal pain, diarrhea,
and vomiting, severe respiratory illness (e.g., shortness of breath,

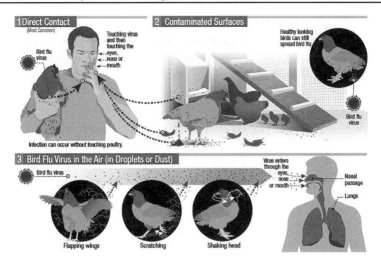

Figure 10.1. *Avian Influenza Transmission*

difficulty breathing, pneumonia, acute respiratory distress, viral pneumonia, respiratory failure), neurologic changes (altered mental status, seizures), and the involvement of other organ systems. Asian lineage H7N9 and HPAI Asian lineage *H5N1* viruses have been responsible for most human illness worldwide to date, including most serious illnesses and highest mortality.

Detecting Avian Influenza A Virus Infection in Humans

Avian influenza A virus infection in people cannot be diagnosed by clinical signs and symptoms alone; laboratory testing is needed. Avian influenza A virus infection is usually diagnosed by collecting a swab from the upper respiratory tract (nose or throat) of the sick person. (Testing is more accurate when the swab is collected during the first few days of illness.) This specimen is sent to a laboratory; the laboratory looks for avian influenza A virus either by using a molecular test, by trying to grow the virus or both. (Growing avian influenza A viruses should only be done in laboratories with high levels of biosafety.)

For critically ill patients, collection and testing of lower respiratory tract specimens also may lead to a diagnosis of avian influenza virus infection. However, for some patients who are no longer very sick or who have fully recovered, it may be difficult to detect the avian influenza A virus in the specimen. Sometimes it may still be possible to diagnose avian influenza A virus infection by looking for evidence of antibodies the body has produced in response to the virus. This is not always an option because it requires two blood specimens (one taken during the first week of illness and another taken 3–4 weeks later). Also, it can take several weeks to verify the results, and testing must be performed in a special laboratory, such as at the Centers for Disease Control and Prevention (CDC).

Treating Avian Influenza A Virus Infections in Humans

CDC currently recommends a neuraminidase inhibitor for the treatment of human infection with avian influenza A viruses. CDC has posted avian influenza guidance for healthcare professionals and laboratorians, including guidance on the use of antiviral medications for the treatment of human infections with novel influenza viruses associated with severe disease. Analyses of available avian influenza viruses circulating worldwide suggest that most viruses are susceptible to oseltamivir, peramivir, and zanamivir. However, some evidence of antiviral resistance has been reported in Asian H5N1 and Asian H7N9 viruses isolated from some human cases. Monitoring for antiviral resistance among avian influenza A viruses is crucial and ongoing.

Preventing Human Infection with Avian Influenza A Viruses

The best way to prevent infection with avian influenza A viruses is to avoid sources of exposure. Most human infections with avian influenza A viruses have occurred following direct or close contact with infected poultry.

People who have had contact with infected birds may be given influenza antiviral drugs preventatively. While antiviral drugs are most often used to treat influenza, they also can be used to prevent infection in someone who has been exposed to influenza viruses. When used to prevent seasonal influenza, antiviral drugs are 70–90 percent effective. CDC has posted interim guidance for clinicians and public health professionals in the United States regarding follow-up and influenza antiviral chemoprophylaxis of persons exposed to birds infected with avian influenza A viruses.

Seasonal influenza vaccination will not prevent infection with avian influenza A viruses, but can reduce the risk of coinfection with human and avian influenza A viruses. It's also possible to make a vaccine that can protect people against avian influenza viruses. For example, the United States government maintains a stockpile of vaccines to protect against some Asian avian influenza A H5N1 viruses. The stockpiled vaccine could be used if similar H5N1 viruses were to begin transmitting easily from person to person. Since influenza viruses change, CDC continues to make new candidate vaccine viruses as needed. Creating a candidate vaccine virus is the first step in producing a vaccine.

Section 10.2

Severe Acute Respiratory Syndrome (SARS)

This section includes text excerpted from "Severe Acute Respiratory Syndrome (SARS)—SARS Basics Fact Sheet," Centers for Disease Control and Prevention (CDC), December 6, 2017.

Severe acute respiratory syndrome (SARS) is a viral respiratory illness caused by a coronavirus, called SARS-associated coronavirus (SARS-CoV). SARS was first reported in Asia in February 2003. Over the next few months, the illness spread to more than two dozen countries in North America, South America, Europe, and Asia before the SARS global outbreak of 2003 was contained.

The SARS Outbreak of 2003

According to the World Health Organization (WHO), a total of 8,098 people worldwide became sick with SARS during the 2003 outbreak. Of these, 774 died. In the United States, only eight people had laboratory evidence of SARS-CoV infection. All of these people had traveled to other parts of the world where SARS was spreading. SARS did not spread more widely in the community in the United States.

Symptoms of SARS

In general, SARS begins with a high fever (temperature greater than 100.4°F [>38.0°C]). Other symptoms may include a headache, an overall feeling of discomfort, and body aches. Some people also have mild respiratory symptoms at the outset. About 10–20 percent of patients have diarrhea. After 2–7 days, SARS patients may develop a dry cough. Most patients develop pneumonia.

How SARS Spreads

The main way that SARS seems to spread is by close person-to-person contact. The virus that causes SARS is thought to be transmitted most readily by respiratory droplets (droplet spread) produced when an infected person coughs or sneezes. Droplet spread can happen when droplets from a cough or sneeze of an infected person have propelled a short distance (generally up to 3 feet) through the air and deposited on the mucous membranes of the mouth, nose, or eyes of persons who are nearby. The virus also can spread when a person touches a surface or object contaminated with infectious droplets and then touches his or her mouth, nose, or eye(s). In addition, it is possible that the SARS virus might spread more broadly through the air (airborne spread) or by other ways that are not now known.

What Does "Close Contact" Mean?

In the context of SARS, close contact means having cared for or lived with someone with SARS or having direct contact with respiratory secretions or body fluids of a patient with SARS. Examples of close contact include kissing or hugging, sharing eating or drinking utensils, talking to someone within 3 feet, and touching someone directly. Close contact does not include activities like walking by a person or briefly sitting in a waiting room or office.

Steps to Protect Yourself and the People around You

If you have SARS, or you have close contact with someone who does, follow these instructions:

If you think you (or someone in your family) might have SARS, you should:

- Call your healthcare provider as soon as possible. Call ahead and alert the healthcare provider before your visit so that precautions can be taken to keep from exposing other people.

- Cover your mouth and nose with a tissue when coughing or sneezing.

- Be careful not to expose others. If you have been exposed to SARS and become ill with any symptoms, limit your activities outside the home. Avoid public transportation (e.g., bus, taxi). Do not go to work, school, out-of-home child care, church, or activities in other public areas until after you are told that you do not have SARS.

- Follow any other instructions provided by local health authorities.

If you have SARS and are being cared for at home, you should:

- Follow the instructions given by your healthcare provider.

- Limit your activities outside the home except as necessary for medical care. For example, do not go to work, school, or public areas. If you must leave the home, wear a mask, if tolerated. Do not use public transportation.

- Wash your hands often and well, especially after you blow your nose.

- Cover your mouth and nose with a tissue when you sneeze or a cough.

- If possible, wear a surgical mask when around other people in your home. If you can't wear a mask, the members of your household should wear one when they are around you.

- Don't share silverware, towels, or bedding with anyone in your home until these items have been washed with soap and hot water.

- Be sure that surfaces (counters, tabletops, doorknobs, bathroom fixtures, etc.) that have been contaminated by your body fluids (sweat, saliva, mucus, vomit, or urine) are cleaned with a household disinfectant used according to the manufacturer's instructions. Be sure that the person who cleans the surfaces wears disposable gloves during all cleaning activities. Disposable gloves should be thrown out after use and should not be reused.

- Follow these instructions for 10 days after your fever and respiratory symptoms have gone away or until the health department says you can return to normal activities.

If you are caring for someone at home who has SARS, you should:

- Be sure that you understand and can help the SARS patient follow the healthcare provider's instructions for medication and care.

- Be sure that all members of your household are washing their hands frequently with soap and hot water or using an alcohol-based hand rub.

- Wear disposable gloves if you will have direct contact with body fluids of a SARS patient. However, wearing gloves is not a substitute for good hand hygiene. After contact with body fluids of a SARS patient, remove the gloves, throw them out, and wash your hands. Do not wash or reuse the gloves.

- Encourage the person with SARS to cover his or her mouth and nose with a tissue when coughing or sneezing. If possible, the person with SARS should wear a surgical mask during close contact with other people in the home. If the person with SARS cannot wear a surgical mask, other members of the household should wear one when in the room with that person.

- Do not use silverware, towels, bedding, clothing, or other items that have been used by the person with SARS until these items have been washed with soap and hot water.

- Clean surfaces in the patient's room and the bathroom fixtures used by the patient daily, with a household disinfectant used according to the manufacturer's instructions. When cleaning, wear disposable gloves, and dispose of them after use. Or, use household utility gloves.

- Limit the number of persons in the household to those who are essential for patient support. Other household members should either be relocated or minimize contact with the patient in the home. This is particularly important for persons at risk of serious complications of SARS (e.g., persons with underlying heart or lung disease, diabetes mellitus, older age).

- Unexposed persons who do not have an essential need to be in the home should not visit.

- Follow these instructions for 10 days after the sick person's fever and respiratory symptoms have gone away or until the health department says the SARS patient can return to normal activities.

- For 10 days after your last exposure to the person with SARS, be vigilant for fever (i.e., measure your temperature twice daily), respiratory symptoms, and other early symptoms of SARS. Common early symptoms include chills, body aches, and headache. In some patients, body aches and headache may appear 12–24 hours before fever. Diarrhea, sore throat, and runny nose may also be early symptoms of SARS. If you do not have any of these symptoms, you do not need to limit your activities outside the home. You may go to work, school, out-of-home child care, church, or activities in other public areas.

- Follow any other instructions provided by local health authorities.

- If you start feeling sick, especially if you develop a fever, respiratory symptoms, or other early symptoms of SARS, contact your healthcare provider immediately, and tell the healthcare provider that you have had close contact with a SARS patient.

Section 10.3

West Nile Virus

This section includes text excerpted from "West Nile Virus," Centers for Disease Control and Prevention (CDC), February 21, 2018.

West Nile is a virus most commonly spread to people by mosquito bites. In North America, cases of West Nile virus (WNV) occur during mosquito season, which starts in the summer and continues through fall. WNV cases have been reported in all of the continental United States. There are no vaccines to prevent or medications to treat WNV. Fortunately, most people infected with WNV do not have symptoms. About 1 in 5 people who are infected develop a fever and other symptoms. About 1 out of 150 infected people develop a serious, sometimes fatal, illness. You can reduce your risk of WNV by using insect repellent and wearing long-sleeved shirts and long pants to prevent mosquito bites.

Transmission

WNV is most commonly spread to people by the bite of an infected mosquito.

Mosquitoes become infected when they feed on infected birds. Infected mosquitoes then spread WNV to people and other animals by biting them.

123

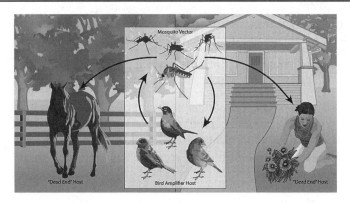

Figure 10.2. *Transmission of West Nile Virus*

In a very small number of cases, WNV has been spread through:

- Exposure in a laboratory setting

- Blood transfusion and organ donation

- Mother to baby, during pregnancy, delivery, or breastfeeding

WNV is not spread:

- Through coughing, sneezing, or touching

- By touching live animals

- From handling live or dead infected birds. Avoid bare-handed contact when handling any dead animal. If you are disposing of a dead bird, use gloves or double plastic bags to place the carcass in a garbage can.

- Through eating infected birds or animals. Always follow instructions for fully cooking meat from either birds or mammals.

Symptoms, Diagnosis, and Treatment

Symptoms

No symptoms in most people. Most people (8 out of 10) infected with WNV do not develop any symptoms.

Febrile illness (fever) in some people. About 1 in 5 people who are infected develop a fever with other symptoms such as a headache, body aches, joint pains, vomiting, diarrhea, or rash. Most people with this type of WNV disease recover completely, but fatigue and weakness can last for weeks or months.

Serious symptoms in a few people. About 1 in 150 people who are infected develop a severe illness affecting the central nervous system (CNS) such as encephalitis (inflammation of the brain) or meningitis (inflammation of the membranes that surround the brain and spinal cord).

- Symptoms of severe illness include high fever, headache, neck stiffness, stupor, disorientation, coma, tremors, convulsions, muscle weakness, vision loss, numbness, and paralysis.

- Severe illness can occur in people of any age; however, people over 60 years of age are at greater risk. People with certain medical conditions, such as cancer, diabetes, hypertension, kidney disease, and people who have received organ transplants, are also at greater risk.

- Recovery from severe illness might take several weeks or months. Some effects to the CNS might be permanent.

- About 1 out of 10 people who develop severe illness affecting the CNS die.

Diagnosis

- See your healthcare provider if you develop the symptoms described above.

- Your healthcare provider can order tests to look for WNV infection.

Treatment

- No vaccine or specific antiviral treatments for WNV infection are available.

- Over-the-counter (OTC) pain relievers can be used to reduce fever and relieve some symptoms.

- In severe cases, patients often need to be hospitalized to receive supportive treatment, such as intravenous fluids, pain medication, and nursing care.

- If you think you or a family member might have WNV disease, talk with your healthcare provider.

Prevention

The most effective way to avoid West Nile virus disease is to prevent mosquito bites. Be aware of the WNV activity in your area and take action to protect yourself and your family.

Use Insect Repellent

Use U.S. Environmental Protection Agency (EPA) registered insect repellents with one of the active ingredients below. When used as directed, EPA registered insect repellents are proven safe and effective, even for pregnant and breastfeeding women.

- N,N-Diethyl-meta-toluamide (DEET)

- Picaridin (known as KBR 3023 and icaridin outside the U.S.)

- IR3535

- Oil of lemon eucalyptus (OLE) or para-menthane-diol (PMD)

- 2-undecanone

Tips for Everyone

- Always follow the product label instructions.

- Re-apply insect repellent as directed.

    - Do not spray repellent on the skin under clothing.

    - If you are also using sunscreen, apply sunscreen first and insect repellent second.

Tips for Babies and Children

- Always follow instructions when applying insect repellent to children.

- Do not use insect repellent on babies younger than 2 months old.

- Do not apply an insect repellent onto a child's hands, eyes, mouth, and cut or irritated skin.

    - **Adults.** Spray insect repellent onto your hands and then apply to a child's face.

- Do not use products containing oil of lemon eucalyptus (OLE) or para-menthane-diol (PMD) on children under 3 years old.

Natural Insect Repellents (Repellents Not Registered with EPA)

Not much is known about the effectiveness of non-EPA registered insect repellents, including some natural repellents.

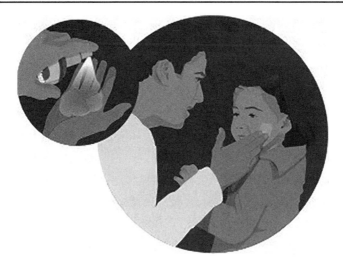

Figure 10.3. *How to Apply Insect Repellent*

To protect yourself against diseases spread by mosquitoes, the Centers for Disease Control and Prevention (CDC) and the FDA recommend using an EPA registered insect repellent.

Choosing an EPA registered repellent ensures the EPA has evaluated the product for effectiveness.

Protect Your Baby or Child

• Dress your child in clothing that covers arms and legs.

• Cover crib, stroller, and baby carrier with mosquito netting.

Wear Long Sleeved Shirts and Long Pants

• Treat items, such as boots, pants, socks, and tents, with permethrin* or buy permethrin-treated clothing and gear.

    • Permethrin-treated clothing will protect you from multiple items of washing. See product information to find out how long the protection will last.

    • If treating items yourself, follow the product instructions.

    • Do not use permethrin products directly on the skin.

In some places, such as Puerto Rico, where permethrin products have been used for years in mosquito control efforts, mosquitoes have become resistant to it. In areas with high levels of resistance, use of permethrin is not likely to be effective.

Take Steps to Control Mosquitoes inside and outside Your Home

- Use screens on windows and doors. Repair holes in screens to keep mosquitoes outside.

- Use air conditioning when available.

  - Sleep under a mosquito bed net if air-conditioned or screened rooms are not available or if sleeping outdoors.

- Once a week, empty and scrub, turn over, cover, or throw out items that hold water, such as tires, buckets, planters, toys, pools, birdbaths, flowerpots, or trash containers. Check inside and outside your home. Mosquitoes lay eggs near water.

Chapter 11

Reproductive Issues and the Environment

Chapter Contents

Section 11.1

Fertility

This section includes text excerpted from "Reproductive and
Birth Outcomes," Centers for Disease Control and
Prevention (CDC), January 10, 2017.

More than three million healthy babies are born annually in the
United States. While most women have a normal term pregnancy and
deliver a normal infant, a safe and healthy pregnancy is not experienced by all women. Certain genetic, behavioral, social, and environmental factors can affect the parents' ability to conceive, carry, and
deliver a healthy, full-term baby.

The understanding of risk factors for reproductive problems has
increased over the past decades. However, there is still much not
known. In order to understand better the role that environmental exposures play in reproductive and infant health problems, the National
Environmental Public Health Tracking Network (Tracking Network)
collects and displays data on reproductive and birth outcomes including
fertility and infertility, premature birth, infant deaths, birthweight,
and sex ratio.

Fertility and Infertility and the Environment

According to data from the National Survey of Family Growth
(NSFG), 11 percent of U.S. couples had impaired fertility from 2006–
2010. Waiting to have a child until later in life and existing medical
conditions are not the only causes of male and female infertility. It
is believed that environmental contaminants may cause infertility
by creating other health conditions. For example, some research
suggests that environmental contaminants can affect a woman's
menstruation and ovulation. Low-level exposures to compounds such
as phthalates, polychlorinated biphenyls (PCBs), dioxin, and pesticides are suspected risk factors. Much more research needs to be
done to find out how environmental contaminants may be affecting
human fertility.

Exposure and Risk

For many people who want to start a family, the dream of having a child is not easily realized. About 6 percent of women in the United States ages 15–44 years have difficulty getting pregnant or staying pregnant. Infertility is a problem that can affect both men and women. It can be caused by many factors that may include the following:

- Age
- Stress
- Poor diet
- Genetics
- Nutrition
- Behavior
- Some medicines
- Athletic training
- Being overweight or underweight
- Tobacco use
- Alcohol consumption
- Sexually transmitted diseases (STDs)
- Health problems that cause hormonal changes

The amount and quality of a man's sperm can be affected by:

- Environmental toxins
- Alcohol
- Illegal drugs
- Tobacco use
- Some medicines
- Radiation treatment or chemotherapy for cancer
- Age

Prevention

Most healthy women younger than 30 years of age should not worry about infertility unless they have been trying to conceive for at least a year. At this point, women and their partners should talk with their doctors about a fertility evaluation. A woman's chances of conceiving decreases quickly every year after the age of 30. Women in this age group who have been trying to conceive for six months should also talk with their doctors about having a complete and timely fertility evaluation.

Some health issues increase a woman's chances of having fertility problems. Women with the following issues should consult their doctors:

- Irregular or no menstrual periods

- Very painful periods

- Endometriosis

- Pelvic inflammatory disease (PID)

- More than one miscarriage

No matter what age, a woman should always talk to her doctor before trying to get pregnant. Doctors can help women prepare their body for a healthy baby. They can also answer questions on fertility and give advice on conceiving.

Section 11.2

Endocrine Disruptors and Reproductive Disorders

This section includes text excerpted from "Endocrine Disruptors," National Institute of Environmental Health Sciences (NIEHS), August 28, 2017.

Endocrine disruptors are chemicals that may interfere with the body's endocrine system and produce adverse developmental, reproductive, neurological, and immune effects in both humans and wildlife. A wide range of substances, both natural and artificial, are thought to cause endocrine disruption, including pharmaceuticals, dioxin and dioxin-like compounds, polychlorinated biphenyls (PCB), dichloro-diphenyl-trichloroethane (DDT) and other pesticides, and plasticizers such as bisphenol A.

Endocrine disruptors may be found in many everyday products—including plastic bottles, metal food cans, detergents, flame retardants, food, toys, cosmetics, and pesticides. The National Institute of Environmental Health Sciences (NIEHS) supports studies to determine whether exposure to endocrine disruptors may result in human health effects including lowered fertility and an increased incidence of endometriosis and some cancers. Research shows that endocrine disruptors may pose the greatest risk during prenatal and early postnatal development when organ and neural systems are forming.

How Do Endocrine Disruptors Work?

From animal studies, researchers have learned much about the mechanisms through which endocrine disruptors influence the endocrine system and alter hormonal functions.

Endocrine disruptors can:

- Mimic or partly mimic naturally occurring hormones in the body like estrogens (the female sex hormone), androgens (the male sex hormone), and thyroid hormones, potentially producing overstimulation

- Bind to a receptor within a cell and block the endogenous hormone from binding. The normal signal then fails to occur and the body fails to respond properly. Examples of chemicals that block or antagonize hormones are antiestrogens and antiandrogens.

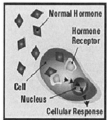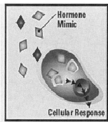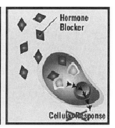

Figure 11.1. *Response of Endocrine Disruptor*

When absorbed in the body, an endocrine disruptor can decrease or increase normal hormone levels (left), mimic the body's natural hormones (middle), or alter the natural production of hormones (right).

- Interfere or block the way natural hormones or their receptors are made or controlled, for example, by altering their metabolism in the liver

What Are Some Examples of Endocrine Disruptors?

A wide and varied range of substances is thought to cause endocrine disruption.

Chemicals that are known endocrine disruptors include diethylstilbestrol (the synthetic estrogen DES), dioxin and dioxin-like compounds, PCBs, DDT, and some other pesticides.

Bisphenol A (BPA) is a chemical produced in large quantities for use primarily in the production of polycarbonate plastics and epoxy resins. The NTP Center for the Evaluation of Risks to Human Reproduction (NTP-CERHR) completed a review of BPA. NTP expressed "some concern for effects on the brain, behavior, and prostate gland in fetuses, infants, and children at current human exposures to bisphenol A."

Di(2-ethylhexyl) phthalate (DEHP) is a high production volume chemical used in the manufacture of a wide variety of consumer food packaging, some children's products, and some polyvinyl chloride (PVC) medical devices. NTP found that DEHP may pose a risk to human development, especially critically ill male infants.

Phytoestrogens are naturally occurring substances in plants that have hormone-like activity. Examples of phytoestrogens are genistein and daidzein, which can be found in soy-derived products.

Chapter 12

The Link between Autism and the Environment

Chapter Contents

Section 12.1

Impact of Environment on Autism

This section includes text excerpted from "Autism,"
National Institute of Environmental Health
Sciences (NIEHS), August 28, 2017.

Autism, also known as autism spectrum disorder (ASD), is a disorder that causes impairment in social interaction, as well as the
presence of repetitive, restricted behaviors and interests. It is usually
first diagnosed in early childhood.

The term spectrum refers to the wide range of symptoms, skills,
and levels of impairment that those with ASD can have. Some are
mildly impaired by their symptoms, while others are severely disabled.
According to the Centers for Disease Control and Prevention (CDC),
ASD affects roughly 1 in 68 children.

Symptoms of Autism

Although people with autism have a range of symptoms that vary
in severity, they all have difficulties communicating and interacting
with others and show restricted and repetitive patterns of behavior
and interests. Most symptoms are noticeable by the time a child is
2–3 years old, but many children are not diagnosed until later. Early
intensive behavioral intervention can improve communication, learning, and social skills in children with autism.

Autism affects people for their entire lives and often comes with
other conditions, such as epilepsy, sleep disturbances, and gastrointestinal (GI) problems. Currently, no drugs have proven effective for
treating core autism symptoms.

Diagnosis of Autism

In the American Psychiatric Association (APA) updated the criteria
for diagnosing ASD in the fifth edition of the *Diagnostic and Statistical
Manual of Mental Disorders* (DSM-5).

The new DSM-5 criteria encourage diagnosis prior to school age.
Children with ASD must show symptoms from early childhood,

136

although the symptoms may not be recognized until later. Sometimes symptoms are not evident until children are old enough to be in social situations that challenge their capacity to respond.

Causes of Autism

Although studies indicate that the rate of ASD is rising, the causes of these disorders are not well understood. Over time, scientists have found that rare gene changes, or mutations, as well as small common genetic variations, are associated with ASD, thus implying a genetic component. However, a growing area of research indicates that ASD may be caused by an interaction of genetic and environmental factors.

For example, one hypothesis states that ASD may be triggered by a mother's exposure to environmental agents while pregnant. These exposures, in turn, could cause or contribute to the child's development of ASD.

Environmental Factors That May Be Associated with Autism

The clearest evidence for environmental risk factors in ASD involves events before and during birth. They may include:

- Advanced parental age at the time of conception

- Prenatal exposure to air pollution

- Maternal obesity or diabetes

- Extreme prematurity and very low birth weight

- Any birth difficulty leading to periods of prenatal oxygen deprivation to the baby's brain

- Prenatal exposure to certain pesticides

Again, however, these factors alone are unlikely to cause ASD. Rather, they appear to increase a child's chances of developing ASD, when combined with the aforementioned genetic factors.

Environmental Factors Play a Role in Autism

Air Pollution

Work supported by National Institute of Environmental Health Sciences (NIEHS) indicates that early-life exposure to air pollution is a risk factor for autism.

- A study reported that children living near a freeway at birth were twice as likely to develop autism. A distance of 1,014 feet, or a little less than 3.5 football fields, was considered near a freeway.

- Building on those findings, researchers reported an increased risk of autism associated with exposure to traffic-related air pollution and regional air pollutants in 2013.

- A study pointed to a likely gene-environment interaction. Children whose genetic makeup causes them to be more susceptible to the health effects of high levels of air pollution showed the highest risk for autism.

Prenatal Conditions

Researchers funded by NIEHS discovered that problems with the immune system, as well as maternal conditions during pregnancy, are linked with higher autism risk.

- Researchers found that some mothers of autistic children have antibodies that may interfere with fetal brain development in ways that could lead to autism.

- Maternal diabetes and obesity may have a role in autism. These metabolic conditions, which are associated with inflammation, both have strong links to the likelihood of having a child with autism or another developmental disability.

- Additional studies have shown that maternal inflammation during pregnancy may be linked to autism. Elevated levels of inflammation, which can come from an infection, were assessed by measuring C-reactive protein in the mother's blood. This finding may help to identify preventive strategies.

Nutrition

According to the National Institute of Environmental Health Sciences (NIEHS)-funded research, prenatal vitamins may help lower autism risk.

- Women were less likely to have a child with autism if they took a daily prenatal vitamin during the three months before pregnancy and the first month of pregnancy, compared to women not taking the supplements. This was more evident in genetically susceptible women or children, suggesting that a gene-environment interaction could be responsible.

- A later study identified folic acid as the source of protective effects of prenatal vitamins. Women who consumed the daily recommended dosage during the first month of pregnancy had a reduced risk of having a child with autism.

Mercury and Other Contaminants

There continues to be concern about autism and mercury exposure.

- Eating fish is the primary way that we are exposed to organic mercury. A study examined people in the Republic of Seychelles, where fish consumption is high. The study found no association between prenatal organic mercury exposure and autism behaviors.

- Scientists can test for exposure to organic mercury with blood tests. Researchers found that after adjusting for dietary and other mercury sources, children with autism had blood mercury levels that were similar to those in children without autism.

- Researchers are also studying other contaminants, such as Bisphenol A (BPA), phthalates, heavy metals, flame retardants, polychlorinated biphenyls (PCBs), and pesticides, to see if they affect early brain development and play a role in autism.

- No link between autism and vaccines containing thimerosal, a mercury-based compound, has been found

Section 12.2

Vaccinations, Thimerosal, and Autism

This section includes text excerpted from "Vaccines, Blood and Biologics—Thimerosal in Vaccines Questions and Answers," U.S. Food and Drug Administration (FDA), February 5, 2018.

Preservatives and Vaccines

Preservatives are compounds that kill or prevent the growth of microorganisms, such as bacteria or fungi. They are used in vaccines to prevent bacterial or fungal growth in the event that the vaccine is accidentally contaminated, as might occur with repeated puncture of multi-dose vials. Vaccines, both in the United States and throughout other parts of the world, are commonly packaged in multidose vials. In some cases, preservatives are added during manufacture to prevent microbial growth; with changes in manufacturing technology, however, the need to add preservatives during the manufacturing process has decreased markedly.

Preservatives have been used in vaccines for over 70 years. The requirement for a preservative in multidose, multi-entry vials was placed into the Code of Federal Regulations (21 CFR 610.15) in January 1968. There are exceptions to this requirement for preservative, primarily involving the live-attenuated viral vaccines.

The general need for preservatives in multidose vials has been underscored by cases in which multidose vials that did not contain preservatives become contaminated during use and caused fatal infections in vaccine recipients.

Thimerosal

Thimerosal is a preservative that has been used in some vaccines since the 1930's when it was first introduced. It is 49.6 percent mercury by weight and is metabolized or degraded into ethylmercury, and thiosalicylate. At concentrations found in vaccines, it meets the requirements for a preservative as set forth by the United States Pharmacopeia (USP); that is, it kills the specified challenge organisms and is able to prevent the growth of the challenge fungi. Prior to its introduction in the 1930's, data were available in several animal species and humans providing evidence for its safety and effectiveness as a preservative. Since then, thimerosal has a long record of safe and effective use preventing bacterial and fungal contamination of vaccines, with no ill effects established other than minor local reactions at the site of injection.

As a vaccine preservative, thimerosal is used in concentrations of 0.003–0.01 percent. A vaccine containing 0.01 percent thimerosal as a preservative contains 50 micrograms of thimerosal per 0.5 ml dose or approximately 25 micrograms of mercury per 0.5 mL dose. The use of mercury-containing preservatives in vaccines has declined over the past three decades.

The U.S. Food and Drug Administration (FDA) is continuing its efforts toward reducing or removing thimerosal from all existing vaccines. Much progress has been made to date. FDA has been actively working with manufacturers, particularly those that manufacture childhood vaccines, to reach the goal of eliminating thimerosal from vaccines, and has been collaborating with another public health service (PHS) agencies to further evaluate the potential health effects of thimerosal. In this regard, all vaccines routinely recommended for children 6 years of age or younger and marketed in the United States contain no thimerosal or only trace amounts (1 microgram or less mercury per dose), with the exception of inactivated influenza vaccine, which was first recommended by the Advisory Committee on Immunization Practices (ACIP) in 2004 for routine use in children 6–23 months of age.

Progress in Elimination of Thimerosal from Vaccines

Great progress has been made in removing thimerosal from vaccines. Manufacturers have been able to accomplish this goal through changing their manufacturing processes, including a switch from multidose vials, which generally require a preservative, to single-dose vials or syringes. Since 2001, all vaccines manufactured for the U.S. market and routinely recommended for children ≤ 6 years of age have contained no thimerosal or only trace amounts (≤ 1 microgram of mercury per dose remaining from the manufacturing process), with the exception of inactivated influenza vaccine. In addition, all of the routinely recommended vaccines that had been previously manufactured with thimerosal as a preservative (some formulations of Diphtheria, Tetanus, Pertussis (DTaP), Haemophilus influenza B conjugate (Hib),

141

and hepatitis B vaccines) had reached the end of their shelf life by January 2003.

In the past, prior to the initiative to reduce or eliminate thimerosal from childhood vaccines, the maximum cumulative exposure to mercury via routine childhood vaccinations during the first six months of life was 187.5 micrograms. With the introduction of thimerosal preservative-free formulations of DTaP, hepatitis B, and HiB, the maximum cumulative exposure from these vaccines decreased to less than three micrograms of mercury in the first 6 months of life. With the addition of influenza vaccine to the recommended vaccines, an infant could receive a thimerosal-containing influenza vaccine at 6–7 months of age. This would result in a maximum exposure or 28 micrograms via routine childhood vaccinations. This level is well below the environmental protection agency (EPA) calculated exposure guideline for methylmercury of 65 micrograms for a child in the 5th percentile body weight during the first 6 months of life.

Currently, all hepatitis vaccines manufactured for the U.S. market contain either no thimerosal or only trace amounts. Also, DT, Td, and Tetanus Toxoid vaccines are now available in formulations that contain no thimerosal or only trace amounts.

Furthermore, all new vaccines licensed free of thimerosal as a preservative. Inactivated influenza vaccine was added to the routinely recommended vaccines for children 6–23 months of age. The FDA has approved thimerosal preservative-free formulations (containing either no or only trace amounts of thimerosal) for the inactivated influenza vaccines. These influenza vaccines continue to be marketed in both the preservative free and thimerosal preservative-containing formulations. In addition, the FDA licensed GlaxoSmithKline's inactivated influenza vaccine, which contains 1.25 micrograms mercury per dose. Of the three licensed inactivated influenza vaccines, Fluzone is the only one approved for use in children down to 6 months of age. Fluvirin is approved for individuals 4 years of age and older, and Fluarix is approved for individuals 18 years of age and older. The live attenuated influenza vaccine (FluMist), which contains no thimerosal, is approved for individuals 5–49 years of age. Based on an estimated annual birth cohort in the United States of 4 million, there are 6 million infants and children between the ages of 6–23 months, most of whom would need two doses each. Thus, the amount of thimerosal preservative-free vaccine that is available based on current manufacturing capacity is well below the number of doses needed to fully vaccinate this age group.

Vaccines That Are "Thimerosal-Free," "Thimerosal-Reduced," and "Preservative-Free"

Thimerosal may be added at the end of the manufacturing process to act as a preservative to prevent bacterial or fungal growth in the event that the vaccine is accidentally contaminated, as might occur with repeated puncture of multi-dose vials. When thimerosal is used as the preservative in vaccines, it is present in concentrations up to 0.01 percent (50 micrograms thimerosal per 0.5 mL dose or 25 micrograms mercury per 0.5 mL dose). In some cases, thimerosal is used during the manufacturing process and is present in small amounts in the final vaccine (1 microgram mercury or less per dose).

The term "preservative-free" indicates that no preservative (thimerosal or otherwise) is used in the vaccine; however, traces used during the manufacturing process may be present in the final formulation. For example, some vaccines may be preservative free but may contain traces of thimerosal (1 microgram mercury or less per dose); in such settings, this information is noted in the package insert. Similarly, the term "thimerosal-reduced" usually indicates that thimerosal is not added as a vaccine preservative, but trace amounts (1 microgram mercury per dose or less) may remain from use in the manufacturing process. Such trace amounts are not felt to be clinically significant, nor would they result in exposure exceeding any federal guideline for mercury exposure. Vaccines may be termed "thimerosal-free" if no thimerosal can be measured; i.e., thimerosal content is below the limit of detection.

Concerns Due to Exposure to Mercury

Mercury is an element that is dispersed widely around the earth. Most of the mercury in the water, soil, plants, and animals are found as inorganic mercury salts. Mercury accumulates in the aquatic food chain, primarily in the form of the methylmercury, an organomercurial. Methylmercury is more easily absorbed and is less readily eliminated from the body than inorganic mercury. Exposure to one chemical with mercury, i.e., methylmercury, has been shown to pose a variety of health risks to humans. Extremely high levels, such as that observed in poisoning episodes in Japan and Iraq has caused neurological damage and death. The fetus is considered more sensitive to health effects of methylmercury than adults. In recent years some studies have found adverse health effects of methylmercury at levels previously thought to be safe. Other studies, however, have shown conflicting results.

143

It is important to note that the preservative thimerosal contains ethylmercury, a related though distinct chemical from methylmercury. Moreover, studies in animal models exposed to thimerosal-containing vaccines or oral methylmercury suggest that methylmercury may not be a suitable reference to assess the risk from exposure to thimerosal. In addition, data from studies in human infants that were given routine immunizations with thimerosal-containing vaccines showed that mercury levels in blood and urine were uniformly below safety guidelines for methylmercury and that unlike methylmercury excretory profiles, infants excreted significant amounts of mercury in stool after thimerosal (ethylmercury) exposure, thus removing mercury from their bodies.

Child Safety Upon Receiving an Influenza Vaccine That Contains Thimerosal

There is no convincing evidence of harm caused by the small doses of thimerosal preservative in influenza vaccines, except for minor effects like swelling and redness at the injection site.

Researchers suggest that healthy children under the age of 2 are more likely than older children and as likely as people over the age of 65 to be hospitalized with flu complications. Therefore, vaccination with thimerosal preservative-containing influenza vaccine and thimerosal reduced influenza vaccine is encouraged when feasible in children, including those that are 6–23 months of age.

Pregnant Women Safety Upon Receiving an Influenza Vaccine That Contains Thimerosal

A study of influenza vaccination examining over 2,000 pregnant women demonstrated no adverse fetal effects associated with influenza vaccine. Case reports and limited studies indicate that pregnancy can increase the risk for serious medical complications of influenza. One study found that out of every 10,000 women in their third trimester of pregnancy during an average flu season, 25 will be hospitalized for flu-related complications.

Additionally, influenza-associated excess deaths among pregnant women have been documented during influenza pandemics. Because pregnant women are at increased risk for influenza-related complications and because a substantial safety margin has been incorporated into the health guidance values for organic mercury exposure, the benefits of thimerosal reduced influenza vaccine or thimerosal preservative-containing influenza vaccine outweighs the theoretical risk, if any, of thimerosal.

Thimerosal Content in Other Vaccines and Biological Products Given to Infants, Children, and Pregnant Women

The FDA is in discussions with manufacturers of influenza vaccine regarding their capacity to further increase the supply of preservative-free formulations. Of note, all hepatitis B vaccines for the United States, including for adults, are now available only as thimerosal-free or thimerosal reduced containing formulations.

Tetanus and Diphtheria toxoids (Td) which are indicated for children 7 years of age or older and adults, is now also available in thimerosal-free formulations. In addition, all vaccines licensed since 1999 with the exception of inactivated influenza vaccine have not contained thimerosal as a preservative. Also, all immune globulin preparations including hepatitis B immune globulin and Rho(D) immune globulin preparations are manufactured without thimerosal.

Section 12.3

Baby Teeth Link Autism and Heavy Metals

This section includes text excerpted from "Baby Teeth Link Autism and Heavy Metals, NIH Study Suggests," National Institute of Environmental Health Sciences (NIEHS), June 1, 2017.

Baby teeth from children with autism contain more toxic lead and less of the essential nutrients zinc and manganese, compared to teeth from children without autism, according to an innovative study funded by the National Institute of Environmental Health Sciences (NIEHS), part of the National Institutes of Health (NIH). The researchers studied twins to control genetic influences and focus on possible environmental contributors to the disease. The findings, published in the journal *Nature Communications*, suggest that differences in early-life

145

exposure to metals, or more importantly how a child's body processes them, may affect the risk of autism.

The differences in metal uptake between children with and without autism were especially notable during the months just before and after the children were born. The scientists determined this by using lasers to map the growth rings in baby teeth generated during different developmental periods.

The researchers observed higher levels of lead in children with autism throughout development, with the greatest disparity, observed during the period following birth. They also observed lower uptake of manganese in children with autism, both before and after birth. The pattern was more complex for zinc. Children with autism had lower zinc levels earlier in the womb, but these levels then increased after birth, compared to children without autism.

The researchers note that replication in larger studies is needed to confirm the connection between metal uptake and autism.

"We think autism begins very early, most likely in the womb, and research suggests that our environment can increase a child's risk. But by the time children are diagnosed at age 3–4, it's hard to go back and know what the moms were exposed to," said Cindy Lawler, Ph.D., head of the NIEHS Genes, Environment, and Health Branch (GEH). "With baby teeth, we can actually do that."

Patterns of metal uptake were compared using teeth from 32 pairs of twins and 12 individual twins. The researchers compared patterns in twins where only one had autism, as well as in twins where both or neither had autism. Smaller differences in the patterns of metal uptake occurred when both twins had autism. Larger differences occurred in twins where only one sibling had autism.

The findings build on prior research showing that exposure to toxic metals, such as lead, and deficiencies of essential nutrients, like manganese, may harm brain development while in the womb or during early childhood. Although manganese is an essential nutrient, it can also be toxic at high doses. Exposure to both lead and high levels of manganese has been associated with autism traits and severity.

The study was led by Manish Arora, Ph.D., an environmental scientist and dentist at the Icahn School of Medicine at Mount Sinai in New York. With support from NIEHS, Arora and colleagues had previously developed a method that used naturally shed baby teeth to measure children's exposure to lead and other metals while in the womb and during early childhood. The researchers use lasers to extract precise layers of dentine, the hard substance beneath tooth enamel, for metal analysis. The team previously showed that the amount of

146

lead in different layers of dentine corresponds to lead exposure during different developmental periods.

Arora said that autism is a condition where both genes and environment play a role, but figuring out which environmental exposures may increase risk has been difficult.

"What is needed is a window into our fetal life," he said. "Unlike genes, our environment is constantly changing, and our body's response to environmental stressors not only depends on just how much we were exposed to but at what age we experienced that exposure."

Prior studies relating toxic metals and essential nutrients to autism have faced key limitations, such as estimating exposure based on blood levels after autism diagnosis rather than before, or not being able to control for differences that could be due to genetic factors.

"A lot of studies have compared current lead levels in kids that are already diagnosed," said Lawler. "Being able to measure something the children were exposed to long before the diagnosis is a major advantage."

The method of using baby teeth to measure past exposure to metals also holds promise for other disorders, such as attention deficit hyperactivity disorder (ADHD). "There is growing excitement about the potential of baby teeth as a rich record of a child's early life exposure to both helpful and harmful factors in the environment," said David Balshaw, Ph.D., head of the NIEHS Exposure, Response, and Technology Branch (ERTB), which supported the development of the tooth method.

Part Three

Outdoor Environmental Hazards: Air, Water, and Soil

Chapter 13

Air Pollution

Chapter Contents

Section 13.1

Ozone (Smog)

This section includes text excerpted from "Air Quality Guide for Ozone," AirNow, U.S. Environmental Protection Agency (EPA), August 3, 2016.

Ozone is a colorless gas that can be good or bad, depending on where it is. Ozone in the stratosphere is good because it shields the earth from the sun's ultraviolet rays. Ozone at ground level, where we breathe, is bad because it can harm human health.

Ozone forms when two types of pollutants volatile organic compounds (VOCs) and oxides of nitrogen (NO_x) react in sunlight. These pollutants come from sources such as vehicles, industries, power plants, and products such as solvents and paints.

Table 13.1. Air Quality Guide for Ozone

Air Quality Index (0–500)	Who Needs to Be Concerned?	What Should I Do?
Good (0–50)	It's a great day to be active outside.	
Moderate (51–100)	Some people who may be unusually sensitive to ozone.	Unusually sensitive people: Consider reducing prolonged or heavy outdoor exertion. Watch for symptoms such as coughing or shortness of breath. These are signs to take it a little easier. Everyone else: It's a good day to be active outside.
Unhealthy for Sensitive Groups (101–150)	Sensitive groups include people with lung disease such as asthma, older adults, children and teenagers, and people who are active outdoors.	Sensitive groups: Reduce prolonged or heavy outdoor exertion. Take more breaks, do less intense activities. Watch for symptoms such as coughing or shortness of breath. Schedule outdoor activities in the morning when ozone is lower.

Table 13.1. Continued

Air Quality Index (0–500)	Who Needs to Be Concerned?	What Should I Do?
		People with asthma should follow their asthma action plans and keep quick-relief medicine handy.
Unhealthy (151–200)	Everyone	Sensitive groups: Avoid prolonged or heavy outdoor exertion. Schedule outdoor activities in the morning when ozone is lower. Consider moving activities indoors. People with asthma, keep quick-relief medicine handy.

Everyone else: Reduce prolonged or heavy outdoor exertion. Take more breaks, do less intense activities. Schedule outdoor activities in the morning when ozone is lower. |
| Very Unhealthy (201–300) | Everyone | Sensitive groups: Avoid all physical activity outdoors. Move activities indoors or reschedule to a time when air quality is better. People with asthma, keep quick-relief medicine handy.

Everyone else: Avoid prolonged or heavy outdoor exertion. Schedule outdoor activities in the morning when ozone is lower. Consider moving activities indoors. |
| Hazardous (301–500) | Everyone | Avoid all physical activity outdoors. |

Note. *If you don't have an air conditioner, staying inside with the windows closed may be dangerous in extremely hot weather. In these cases, seek alternative shelter.*

Ozone Can Be a Problem

Ozone can cause a number of health problems, including coughing, breathing difficulty, and lung damage. Exposure to ozone can make the lungs more susceptible to infection, aggravate lung diseases, increase the frequency of asthma attacks, and increase the risk of early death from heart or lung disease.

Even healthy adults can experience ozone's harmful effects, but some people may be at greater risk. They include:

- People with lung disease such as asthma

- Children, including teenagers, because their lungs are still developing and they breathe more air per pound of body weight than adults

- Older adults

- People who are active outdoors, including outdoor workers

Steps to Protect Yourself

Use the Air Quality Index (AQI) to plan outdoor activities. To keep the AQI handy, sign up for EnviroFlash emails, get the free AirNow app, or install the free widget. Find all of these tools at www.airnow. gov.

Stay healthy. Exercise, eat a balanced diet and keep asthma under control with your asthma action plan. When you see that the AQI is unhealthy, take simple steps to reduce your exposure:

- Choose a less strenuous activity

- Take more breaks during outdoor activity

- Reschedule activities in the morning or to another day

- Move your activity inside where ozone levels are usually lower

Can I Help Reduce Ozone?

Yes! Here are a few tips.

- Turn off lights you are not using.

- Drive less—carpool, use public transportation, bike or walk.

- Keep your engine tuned, and don't let your engine idle.

- When refueling—stop when the pump shuts off, avoid spilling fuel, and tighten your gas cap.

- Inflate tires to the recommended pressure.

- Use low VOC paint and cleaning products, and seal and store them so they can't evaporate.

- Watch for Air Quality Action Days in your area.

Section 13.2

Particle Pollution

This section includes text excerpted from "Particle Pollution and Your Patients' Health—What Is Particle Pollution?" U.S. Environmental Protection Agency (EPA), August 14, 2017.

Particle pollution, also known as particulate matter or PM, is a general term for a mixture of solid and liquid droplets suspended in the air. Particle pollution comes in many sizes and shapes and can be made up of a number of different components, including acids (such as sulfuric acid), inorganic compounds (such as ammonium sulfate $((NH_4)_2SO_4)$, ammonium nitrate (NH_4NO_3), and sodium chloride (NaCl)), organic chemicals, soot, metals, soil or dust particles, and biological materials (such as pollen and mold spores).

The air we breathe indoors and outdoors always contains particle pollution. Some particles, such as dust, dirt, soot, or smoke, are large enough to be seen with the naked eye. Others are so small they can only be detected using an electron microscope.

The diameter of both fine and coarse particle pollution is smaller than the diameter of a human hair. Particles that are 10 micrometers (μm) in diameter or smaller pose the greatest problems. These smaller particles generally pass through the nose and throat and enter the lungs. Once inhaled, these particles can affect the lungs and heart and cause serious health effects in individuals at greatest risk, such as people with heart or lung disease, people with diabetes, older adults and children (up to 18 years of age). Larger particles (>10 μm) are generally of less concern because they usually do not enter the lungs, although they can still irritate the eyes, nose, and throat.

Particles of concern can be grouped into two main categories:

- **Coarse particles** (also known as PM10-2.5): particles with diameters generally larger than 2.5 μm and smaller than, or equal to, 10 μm in diameter. Note that the term **large coarse particles** in this course refer to particles greater than 10 μm in diameter.

155

- **Fine particles** (also known as PM2.5): particles generally 2.5 μm in diameter or smaller. This group of particles also encompasses **ultrafine** and **nanoparticles** which are generally classified as having diameters less than 0.1 μm.

Note that PM10 is a term that encompasses coarse, fine and ultrafine particle fractions.

Fine and coarse particles differ by their sources, composition, dosimetry (deposition and retention in the respiratory system), and health effects as observed in scientific studies. Though it is often hypothesized that specific components or sources may be responsible for particle pollution-related mortality and morbidity, the available evidence is not sufficient to allow differentiation of those components or sources that are more closely related to specific health outcomes. Rather, the overall evidence indicates that many particle pollution components can be linked with such effects. This course will mainly focus on the health effects of fine particles because the scientific evidence of health effects is much stronger than for other size fractions.

Source of Particle Pollution

Some particles, known as primary particles, are emitted directly from a source, such as construction sites, unpaved roads, smokestacks or fires. Other particles, known as secondary particles, form in complicated atmospheric reactions involving chemicals such as sulfur dioxides and nitrogen oxides that are emitted from power plants, industries, and automobiles. Secondary particles make up most of the fine particle pollution in the United States.

Cooking, smoking, dusting, and vacuuming can also produce particle pollution, particularly in indoor settings. Particles produced by combustion are more likely to be fine particles, while particles of crustal (earth) and biological origin are more likely to be coarse particles.

The Problem of Particle Pollution

Particle pollution is found everywhere—not just in haze, smoke, and dust, but also in the air that looks clean. Particle pollution can occur year-round and presents air quality problems at concentrations found in many major cities throughout the United States.

Some particles can remain in the atmosphere for days to weeks. Consequently, particle pollution generated in one area can travel hundreds or thousands of miles and influence the air quality of regions far from the original source.

Particle pollution levels can be especially high in the following circumstances:

- Near busy roads, in urban areas (especially during rush hour), and in industrial areas

- When there is smoke in the air from wood stoves, fireplaces, campfires, or wildfires

- When the weather is calm, allowing air pollution to build up. For example, hot humid days with stagnant air have much higher particle concentrations than days with air partially "scrubbed" by rain or snow.

Because of their small size, fine particles outdoors can penetrate into homes and buildings. Therefore, high outdoor particle pollution levels can elevate indoor particle pollution concentrations. Fine particle pollution often has a seasonal pattern. Fine particle concentrations in the eastern half of the United States are typically higher from July through September, when sulfates are more readily formed from sulfur dioxide (SO_2) emissions from power plants in that region and contribute to the formation of fine particles.

Fine particle concentrations tend to be higher from October through December in many areas of the West, in part because fine particle nitrates are more readily formed in cooler weather and due to the wood stove and fireplace use. In some locations, such as mountainous areas where wood is burned for heat, particle pollution levels can be especially high during wintertime inversions. An inversion traps the smoke close to the ground, allowing particle pollution levels to increase before the inversion lifts.

Section 13.3

Acid Rain

This section includes text excerpted from "What Is Acid Rain?" U.S. Environmental Protection Agency (EPA), March 7, 2017.

Acid rain, or acid deposition, is a broad term that includes any form of precipitation with acidic components, such as sulfuric or nitric acid that fall to the ground from the atmosphere in wet or dry forms. This can include rain, snow, fog, hail or even dust that is acidic.

Causes of Acid Rain

Acid rain results when sulfur dioxide (SO_2) and nitrogen oxides (NO_X) are emitted into the atmosphere and transported by wind and air currents. The SO_2 and NO_X react with water, oxygen and other chemicals to form sulfuric and nitric acids. These then mix with water and other materials before falling to the ground.

While a small portion of the SO_2 and NO_X that cause acid rain is from natural sources such as volcanoes, most of it comes from the burning of fossil fuels. The major sources of SO_2 and NO_X in the atmosphere are:

- Burning of fossil fuels to generate electricity. Two-thirds of SO_2 and one-fourth of NO_X in the atmosphere come from electric power generators.

- Vehicles and heavy equipment

- Manufacturing, oil refineries, and other industries

- Winds can blow SO_2 and NO_X over long distances and across borders making acid rain a problem for everyone and not just those who live close to these sources

Forms of Acid Deposition

Wet Deposition

Wet deposition is what we most commonly think of as acid rain. The sulfuric and nitric acids formed in the atmosphere fall to the ground mixed with rain, snow, fog, or hail.

Dry Deposition

Acidic particles and gases can also deposit from the atmosphere in the absence of moisture as dry deposition. The acidic particles and gases may deposit to surfaces (water bodies, vegetation, buildings) quickly or may react during atmospheric transport to form larger particles that can be harmful to human health. When the accumulated acids are washed off a surface by the next rain, this acidic water flows over and through the ground, and can harm plants and wildlife, such as insects and fish.

The amount of acidity in the atmosphere that deposits to earth through dry deposition depends on the amount of rainfall an area receives. For example, in a desert area, the ratio of dry to wet deposition is higher than an area that receives several inches of rain each year.

Measuring Acid Rain

Acidity and alkalinity are measured using a potential of hydrogen (pH) scale for which 7.0 is neutral. The lower a substance's pH (less than 7), the more acidic it is; the higher a substance's pH (greater than 7), the more alkaline it is. Normal rain has a pH of about 5.6; it is slightly acidic because carbon dioxide (CO_2) dissolves into it forming weak carbonic acid. Acid rain usually has a pH between 4.2–4.4.

Policymakers, research scientists, ecologists, and modelers rely on the National Atmospheric Deposition Program (NADP) National Trends Network (NTN) for measurements of wet deposition. The NADP/NTN collects acid rain at more than 250 monitoring sites throughout the United States, Canada, Alaska, Hawaii, and the U.S. Virgin Islands. Unlike wet deposition, dry deposition is difficult and expensive to measure. Dry deposition estimates for nitrogen and sulfur pollutants are provided by the Clean Air Status and Trends Network (CASTNET). Air concentrations are measured by CASTNET at more than 90 locations.

When acid deposition is washed into lakes and streams, it can cause some to turn acidic. The Long-Term Monitoring (LTM) Network measures and monitors surface water chemistry at over 280 sites to provide valuable information on aquatic ecosystem health and how water bodies respond to changes in acid causing emissions and acid deposition.

Effects of Acid Rain

The Effects of Acid Rain on Ecosystems

An ecosystem is a community of plants, animals and other organisms along with their environment including the air, water, and soil. Everything in an ecosystem is connected. If something harms one part of an ecosystem—one species of plant or animal, the soil or the water—it can have an impact on everything else.

Effects of Acid Rain on Fish and Wildlife

The ecological effects of acid rain are most clearly seen in aquatic environments, such as streams, lakes, and marshes where it can be harmful to fish and other wildlife. As it flows through the soil, acidic rainwater can leach aluminum from soil clay particles and then flow into streams and lakes. The more acid that is introduced into the ecosystem, the more aluminum is released.

Some types of plants and animals are able to tolerate acidic waters and moderate amounts of aluminum. Others, however, are acid sensitive and will be lost as the pH declines. Generally, the young of most species are more sensitive to environmental conditions than adults. At pH 5, most fish eggs cannot hatch. At lower pH levels, some adult fish die. Some acidic lakes have no fish. Even if a species of fish or animal can tolerate moderately acidic water, the animals or plants it eats might not. For example, frogs have a critical pH around 4, but the mayflies they eat are more sensitive and may not survive pH below 5.5.

Effects of Acid Rain on Plants and Trees

Dead or dying trees are a common sight in areas affected by acid rain. Acid rain leaches aluminum from the soil. That aluminum may be harmful to plants as well as animals. Acid rain also removes minerals and nutrients from the soil that trees need to grow.

At high elevations, acidic fog and clouds might strip nutrients from trees' foliage, leaving them with brown or dead leaves and needles. The trees are then less able to absorb sunlight, which makes them weak and less able to withstand freezing temperatures.

Buffering Capacity

Many forests, streams, and lakes that experience acid rain doesn't suffer effects because the soil in those areas can buffer the acid rain by neutralizing the acidity in the rainwater flowing through it. This capacity depends on the thickness and composition of the soil and the type of bedrock underneath it. In areas such as mountainous parts of the Northeast United States, the soil is thin and lacks the ability to adequately neutralize the acid in the rainwater. As a result, these areas are particularly vulnerable and the acid and aluminum can accumulate in the soil, streams, or lakes.

Episodic Acidification

Melting snow and heavy rain downpours can result in what is known as episodic acidification. Lakes that do not normally have a high level of acidity may temporarily experience effects of acid rain when the melting snow or downpour brings greater amounts of acidic deposition and the soil can't buffer it. This short duration of higher acidity (i.e., lower pH) can result in a short-term stress on the ecosystem where a variety of organisms or species may be injured or killed.

Nitrogen Pollution

It's not just the acidity of acid rain that can cause problems. Acid rain also contains nitrogen, and this can have an impact on some ecosystems. For example, nitrogen pollution in our coastal waters is partially responsible for declining fish and shellfish populations in some areas. In addition to agriculture and wastewater, much of the nitrogen produced by human activity that reaches coastal waters comes from the atmosphere.

Effects of Acid Rain on Materials

Not all acidic deposition is wet. Sometimes dust particles can become acidic as well, and this is called dry deposition. When acid rain and dry acidic particles fall to earth, the nitric and sulfuric acid that makes the particles acidic can land on statues, buildings, and other manmade structures, and damage their surfaces. The acidic particles corrode metal and cause paint and stone to deteriorate more quickly. They also dirty the surfaces of buildings and other structures such as monuments.

The consequences of this damage can be costly:

- damaged materials that need to be repaired or replaced

- increased maintenance costs

- loss of detail on stone and metal statues, monuments, and tombstones

Other Effects of SO_2 and NO_X

Visibility

In the atmosphere, SO_2 and NO_X gases can be transformed into sulfate and nitrate particles, while some NO_X can also react with other pollutants to form ozone. These particles and ozone make the air hazy and difficult to see through. This affects our enjoyment of national parks that we visit for the scenic view such as Shenandoah and the Great Smoky Mountains.

Human Health

Walking in the acid rain, or even swimming in a lake affected by acid rain, is no more dangerous to humans than walking in the normal rain or swimming in nonacidic lakes. However, when the pollutants that cause acid rain—SO_2 and NO_X, as well as sulfate and nitrate particles—are in the air, they can be harmful to humans.

SO_2 and NO_X react in the atmosphere to form fine sulfate and nitrate particles that people can inhale into their lungs. Many scientific studies have shown a relationship between these particles and effects on heart function, such as heart attacks resulting in death for people with increased heart disease risk, and effects on lung function, such as breathing difficulties for people with asthma.

Chapter 14

Climate Change and Extreme Heat

Chapter Contents

Section 14.1

Climate Change: Overview

This section includes text excerpted from "Climate
Change Science—Overview of Climate Change Science,"
U.S. Environmental Protection Agency (EPA), September 29, 2016.

Earth's climate is changing. Multiple lines of evidence show changes in our weather, oceans, ecosystems, and more. Natural causes alone cannot explain all of these changes. Human activities are contributing to climate change, primarily by releasing billions of tons of carbon dioxide (CO_2) and other heat-trapping gases, known as greenhouse gases, into the atmosphere every year.

Climate changes will continue into the future. The more greenhouse gases we emit, the larger future climate changes will be. Changes in the climate system affect our health, environment, and economy. We can prepare for some of the impacts of climate change to reduce their effects on our well-being.

Earth's Climate Is Changing

The global average temperature has increased by more than 1.5°F since the late 1800s. Some regions of the world have warmed by more than twice this amount. The buildup of greenhouse gases in our atmosphere and the warming of the planet are responsible for other changes, such as:

- Changing temperature and precipitation patterns

- Increases in ocean temperatures, sea level, and acidity

- Melting of glaciers and sea ice

- Changes in the frequency, intensity, and duration of extreme weather events

- Shifts in ecosystem characteristics, like the length of the growing season, the timing of flower blooms, and migration of birds

- Increasing effects on human health and well-being

Climate Change versus Global Warming

The term "climate change" is sometimes used interchangeably with the term "global warming." However, the terms do not refer entirely to the same thing.

Global warming refers to the ongoing rise in global average temperature near Earth's surface. It is caused mostly by increasing concentrations of greenhouse gases in the atmosphere. Global warming is causing climate patterns to change. However, global warming itself represents only one aspect of climate change.

Climate change refers to any significant change in the measures of climate lasting for an extended period of time. In other words, climate change includes major changes in temperature, precipitation, or wind patterns, among others, that occur over several decades or longer. Climate change can occur at the global, continental, regional, and local levels. Climate change may refer to natural changes in climate or changes caused by human activities.

Weather versus Climate

The difference between weather and climate is primarily a matter of time and geography. Weather refers to the conditions of the atmosphere over a short period of time, such as hours or days, and typically for a local area. Climate refers to the behavior of the atmosphere over a longer period of time, and usually for a large area.

Familiar examples of weather characteristics include the daily temperature, humidity, or the amount of precipitation produced by a storm. Weather also includes severe weather conditions such as hurricanes, tornadoes, and blizzards. Because of the dynamic nature of the atmosphere, it is not possible to predict weather conditions in specific location months or years in advance.

Climate is typically defined based on 30-year averages of weather. Climate represents our expectations for the weather. For example, climate tells us how warm we expect a typical summer to be, how much rainfall would correspond to a wetter-than-average spring, or how frequently we expect a snowy winter to occur. Scientists can compare long-term observations of the climate to detect the influence of greenhouse gases on climate conditions.

Natural Causes Alone Cannot Explain Climate Changes

Natural processes such as changes in the sun's energy, shifts in ocean currents, and others affect Earth's climate. However, they do not explain the warming that we have observed over the last half-century.

Human Causes Can Explain These Changes

Most of the warming of the past half-century has been caused by human emissions of greenhouse gases. Greenhouse gases come from a variety of human activities, including burning fossil fuels for heat and energy, clearing forests, fertilizing crops, storing waste in landfills, raising livestock, and producing some kinds of industrial products.

Greenhouse gas emissions are not the only way that people can change the climate. Activities such as agriculture or road construction can change the reflectivity of Earth's surface, leading to local warming or cooling. This effect is observed in urban centers, which are often warmer than surrounding, less populated areas. Emissions of small particles, known as aerosols, into the air can also lead to reflection or absorption of the sun's energy.

The Extent of Future Climate Change Depends on Us

The extent of the change will depend on how much, and how quickly, we can reduce greenhouse gas emissions. During the 21st century, global warming is projected to continue and climate changes are likely to intensify. Scientists have used climate models to project different aspects of future climate, including temperature, precipitation, snow and ice, ocean level, and ocean acidity. Depending on future emissions of greenhouse gases and how the climate responds, average global temperatures are projected to increase worldwide by 0.5–8.6°F by 2100, with a likely increase of at least 2.0°F for all scenarios except the one representing the most aggressive mitigation of greenhouse gas emissions.

Climate Change Impacts Our Health, Environment, and Economy

Climate change affects our environment and natural resources and impacts our way of life in many ways. For example:

- Warmer temperatures increase the frequency, intensity, and duration of heat waves, which can pose health risks, particularly for young children and the elderly

166

- Climate change can also impact human health by worsening air and water quality, increasing the spread of certain diseases, and altering the frequency or intensity of extreme weather events

- Rising sea levels threaten coastal communities and ecosystems

- Changes in the patterns and amount of rainfall, as well as changes in the timing and amount of streamflow, can affect water supplies and water quality and the production of hydroelectricity

- Changing ecosystems influence geographic ranges of many plants and animal species and the timing of their lifecycle events, such as migration and reproduction

- Increases in the frequency and intensity of extreme weather events, such as heat waves, droughts, and floods, can increase losses to property, cause costly disruptions to society, and reduce the availability and affordability of insurance

We can prepare for some of the likely climate change impacts to reduce their effect on ecosystems and human well-being. Making such preparations is known as adaptation. Examples of adaptation include strengthening water conservation programs, upgrading stormwater systems, developing early warning systems for extreme heat events, and preparing for stronger storms through better emergency preparation and response strategies.

Section 14.2

Extreme Heat and Its Implications

This section includes text excerpted from "Natural Disasters and Severe Weather—About Extreme Heat," Centers for Disease Control and Prevention (CDC), June 19, 2017.

What Is Extreme Heat?

Extreme heat is defined as summertime temperatures that are much hotter and/or humid than average. Because some places are hotter than others, this depends on what's considered average for a particular location at that time of year. Humid and muggy conditions can make it seem hotter than it really is.

Causes of Heat-Related Illness

Heat-related illnesses, like heat exhaustion or heat stroke, happen when the body is not able to properly cool itself. While the body normally cools itself by sweating, during extreme heat, this might not be enough. In these cases, a person's body temperature rises faster than it can cool itself down. This can cause damage to the brain and other vital organs.

Some factors that might increase your risk of developing a heat-related illness include:

- High levels of humidity
- Obesity
- Fever
- Dehydration

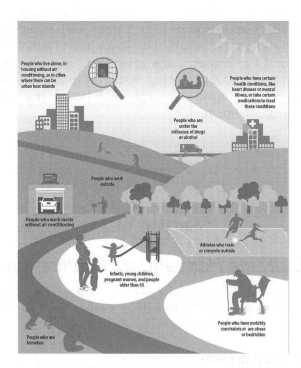

Figure 14.1. *Extreme Heat: Who's at Risk?* (Source: "Climate Change and Extreme Heat: What You Can Do to Prepare," U.S. Environmental Protection Agency (EPA).)

* Prescription drug use
* Heart disease
* Mental illness

* Poor circulation
* Sunburn
* Alcohol use

Who Is Most at Risk?

Older adults, the very young, and people with mental illness and chronic diseases are at highest risk. However, even young and healthy people can be affected if they participate in strenuous physical activities during hot weather.

Summertime activity, whether on the playing field or the construction site, must be balanced with actions that help the body cool itself to prevent heat-related illness.

Warning Signs and Symptoms of Heat-Related Illness

Heat Stroke

What to look for:

* High body temperature (103°F or higher)

* Hot, red, dry, or damp skin

* Fast, strong pulse

* A headache

* Dizziness

* Nausea

* Confusion

* Losing consciousness (passing out)

What to do:

* Call 911 right away-heat stroke is a medical emergency

* Move the person to a cooler place

* Help lower the person's temperature with cool cloths or a cool bath

* Do not give the person anything to drink

Heat Exhaustion

What to look for:

- Heavy sweating
- Cold, pale, and clammy skin
- Fast, weak pulse
- Nausea or vomiting
- Muscle cramps
- Tiredness or weakness
- Dizziness
- A headache
- Fainting (passing out)

What to do:

- Move to a cool place
- Loosen your clothes
- Put cool, wet cloths on your body or take a cool bath
- Sip water

Get medical help right away if:

- You are throwing up
- Your symptoms get worse
- Your symptoms last longer than 1 hour

Heat Cramps

What to look for:

- Heavy sweating during intense exercise
- Muscle pain or spasms

What to do:

- Stop physical activity and move to a cool place
- Drink water or a sports drink
- Wait for cramps to go away before you do any more physical activity

Get medical help right away if:

- Cramps last longer than 1 hour
- You're on a low-sodium diet
- You have heart problems

Sunburn

What to look for:

- Painful, red, and warm skin
- Blisters on the skin

What to do:

- Stay out of the sun until your sunburn heals
- Put cool cloths on sunburned areas or take a cool bath
- Put moisturizing lotion on sunburned areas
- Do not break blisters

Heat Rash

What to look for:

- Red clusters of small blisters that look like pimples on the skin (usually on the neck, chest, groin, or in elbow creases)

What to do:

- Stay in a cool, dry place
- Keep the rash dry
- Use powder (like baby powder) to soothe the rash

Tips for Preventing Heat-Related Illness

Stay Cool

Wear appropriate clothing. Choose lightweight, light-colored, and loose-fitting clothing.

Stay cool indoors. Stay in an air-conditioned place as much as possible. If your home does not have air conditioning, go to the shopping mall or public library—even a few hours spent in air conditioning can help your body stay cooler when you go back into the heat. Call your local health department to see if there are any heat-relief shelters in your area.

- **Keep in mind.** Electric fans may provide comfort, but when the temperature is in the high 90s, they will not prevent heat-related illness. Taking a cool shower or bath or moving to an air-conditioned place is a much better way to cool off. Use your stove and oven less to maintain a cooler temperature in your home.

Schedule outdoor activities carefully. Try to limit your outdoor activity to when it's coolest, like morning and evening hours. Rest often in shady areas so that your body has a chance to recover.

Pace yourself. Cut down on exercise during the heat. If you're not accustomed to working or exercising in a hot environment, start slowly and pick up the pace gradually. If exertion in the heat makes your heart pound and leaves you gasping for breath, STOP all activity. Get into a cool area or into the shade, and rest, especially if you become lightheaded, confused, weak, or faint.

Wear sunscreen. Sunburn affects your body's ability to cool down and can make you dehydrated. If you must go outdoors, protect yourself from the sun by wearing a wide-brimmed hat, sunglasses, and by putting on sunscreen of sun protection factor (SPF) 15 or higher 30 minutes prior to going out. Continue to reapply it according to the package directions.

- **Tip.** Look for sunscreens that say "broad spectrum" or "ultraviolet A (UVA)/ultraviolet B (UVB) protection" on their labels these products work best.

Do not leave children in cars. Cars can quickly heat up to dangerous temperatures, even with a window cracked open. While anyone left in a parked car is at risk, children are especially at risk of getting a heat stroke or dying. When traveling with children, remember to do the following:

- Never leave infants, children or pets in a parked car, even if the windows are cracked open.

- To remind yourself that a child is in the car, keep a stuffed animal in the car seat. When the child is buckled in, place the stuffed animal in the front with the driver.

- When leaving your car, check to be sure everyone is out of the car. Do not overlook any children who have fallen asleep in the car.

Avoid hot and heavy meals. They add heat to your body!

Stay Hydrated

Drink plenty of fluids. Drink more fluids, regardless of how active you are. Don't wait until you're thirsty to drink.

- **Warning.** If your doctor limits the amount you drink or has you on water pills, ask how much you should drink while the weather is hot.

- **Stay away from very sugary or alcoholic drinks.** These actually cause you to lose more body fluid. Also avoid very cold drinks, because they can cause stomach cramps.

- **Replace salt and minerals.** Heavy sweating removes salt and minerals from the body that need to be replaced. A sports drink can replace the salt and minerals you lose in sweat.

  - If you are on a low-salt diet, have diabetes, high blood pressure, or other chronic conditions, talk with your doctor before drinking a sports beverage or taking salt tablets.

- **Keep your pets hydrated.** Provide plenty of fresh water for your pets, and leave the water in a shady area.

Stay Informed

Check for updates. Check your local news for extreme heat alerts and safety tips and to learn about any cooling shelters in your area.

Know the signs. Learn the signs and symptoms of heat-related illnesses and how to treat them.

Use a buddy system. When working in the heat, monitor the condition of your co-workers and have someone do the same for you. Heat-induced illness can cause a person to become confused or lose consciousness. If you are 65 years of age or older, have a friend or relative call to check on you twice a day during a heat wave. If you know someone in this age group, check on them at least twice a day.

Monitor those at high risk. Although anyone at any time can suffer from heat-related illness, some people are at greater risk than others:

- Infants and young children

- People 65 years of age or older

- People who are overweight

- People who overexert during work or exercise

- People who are physically ill, especially with heart disease or high blood pressure, or who take certain medications, such as for depression, insomnia, or poor circulation

Visit adults at risk at least twice a day and closely watch them for signs of heat exhaustion or heat stroke. Infants and young children, of course, need much more frequent watching.

Chapter 15

Noise Pollution

Hearing Loss: A Chronic Health Condition

Hearing loss is the third most common chronic health condition in the United States. Almost twice as many people report hearing loss as report diabetes or cancer. Noise exposure away from your job can damage your hearing just as much as working in a noisy place. Being around too much loud noise—like using a leaf blower or going to loud concerts—can cause permanent hearing loss. And once it's gone, you can't get it back! You can have hearing loss before you even notice you're having problems. Noise is measured in what are called decibels (dB). Over time, listening to loud sounds at high dB levels can cause hearing loss—or other hearing problems like a ringing sound in your ear that won't go away. The louder a sound is, and the longer you are exposed to it, the more likely it will damage your hearing. The more often you are exposed to loud sounds over time, the more damage occurs. It's important for healthcare providers to ask about hearing and to screen those who are at risk.

Facts at a Glance

- About 40 million U.S. adults aged 20–69 years have a noise-induced hearing loss.

This chapter includes text excerpted from "Too Loud! For Too Long!" Centers for Disease Control and Prevention (CDC), February 7, 2017.

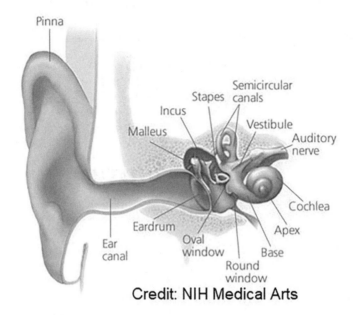

Credit: NIH Medical Arts

Figure 15.1. *Parts of the Inner Ear* (Source: "Noise-Induced Hearing Loss," National Institute on Deafness and Other Communication Disorders (NIDCD).)

- More than 1 in 2 U.S. adults with hearing damage from noise do not have noisy jobs.
- About 1 in 4 U.S. adults who report excellent to good hearing already have hearing damage.

Problem

Many people are exposed to noise that damages their hearing. Hearing gets worse over time the more often people are exposed to loud sounds.

- About 53 percent of people ages 20–69 who have hearing damage from noise report no on-the-job exposure.
- About 24 percent of people ages 20–69 who report having excellent hearing have measurable hearing damage.
- About 20 percent of adults with no job exposure to loud sounds have hearing damage.

Hearing loss often gets worse for years before anyone notices or diagnoses it.

• People may not know that activities away from work can damage hearing just as much as noise on the job.

• People delay reporting a hearing loss because they don't know or won't admit they have a problem.

• Less than half (46%) of adults who reported trouble hearing had seen a healthcare provider for their hearing in the past 5 years.

Hearing loss causes many problems.

• Continual exposure to noise can cause stress, anxiety, depression, high blood pressure, heart disease, and many other health problems.

• Some people are at higher risk for hearing loss, including those who:

    • are exposed to loud sounds at home and in the community

    • work in noisy environments (especially noise of 85 dB or more for 8 hours or longer)

    • take medicines that increase their risk

    • are male

    • are age 40 or older

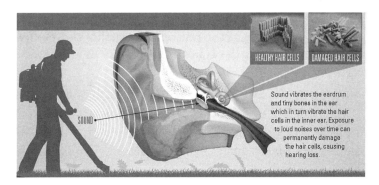

Figure 15.2. *How Noise Causes Permanent Damage*

Graphic showing the silhouette of a man using a blower on a yard. The sound of the blower is shown penetrating a big ear, going to the inner ear to the right of the man, and causing hearing loss. Images of healthy hair cells and damaged hair cells are shown to the right of the big ear.

How Hearing Loss Occurs

Common noises can be loud.

- 70 dB (decibels) washing machine
- 80 dB traffic noise inside a car
- 90 dB leaf blower 2 hours can cause damage
- 100 dB sporting event 14 minutes can cause damage
- 110 dB rock concert 2 minutes can cause damage
- 120 dB siren 1 minute can cause damage
- 85 dB is the approximate point at which extended exposure can cause hearing damage

How Noise Causes Permanent Hearing Damage

Sound vibrates the eardrum and tiny bones in the ear which in turn vibrate the hair cells in the inner ear. Exposure to loud noises over time can permanently damage the hair cells, causing hearing loss.

- Sound
- Healthy hair cells
- Damaged hair cells

How This Problem Is to Be Addressed

The federal government is:

- Monitoring the health of the nation and setting targets for improvement through the Healthy People 2020 hearing objectives
  - Raising public awareness about the health effects of noise-induced hearing loss and how to prevent it
  - Tracking hearing loss and establishing standards to protect hearing in places such as mines, factories, and airports
- Providing information to healthcare providers about effective counseling on the effects of noise exposure and correct use of hearing protection
- Supporting research on the extent of hearing the loss in America, contributing factors, and the most effective prevention strategies

Healthcare providers can:

- Ask patients about exposure to loud noise and trouble hearing, and examine hearing as part of routine care.
- Provide hearing tests when patients show or report hearing problems, or refer them to a hearing specialist.
- Explain how noise exposure can permanently damage hearing.
- Counsel patients on how to protect hearing.

Everyone can:

- Avoid noisy places whenever possible.
- Use earplugs, protective ear muffs, noise canceling headphones when near loud noises.
- Keep the volume down when watching television (TV), listening to music, and using earbuds or headphones.
- Ask your doctor for a hearing checkup and how to protect your hearing from noise.

Chapter 16

Ultraviolet (UV) Radiation

What Is Ultraviolet (UV) Radiation?

All radiation is a form of energy, most of which is invisible to the human eye. Ultraviolet (UV) radiation is only one form of radiation and it is measured on a scientific scale called the electromagnetic (EM) spectrum.

UV radiation is only one type of EM energy you may be familiar with. Radio waves that transmit sound from a radio station's tower to your stereo, or between cell phones; microwaves, like those that heat your food in a microwave oven; visible light that is emitted from the lights in your home; and X-rays like those used in hospital X-ray machines to capture images of the bones inside your body, are all forms of EM energy.

UV radiation is the portion of the EM spectrum between X-rays and visible light.

How Is Radiation Classified on the Electromagnetic Spectrum?

Electromagnetic radiation is all around us, though we can only see some of it. All EM radiation (also called EM energy) is made up of

This chapter contains text excerpted from the following sources: Text beginning with the heading "What Is Ultraviolet (UV) Radiation?" is excerpted from "Radiation-Emitting Products—Ultraviolet (UV) Radiation," U.S. Food and Drug Administration (FDA), December 12, 2017; Text under the heading "Health Effects of UV Radiation" is excerpted from "Health Effects of UV Radiation," U.S. Environmental Protection Agency (EPA), November 14, 2017.

minute packets of energy or 'particles,' called photons, which travel in a wave-like pattern and move at the speed of light. The EM spectrum is divided into categories defined by a range of numbers. These ranges describe the activity level, or how energetic the photons are, and the size of the wavelength in each category.

For example, at the bottom of the spectrum radio waves have photons with low energies, so their wavelengths are long with peaks that are far apart. The photons of microwaves have higher energies, followed by infrared (IR) waves, UV rays, and X-rays. At the top of the spectrum, gamma rays have photons with very high energies and short wavelengths with peaks that are close together.

What Are the Different Types of UV Radiation?

The most common form of UV radiation is sunlight, which produces three main types of UV rays:

- Ultraviolet A (UVA)
- Ultraviolet B (UVB)
- Ultraviolet C (UVC)

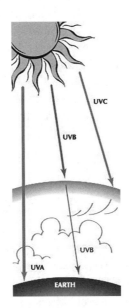

Figure 16.1. *Ultraviolet Radiation (Source: "UV Radiation," U.S. Environmental Protection Agency (EPA).)*

The stratospheric ozone layer screens out much of the sun's harmful UV rays.

(Source: "UV Radiation," U.S. Environmental Protection Agency (EPA).)

UVA rays have the longest wavelengths, followed by UVB, and UVC rays which have the shortest wavelengths. While UVA and UVB rays are transmitted through the atmosphere, all UVC and some UVB rays are absorbed by the Earth's ozone layer. So, most of the UV rays you come in contact with are UVA with a small amount of UVB.

Like all forms of light on the EM spectrum, UV radiation is classified by wavelength. Wavelength describes the distance between the peaks in a series of waves.

- UVB rays have a short wavelength that reaches the outer layer of your skin (the epidermis)

- UVA rays have a longer wavelength that can penetrate the middle layer of your skin (the dermis)

Health Effects of UV Radiation

Ozone layer depletion decreases our atmosphere's natural protection from the sun's harmful UV radiation. Understanding these risks and taking sensible precautions will help you enjoy the sun while reducing your chances of sun-related health problems.

Skin Cancer

Each year, more new cases of skin cancer are diagnosed in the United States than new cases of breast, prostate, lung, and colon cancer combined. One in five Americans will develop skin cancer in their lifetime. One American dies from skin cancer every hour. Unprotected exposure to UV radiation is the most preventable risk factor for skin cancer.

Melanoma

Melanoma, the most serious form of skin cancer, is now one of the most common cancers among adolescents and young adults ages 15–29. While melanoma accounts for about three percent of skin cancer cases, it causes more than 75 percent of skin cancer deaths. UV exposure and sunburns, particularly during childhood, are risk factors for the disease. Not all melanomas are exclusively sun related—other possible influences include genetic factors and immune system deficiencies.

Nonmelanoma Skin Cancers

Nonmelanoma skin cancers are less deadly than melanomas. Nevertheless, they can spread if left untreated, causing disfigurement and more serious health problems. There are two primary types of nonmelanoma skin cancers: basal cell and squamous cell carcinomas. If caught and treated early, these two cancers are rarely fatal.

1. **Basal cell carcinomas** are the most common type of skin cancer tumors. They usually appear as small, fleshy bumps or nodules on the head and neck, but can occur on other skin areas. Basal cell carcinoma grows slowly, and it rarely spreads to other parts of the body. It can, however, penetrate to the bone and cause considerable damage.

2. **Squamous cell carcinomas** are tumors that may appear as nodules or as red, scaly patches. This cancer can develop into large masses, and unlike basal cell carcinoma, it can spread to other parts of the body.

Premature Aging and Other Skin Damage

Other UV-related skin disorders include actinic keratoses and premature aging of the skin. Actinic keratoses are skin growths that occur in body areas exposed to the sun. The face, hands, forearms, and the "V" of the neck are especially susceptible to this type of lesion. Although premalignant, actinic keratoses are a risk factor for squamous cell carcinoma. Look for raised, reddish, rough-textured growths and seek prompt medical attention if you discover them.

Chronic exposure to the sun also causes premature aging, which over time can make the skin become thick, wrinkled, and leathery. Since it occurs gradually, often manifesting itself many years after the majority of a person's sun exposure, premature aging is often regarded as an unavoidable, normal part of growing older. However, up to 90 percent of the visible skin changes commonly attributed to aging are caused by the sun. With proper protection from UV radiation, most premature aging of the skin can be avoided.

Cataracts and Other Eye Damage

Cataracts are a form of eye damage in which a loss of transparency in the lens of the eye clouds vision. If left untreated, cataracts can lead to blindness. Research has shown that UV radiation increases the likelihood of certain cataracts. Although curable with modern eye surgery, cataracts diminish the eyesight of millions of Americans and cost billions of dollars in medical care each year.

Other kinds of eye damage include pterygium (tissue growth that can block vision), skin cancer around the eyes, and degeneration of the macula (the part of the retina where visual perception is most acute). All of these problems can be lessened with proper eye protection. Look for sunglasses, glasses or contact lenses if you wear them, that offer 99–100 percent UV protection.

Immune Suppression

Scientists have found that overexposure to UV radiation may suppress proper functioning of the body's immune system and the skin's natural defenses. For example, the skin normally mounts a defense against foreign invaders such as cancers and infections. But overexposure to UV radiation can weaken the immune system, reducing the skin's ability to protect against these invaders.

Chapter 17

Drinking Water

Chapter Contents

Section 17.1

Drinking Water Contaminants

This section includes text excerpted from "Drinking
Water Contaminants," U.S. Environmental Protection
Agency (EPA), October 2015.

Drinking water sources may contain a variety of contaminants that,
at elevated levels, have been associated with increased risk of a range
of diseases in children, including acute diseases such as gastrointestinal illness, developmental effects such as learning disorders, endocrine
disruption, and cancer. Because children tend to take in more water
relative to their body weight than adults do, children are likely to have
higher exposure to drinking water contaminants.

Drinking water sources include surface water, such as rivers, lakes,
and reservoirs; and groundwater aquifers, which are subsurface layers of porous soil and rock that contain large collections of water.
Groundwater and surface water are not isolated systems and are con-
tinually recharged by each other as well as by rain and other natural
precipitation.

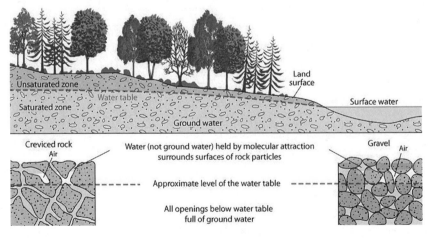

Figure 17.1. *Water Sources* (Source: "Public Water Systems—Water
Sources," Centers for Disease Control and Prevention (CDC).)

Drinking Water Safety Standards

The U.S. Environmental Protection Agency (EPA) and the U.S. Food and Drug Administration (FDA) are both responsible for the safety of drinking water. The FDA regulates bottled drinking water, while the EPA regulates drinking water provided by public water systems. EPA sets enforceable drinking water standards for public water systems, and unless otherwise specified, the term "drinking water" in this text refers to water provided by these systems. The drinking water standards include maximum contaminant levels and treatment technique requirements for more than 90 chemical, radiological, and microbial contaminants, designed to protect people, including sensitive populations such as children, against adverse health effects.

Drinking Water Contaminants and Concern for Children's Health

Several types of drinking water contaminants may be of concern for children's health. Examples include microorganisms, (e.g., *E. coli, Giardia*, and noroviruses), inorganic chemicals (e.g., lead, arsenic, nitrates, and nitrites), organic chemicals (e.g., atrazine, glyphosate, trichloroethylene, and tetrachloroethylene), and disinfection By-Products (e.g., chloroform).

Microbial contaminants, lead, nitrates, and nitrites, arsenic, disinfection by-products, pesticides, and solvents are among the contaminants for which the EPA has set health-based standards. Microbial contaminants include bacteria, viruses, and protozoa that may cause severe gastrointestinal illness. Children are particularly sensitive to microbial contaminants, such as *Giardia, Cryptosporidium, E. coli,* and noroviruses, because their immune systems are less developed than those of most adults.

Lead

Drinking water is a known source of lead exposure among children in the United States, particularly from corrosion of pipes and other elements of the drinking water distribution systems. Exposure to lead via drinking water may be particularly high among very young children who consume baby formula prepared with drinking water that is contaminated by leaching lead pipes. The National Toxicology Program (NTP) has concluded that childhood lead exposure is associated with the reduced cognitive function, reduced academic achievement, and increased attention-related behavioral problems.

Nitrates and Nitrites

Fertilizer, livestock manure, and human sewage can be significant contributors of nitrates and nitrites in groundwater sources of drinking water. High levels of nitrates and nitrites can cause the blood disorder methemoglobinemia (blue baby syndrome) and have been associated with thyroid dysfunction in children and pregnant women. Moderate deficits in maternal thyroid hormone levels during early pregnancy have been linked to reduced childhood intelligence quotient (IQ) scores and other neurodevelopmental effects, as well as unsuccessful or complicated pregnancies.

Arsenic

Arsenic enters drinking water sources from natural deposits in the earth, which vary widely from one region to another, or from agricultural and industrial sources where it is used as a wood preservative and a component of fertilizers, animal feed, and a variety of industrial products. Population studies of health effects associated with arsenic exposure have been conducted primarily in countries such as Bangladesh, Taiwan, and Chile, where arsenic levels in drinking water are generally much higher than in the United States due to high levels of naturally occurring arsenic in groundwater. Long-term consumption of arsenic-contaminated water has been associated with the development of skin conditions and circulatory system problems, as well as increased risk of cancer of the bladder, lungs, skin, kidney, nasal passages, liver, and prostate. In many cases, long-term exposure to arsenic begins during prenatal development or childhood, which increases the risk of mortality and morbidity among young adults exposed to arsenic long term. A review of the literature concluded that epidemiological studies of associations between exposure to arsenic and some adverse health outcomes pertinent to children's health have mixed findings. These include studies of associations between high levels of exposure to arsenic and abnormal pregnancy outcomes, such as spontaneous abortion, still-births, reduced birth weight, and infant mortality, as well as associations between early life exposure to arsenic and increased incidence of childhood cancer and reduced cognitive function.

Contamination of Water

Water can contain microorganisms such as parasites, viruses, and bacteria; the disinfection of drinking water to reduce waterborne infectious disease is one of the major public health advances of the 20th century. The method by which infectious agents are removed or chemically inactivated depends on the type and quality of the drinking water source and the volume of water to be treated. Surface water systems are more exposed than groundwater systems to weather and runoff; therefore, they may be more susceptible to contamination. Surface and groundwater systems use filtration and other treatment methods to physically remove particles.

Disinfectants

Disinfectants, such as chlorine and chloramine, ultraviolet radiation, and ozone are added to drinking water provided by public water systems to kill or neutralize microbial contaminants. However, this process can produce disinfection by-products, which form when chemical disinfectants react with naturally occurring organic matter in water. The most common of these disinfection by-products are chloroform ($CHCl_3$) and other trihalomethanes.

Consumption of drinking water from systems in the United States and other industrialized countries with relatively high levels of disinfection by-products has been associated with bladder cancer and developmental effects in some studies. Some individual epidemiological studies have reported associations between the presence of disinfection by-products in drinking water and increased risk of birth defects, especially neural tube defects and oral clefts; however, articles reviewing the body of literature determined that the evidence is too limited to make conclusions about a possible association between exposure to disinfection by-products and birth defects.

Pesticides

Some of the most widely used agricultural pesticides in the United States, such as atrazine, and glyphosate, are also drinking water contaminants. Pesticides can enter drinking water sources as runoff from crop production in agricultural areas and enter groundwater through abandoned wells on farms. Some epidemiological studies have reported associations between prenatal exposure to atrazine and reduced fetal growth.

Herbicides

The use of glyphosate, a herbicide used to kill weeds, has increased dramatically because of the growing popularity of crops genetically modified to survive glyphosate treatment. Previous safety assessments have concluded that glyphosate does not affect fertility or reproduction in laboratory animal studies. However, more studies in laboratory animals have found that male rats exposed to high levels of glyphosate, either during prenatal or pubertal development, may suffer from reproductive problems, such as delayed puberty, decreased sperm production, and decreased testosterone production. Very few epidemiological human studies have investigated effects of glyphosate exposure on reproductive endpoints. In contrast to the results of animal studies, one such epidemiological study of women living in regions with different levels of exposure to glyphosate found no associations between glyphosate exposure and delayed time to pregnancy.

Industrial Wastes

A variety of other chemical contaminants can enter the water supply after use in industry. Examples include trichloroethylene and tetrachloroethylene (also known as perchloroethylene), which are solvents widely used in industry as degreasers, dry cleaning agents, paint removers, chemical extractors, and components of adhesives and lubricants. Potential health concerns from exposure to trichloroethylene, based on limited epidemiological data and evidence from animal studies, include decreased fetal growth and birth defects, particularly cardiac birth defects. A study conducted in Massachusetts reported associations between birth defects and maternal exposure to drinking water contaminated with high levels of tetrachloroethylene around the time of conception. An additional study reported that older mothers or mothers who had previously miscarried, and who were exposed to high levels of tetrachloroethylene in contaminated drinking water, had a higher risk of delivering a baby with reduced birth weight. However, other studies did not find associations between maternal exposure to tetrachloroethylene and pregnancy loss, gestational age, or birth weight. Studies in laboratory animals indicate that mothers exposed to high levels of tetrachloroethylene can have a spontaneous abortion, and their fetuses can suffer from altered growth and birth defects.

Personal Care Products and Veterinary Medications

The EPA has not determined whether standards are necessary for some drinking water contaminants, such as personal care products. Personal care products, such as cosmetics, sunscreens, and fragrances; and pharmaceuticals, including prescription, over-the-counter (OTC), and veterinary medications, can enter water systems after use by humans or domestic animals and have been measured at very low levels in drinking water sources. Many concentrated animal feeding operations treat livestock with hormones and antibiotics, and can be one significant source of pharmaceuticals in water. Other major sources of pharmaceuticals in water are human waste, manufacturing plants, and hospitals, and other human activities such as showering and swimming. Any potential health implications of long-term exposure to levels of pharmaceuticals and personal care products found in drinking water are unclear.

Naturally Occurring Minerals

Manganese. Manganese is a naturally occurring mineral that can enter drinking water sources from rocks and soil or from human activities. While manganese is an essential nutrient at low doses, chronic exposure to high doses may be harmful, particularly to the nervous system. Many of the reports on adverse effects from manganese exposure are based on inhalation exposures in occupational settings. Fewer studies have examined health effects associated with oral exposure to manganese. However, some epidemiological studies have reported associations between long-term exposure to high levels of manganese in drinking water during prenatal development or childhood and intellectual impairment; decreased nonverbal memory, attention, and motor skills; hyperactivity; and other behavioral effects. Most studies on the health effects of manganese have been conducted in countries where manganese exposure is generally higher than in the United States. However, two individual studies conducted in specific areas of relatively high manganese contamination in the United States reported associations between prenatal or childhood manganese exposure and problems with general intelligence, memory, and behavior. Although there is no health-based regulatory standard for manganese in drinking water, The EPA has set a voluntary standard for manganese as a guideline to assist public water systems in managing their drinking water for aesthetic considerations, such as taste, color, and odor.

Perchlorate. Perchlorate is a naturally occurring and artificial chemical that has been found in surface and groundwater in the United States. Perchlorate is used in the manufacture of fireworks, explosives, flares, and rocket fuel. Perchlorate was detected in just over 4 percent of public water systems in a nationally representative monitoring study conducted. Some infant formulas have been found to contain perchlorate, and the perchlorate content of the formula is increased if it is prepared with perchlorate-contaminated water. Exposure to elevated levels of perchlorate can inhibit iodide uptake into the thyroid gland, possibly disrupting the function of the thyroid and potentially leading to a reduction in the production of thyroid hormone. As noted above, thyroid hormones are particularly important for growth and development of the central nervous system (CNS) in fetuses and infants.

Section 17.2

Agricultural Practices

This section includes text excerpted from "Other Uses and Types of Water—Water Contamination," Centers for Disease Control and Prevention (CDC), October 11, 2016.

Over the past few decades, the increase in population and advances made in farming technology has increased the demand for crops and livestock from the agricultural industry. This growth in agricultural production has resulted in an increase in contaminants polluting soil and waterways. The increase in contaminants has prompted efforts to reduce the number of pollutants in waterways in order to improve overall water quality.

Agricultural Sources

Agriculture in many parts of the world is highly efficient in producing and delivering high-quality products to consumers. However, when agricultural activities are not well-monitored and managed, certain practices can negatively affect water quality.

Agricultural Runoff

According to the U.S. Environmental Protection Agency (EPA), nonpoint source (NPS) pollution is pollution that comes from many diffuse sources, unlike pollution from point sources such as industrial and sewage treatment plants. "Polluted runoff is created by rainfall or snowmelt moving over and through the ground. As the runoff moves, it picks up and carries away natural and human-made pollutants, finally depositing them into watersheds via lakes, rivers, wetlands, coastal waters, and even our underground sources of drinking water."

The National Water Quality Inventory report to U.S. Congress reported that agricultural nonpoint source (NPS) pollution is the leading cause of river and stream impairment and the second leading cause of impairment in lakes, ponds, and reservoirs.

Agricultural activities that cause nonpoint source pollution include:

- Poorly managed animal feeding operations

- Overgrazing

- Overworking the land (for example, plowing too often)

- Poorly managed and ineffective application of pesticides, irrigation water, and fertilizer

Effects

Agricultural water can become contaminated through a variety of ways and can potentially spread bacteria, viruses, and parasites to crops and animals.

Crop Production

Fresh fruits and vegetables come in contact with water during various stages of the production process. Contaminated water that is used during crop production, harvesting, and processing can lead to health issues.

Below is a list of the potential food production points where contaminated water sources can affect crop production:

- **Chemical application.** Crops with contaminated water used for pesticide or herbicide application. Water used for mixing chemicals should be of appropriate quality.

- **Irrigation.** Irrigating crops with contaminated water. Water used for irrigation should be of appropriate quality.

- **Worker hygiene.** Lack of potable water for hand hygiene. There should be an established handwashing and hygiene policy for farm workers.

- **Food processing.** Wash crops in the final wash process with quality water. Water should be of drinking water quality and should not be recycled.

People who consume fruit or vegetables that were exposed to contaminated water are at risk of developing a foodborne illness. Some of the bacteria that are spread through the water within the United States include *E. coli, Salmonella spp., Shigella spp., Cryptosporidium, Giardia, Toxoplasma*, norovirus, and hepatitis A virus. Irrigation of foods imported from international locations can spread these and other microbes (for example, Cyclospora) not usually found in developed countries. Small amounts of any of these organisms can cause foodborne illness. In order to keep microbes out of water sources, growers should use practices that are appropriate for their operation and make sure that they are using the best quality water. Water quality is also important in ensuring post-harvest quality by decreasing decay.

Animal Health

It is important that livestock are provided with adequate amounts of quality water, free of contamination. Contaminated water can contain disease-causing organisms which can rapidly spread if animals are drinking from the same trough. If there is a reason to question the quality of the water that is provided to livestock, it is important to test the water to ensure its safety. There are many chemicals and microorganisms that can be potentially dangerous to livestock. Some chemicals include nitrates, sulfates, and chemicals found in pesticides like dichloro-diphenyl-trichloroethane (DDT), chlordane, and endrin. Certain microorganisms such as blue-green algae, *Cryptosporidium*, or *Staphylococcus*, can be toxic to animals and cause symptoms like diarrhea, lack of coordination, labored breathing, or death. Ill animals can then release millions of infectious microbes into the soil that can further contaminate other water sources.

Section 17.3

Household Wells

This section includes text excerpted from "Private Drinking Water Wells," U.S. Environmental Protection Agency (EPA), February 27, 2018.

More than 15 million households rely on private wells for drinking water in the United States. Private well owners are responsible for the safety of their water.

Testing Wells to Safeguard Your Water

Testing Frequency

Test your private well annually for total coliform bacteria, nitrates, total dissolved solids, and pH levels. If you suspect the presence of other contaminants, you should test for those also. You can also contact your local health department to find out what substances may be common in your area's groundwater.

You may want to test more frequently if small children or elderly adults live in your house or if someone in your house is pregnant or nursing. These segments of the population are often more vulnerable to pollutants than others.

You should also test your private well immediately if:

• There are known problems with groundwater or drinking water in your area

• Conditions near your well have changed significantly i.e., flooding, land disturbances, and new construction or industrial activity)

• You replace or repair any part of your good system

• You notice a change in your water quality (i.e., odor, color, taste)

In addition, well owners should also determine if the groundwater you rely on for household use is under direct influence from surface water. Groundwater under the direct influence of surface water is susceptible to contamination from activities on the surface. Direct influence is determined on a site by site basis under state program criteria.

Identifying Reasons to Test Your Water

The table below lists common conditions or nearby activities that well owners should be aware of and the substance(s) that you should consider testing to ensure your well is safe. Not all of the substances listed pose an immediate or long-term health problem, some impact quality of life only such as appearance, taste, and odor.

Table 17.1. Conditions and Testing

Conditions or Nearby Activities	Test For
Recurring gastrointestinal illness	Coliform bacteria
Household plumbing or service lines that contain lead	pH, lead, copper
Radon in indoor air or region is radon-rich	Radon
Corrosion of pipes, plumbing	Corrosion, pH, lead
Nearby areas of intensive agriculture	Nitrate, nitrite, pesticides, coliform bacteria
Coal or other mining operations nearby	Metals, pH, corrosion
Gas drilling operations nearby	Chloride, sodium, barium, strontium
Dump, junkyard, landfill, factory, gas station or dry-cleaning operation nearby	Volatile organic compounds, total dissolved solids, pH, sulfate, chloride, metals
The odor of gasoline or fuel oil, and near a gas station or buried fuel tanks	Volatile organic compounds
Objectionable taste or smell	Hydrogen sulfide, corrosion, metals
Stained plumbing fixtures, laundry	Iron, copper, manganese
Salty taste and seawater, or a heavily salted roadway nearby	Chloride, total dissolved solids, sodium
Scaly residues, soaps don't lather	Hardness
Rapid wear of water treatment equipment	pH, corrosion
Water softener needed to treat hardness	Manganese, iron
Water appears cloudy, frothy or colored	Color, detergents

Where to Test Your Water

Only use laboratories that are certified to do drinking water testing. To find a certified laboratory in your state, you can contact:

- A state certified laboratory in your state

- Your local health department, which may provide private well testing for free

Test Results

Your water test results should include the concentration of the substances you tested for. It may also include whether the substance concentration exceeds a national primary or secondary drinking water standard.

Treatment

If a contaminant is found to exceed health standards in your sample, contact your public health department for specific steps to follow and have your well re-tested to confirm the contaminant's presence and concentrations. Some problems can be handled quickly. For example, high bacteria concentrations can sometimes be controlled by adding disinfection to a well, such as chlorine, ozone, ultraviolet (UV) light, and electronic radiation.

On-site treatment processes like disinfection, distillation, and filtration may remove the contaminants found in your well water. However, depending on the contaminant, its concentration, and the condition of the well, you may need a new source of water or to drill a new well.

Prevent Water Well Pollution

Protect your water supply by carefully managing activities near the water source. For households using a domestic well, this includes keeping contaminants away from sinkholes and the well itself. Keep hazardous chemicals out of septic systems.

- Slope the area around the well to drain surface runoff away from the well.

- Install a good cap or sanitary seal to prevent unauthorized use of, or entry into, the well.

- Keep accurate records of good maintenance, such as disinfection or sediment removal, that may require the use of chemicals in the well.

- Hire a certified well driller for any new well construction, modification, or abandonment and closure.

- Avoid mixing or using pesticides, fertilizers, herbicides, degreasers, fuels, and other pollutants near the well.

- Do not dispose of wastes in dry wells or in abandoned wells.

- Do not cut off the good casing below the land surface.

- Pump and inspect septic systems as often as recommended by your local health department.

- Never dispose of harsh chemicals, solvents, petroleum products, or pesticides in a septic system or dry well.

- Periodically inspect exposed parts of the well for problems such as:

  - Cracked, corroded or damaged well casing

  - Broken or missing well cap

  - Settling and cracking of surface seals

- Regularly check the integrity of any above ground and underground storage tanks that hold home heating oil, diesel, or gasoline on your property

- Check with your local health department or environmental agency to ensure activities and industry on or near your property are set a safe distance from your well.

Identify Potential Sources of Contamination in Your Community

In addition to the area near your drinking water well, you should be aware of other possible sources of contamination that may already be present in your community or may be moving into the area.

Consult a local expert to find out the physical and chemical properties of the groundwater you rely on and the presence of any potential drinking water contaminants. Such experts may include, but are not limited to:

- Local health department officials

- State environmental agency officials

- Agricultural extension agents

- Nearby public water system officials
- Local professional geologists and civil engineers

Find out about existing and proposed facilities that may pollute your drinking water. Check the local paper for announcements or call your planning or zoning commission to find hearings or zoning appeals on development, construction or industrial projects. Attend these hearings, planning meetings, or zoning appeals. Ask questions to ensure your drinking water will be protected during construction and operation of a facility. Make sure the project has plans for managing stormwater and any wastewater it might produce. Request the project's environmental impact statement to confirm it includes a review of drinking water sources.

Protect Your Water after a Natural Disaster or Emergency

Flooding, earthquakes, landslides, and other natural disasters can impact the safety of your drinking water by allowing contaminants to enter your private well system. If you suspect your drinking water well may be contaminated after a flood or another natural disaster, contact your local or state health department or environmental agency for advice on inspecting and testing your well. If possible, use a contractor with experience in servicing drinking water wells to inspect and test your well.

Water Well Flood Response Steps

- Stay away from the pump while flooded to avoid electric shock.
- Do not drink or wash from the flooded well to avoid becoming sick.
- Get assistance from a well or pump contractor to clean and disinfect your well before turning on the pump.
- After the pump is turned back on, pump the well until the water runs clear to rid the well of flood water.
- If the water does not run clear, get advice from the county or state health department or extension service.

Section 17.4

Lead in Drinking Water

This section includes text excerpted from "Ground
Water and Drinking Water—General Information about
Lead in Drinking Water," U.S. Environmental Protection
Agency (EPA), March 23, 2018.

How Lead Gets into Drinking Water

Lead can enter drinking water when service pipes that contain lead corrode, especially where the water has high acidity or low mineral content that corrodes pipes and fixtures. The most common problem is with brass or chrome-plated brass faucets and fixtures with lead solder, from which significant amounts of lead can enter into the water, especially hot water.

Homes built before 1986 are more likely to have lead pipes, fixtures, and solder. The Safe Drinking Water Act (SDWA) has reduced the maximum allowable lead content—that is, content that is considered "lead-free"—to be a weighted average of 0.25 percent calculated across the wetted surfaces of pipes, pipe fittings, plumbing fittings, and fixtures and 0.2 percent for solder and flux.

Corrosion is a dissolving or wearing away of metal caused by a chemical reaction between water and your plumbing. A number of factors are involved in the extent to which lead enters the water, including:

- the chemistry of the water (acidity and alkalinity) and the types and amounts of minerals in the water

- the amount of lead it comes into contact with

- the temperature of the water

- the amount of wear in the pipes

- how long the water stays in pipes

- the presence of protective scales or coatings inside the plumbing materials

To address corrosion of lead and copper into drinking water, U.S. Environmental Protection Agency (EPA) issued the Lead and Copper

Rule (LCR) under the authority of the SDWA. One requirement of the LCR is corrosion control treatment to prevent lead and copper from contaminating drinking water. Corrosion control treatment means utilities must make drinking water less corrosive to the materials it comes into contact with on its way to consumers' taps.

Health Effects of Exposures to Lead in Drinking Water

Is There a Safe Level of Lead in Drinking Water?

The SDWA requires the EPA to determine the level of contaminants in drinking water at which no adverse health effects are likely to occur with an adequate margin of safety. These nonenforceable health goals, based solely on possible health risks, are called maximum contaminant level goals (MCLGs). The EPA has set the maximum contaminant level goal for lead in drinking water at zero because lead is a toxic metal that can be harmful to human health even at low exposure levels. Lead is persistent, and it can bioaccumulate in the body over time.

Young children, infants, and fetuses are particularly vulnerable to lead because the physical and behavioral effects of lead occur at lower exposure levels in children than in adults. A dose of lead that would have little effect on an adult can have a significant effect on a child. In children, low levels of exposure have been linked to damage to the central and peripheral nervous system, learning disabilities, shorter stature, impaired hearing, and impaired formation and function of blood cells.

The Centers for Disease Control and Prevention (CDC) recommends that public health actions be initiated when the level of lead in a child's blood is 5 micrograms per deciliter (μg/dL) or more.

It is important to recognize all the ways a child can be exposed to lead. Children are exposed to lead in paint, dust, soil, air, and food, as well as drinking water. If the level of lead in a child's blood is at or above the CDC action level of 5 μg/dL, it may be due to lead exposures from a combination of sources. The EPA estimates that drinking water can make up 20 percent or more of a person's total exposure to lead. Infants who consume mostly mixed formula can receive 40–60 percent of their exposure to lead from drinking water.

Children

Even low levels of lead in the blood of children can result in:

- Behavior and learning problems
- Lower IQ and hyperactivity

- Slowed growth

- Hearing problems

- Anemia

In rare cases, ingestion of lead can cause seizures, coma, and even death.

Pregnant Women

Lead can accumulate in our bodies over time, where it is stored in bones along with calcium. During pregnancy, lead is released from bones as maternal calcium and is used to help form the bones of the fetus. This is particularly true if a woman does not have enough dietary calcium. Lead can also cross the placental barrier expose the fetus to lead. This can result in serious effects on the mother and her developing fetus, including:

- Reduced growth of the fetus

- Premature birth

Adults

Lead is also harmful to adults. Adults exposed to lead can suffer from:

- Cardiovascular effects, increased blood pressure and incidence of hypertension

- Decreased kidney function

- Reproductive problems (in both men and women)

Can I Shower in Lead-Contaminated Water?

Yes. Bathing and showering should be safe for you and your children, even if the water contains lead over EPA's action level. Human skin does not absorb lead in water.

This information applies to most situations and to a large majority of the population, but individual circumstances may vary. Some situations, such as cases involving highly corrosive water, may require additional recommendations or more stringent actions. Your local water authority is always your first source for testing and identifying lead contamination in your tap water. Many public water authorities have websites that include data on drinking water quality, including results of lead testing.

What You Can Do?

Find out If Lead Is in Your Drinking Water

First, learn more about the water coming into your home.
EPA requires all community water systems to prepare and deliver an annual water quality report called a *Consumer Confidence Report (CCR)* for their customers by July 1 of each year. Contact your water utility if you'd like to receive a copy of their latest report. If your water comes from a household well or other private water supply, check with your health department, or with any nearby water utilities that use groundwater, for information on contaminants of concern in your area.

Second, you can have your water tested for lead. Homes may have internal plumbing materials containing lead. Since you cannot see, taste, or smell lead dissolved in water, testing is the only sure way of telling whether there are harmful quantities of lead in your drinking water. A list of certified laboratories is available from your state or local drinking water authority. Testing costs between $20 and $100. Contact your water supplier as they may have useful information, including whether the service connector used in your home or area is made of lead.

Reduce Your Exposure to Lead in Drinking Water at Home

- Use only cold water for drinking, cooking and making baby formula. Boiling water does not remove lead from water.

- Regularly clean your faucet's screen (also known as an aerator).

- Consider using a water filter certified to remove lead and know when it's time to replace the filter.

- Before drinking, flush your pipes by running your tap, taking a shower, doing laundry or a load of dishes.

- Contact your water system to learn more about sources of lead and removing lead service lines.

Get Your Child Tested to Determine Lead Levels in His or Her Blood

A family doctor or pediatrician can perform a blood test for lead and provide information about the health effects of lead. State, city or county departments of health can also provide information about how you can have your child's blood tested for lead. The CDC recommends that public health actions be initiated when the level of lead in a child's blood is 5 μg/dL or more.

Find out If Lead in Drinking Water Is an Issue in Your Child's School or Child Care Facility

Children spend a significant part of their days at school or in a child care facility. The faucets that provide water used for consumption, including drinking, cooking lunch, and preparing juice and infant formula, should be tested.

- Protect your children from lead where they learn and play: learn how to test your child, and how to check the condition of schools and child care facilities.

- Know how schools and child care centers can test for lead in drinking water.

Drinking Water Requirements for Lead

EPA's Drinking Water Regulations for Lead

In 1974, Congress passed the SDWA. This law requires EPA to determine the level of contaminants in drinking water at which no adverse health effects are likely to occur with an adequate margin of safety. These nonenforceable health goals, based solely on possible health risks are called MCLGs. The MCLG for lead is zero. The EPA has set this level based on the best available science which shows there is no safe level of exposure to lead.

For most contaminants, EPA sets an enforceable regulation called a maximum contaminant level (MCL) based on the MCLG. MCLs are set as close to the MCLGs as possible, considering cost, benefits and the ability of public water systems to detect and remove contaminants using suitable treatment technologies.

However, because lead contamination of drinking water often results from corrosion of the plumbing materials belonging to water system customers, EPA established a treatment technique rather than an MCL for the lead. A treatment technique is an enforceable procedure or level of technological performance which water systems must follow to ensure control of a contaminant.

The treatment technique regulation for lead (referred to as the Lead and Copper Rule) requires water systems to control the corrosivity of the water. The regulation also requires systems to collect tap samples from sites served by the system that are more likely to have plumbing materials containing lead. If more than 10 percent of tap water samples exceed the lead action level of 15 parts per billion, then water systems are required to take additional actions including:

- Taking further steps optimize their corrosion control treatment (for water systems serving 50,000 people that have not fully optimized their corrosion control)

- Educating the public about lead in drinking water and actions consumers can take to reduce their exposure to lead

- Replacing the portions of lead service lines (lines that connect distribution mains to customers) under the water system's control

EPA issued the Lead and Copper Rule in 1991 and revised the regulation in 2000 and 2007. States may set more stringent drinking water regulations than EPA.

How EPA Requires States and Public Water Systems to Protect Drinking Water

The SDWA requires EPA to establish and enforce standards that public drinking water systems must follow. EPA delegates primary enforcement responsibility (also called primacy) for public water systems to states and tribes if they meet certain requirements.

Section 17.5

Fluoride

This section includes text excerpted from "Community
Water Fluoridation FAQs—About Fluoride," Centers for Disease
Control and Prevention (CDC), November 3, 2015.

About Fluoride

What Is Fluoride, and How Does It Get into Tap Water?

Fluoride is a mineral that occurs naturally and is released from rocks into the soil, water, and air. Almost all water contains some fluoride, but usually not enough to prevent tooth decay.

Fluoride can also be added to drinking water supplies as a public health measure for reducing cavities. Decisions about adding fluoride to drinking water are made at the state or local level.

What Are the Common Sources of Fluoride?

The primary sources for fluoride intake include drinking water in fluoridated communities, toothpaste (if swallowed by young children), beverages and food processed with fluoridated water, dietary prescription supplements that include fluoride (e.g., tablets or drops), and other professional dental products (e.g., mouth rinses, gels, and foams).

Community Water Fluoridation

What Is Community Water Fluoridation?

Almost all water contains some naturally-occurring fluoride, but usually at levels too low to prevent tooth decay. Many communities adjust the fluoride concentration in the water supply to a level known to reduce tooth decay and promote good oral health (often called the optimal level). This practice is known as community water fluoridation and reaches all people who drink that water. Given the dramatic decline in tooth decay during the past 70 years since community water fluoridation was initiated, the Centers for Disease Control and Prevention (CDC) named fluoridation of drinking water to prevent dental caries (tooth decay) as one of ten great public health interventions of the 20th Century.

Does My Public Water System Add Fluoride to the Water?

The best way to find the fluoride level of your local public water system is to contact your water utility provider. Consumers can find the name and contact information of the water utility on the water bill. The U.S. Environmental Protection Agency (EPA) requires that all community water systems provide each customer with an annual report on water quality, including the fluoride content.

If I Am Drinking Water with Fluoride, Why Do I Also Need to Brush with Toothpaste That Contains Fluoride?

Both drinking water and toothpaste with fluoride provide important and complementary benefits. Fluoridated water keeps a low level of fluoride in saliva and dental plaque all day. The much higher concentration of fluoride in toothpaste offers additional benefit. Fluoride slows the activity of bacteria that cause decay and combines with enamel on the tooth surface to make it stronger and better able to resist decay. Together, the two sources offer more protection than using either one alone.

Given That We Get Fluoride from Other Sources, Should Communities Still Fluoridate Water to Prevent Tooth Decay?

Yes. Consuming fluoridated water and other beverages and foods prepared or processed with fluoridated water is still important for prevention of decay in a community. Ingesting fluoridated water throughout the day maintains a low level of fluoride in saliva and plaque that enhances the remineralization of weakened tooth surfaces. Community water fluoridation has been identified as the most cost-effective method of delivering fluoride to all members of the community regardless of age, educational attainment, income level, and the availability of dental care. In studies conducted after other fluoride products, such as toothpaste, were widely available, scientists found additional reductions in tooth decay—up to 25 percent—among people with community water fluoridation as compared to those without fluoridation.

Has the Safety of Community Water Fluoridation Been Evaluated?

The safety and effectiveness of fluoride at levels used in community water fluoridation have been thoroughly reviewed by multinational scientific and public health organizations (United States, Canada, Australia, New Zealand, Great Britain, and the World Health Organization(WHO)) using evidence-based reviews and expert panels. These panels include scientists with expertise in various health and scientific disciplines, including medicine, biophysics, chemistry, toxicological pathology, oral health, and epidemiology.

Experts have weighed the findings and quality of available evidence and concluded that there is no association between water fluoridation and any unwanted health effects other than dental fluorosis.

Are There Any Harmful Health Effects Due to Community Water Fluoridation?

The safety and effectiveness of community water fluoridation continue to be supported by scientific evidence produced by independent scientists and summarized by panels of experts. The independent, nongovernmental Community Preventive Services Task Force (CPSTF) has noted that the research evidence does not demonstrate that community water fluoridation results in any unwanted health effects other than dental fluorosis, a condition that causes primarily cosmetic changes in the appearance of tooth enamel.

Will Using a Home Water Filtration System Take the Fluoride out of My Home's Water?

Removal of fluoride from water is a difficult water treatment action. Most point-of-use treatment systems for homes that are installed on single faucets use activated carbon filtration, which will not remove the fluoride ion. Other treatment systems (such as reverse osmosis, ion exchange, or distillation systems to reduce fluoride levels) vary in their effectiveness to reduce fluoride. Check with the manufacturer of the individual product.

Will Boiling or Freezing Reduce the Fluoride Level in Water?

Fluoride is not released from water when it is boiled or frozen. One exception would be a water distillation system. These systems heat water to the boiling point and then collect water vapor as it evaporates. Water distillation systems are typically used in laboratory installations. For home use, these systems can be expensive and may present safety and maintenance concerns.

Will Water Fluoridation Result in Pipe Corrosion or Increased Lead in Drinking Water?

Water fluoridation will not increase pipe corrosion or cause lead to leach from pipes and household plumbing fixtures. Although lead in public drinking water is typically found to be very low or is below laboratory detection, there are locations where old lead pipes, solder, or plumbing fixtures in old homes may experience leaching of lead into the water. Claims by some that fluoride might result in increased lead leaching from pipes and fixtures have not been substantiated in the peer-reviewed literature.

What Did 2015 Report from the Cochrane Oral Health Group Say about the Effectiveness of Water Fluoridation?

The Cochrane review found that water fluoridation is effective in reducing cavities in primary and permanent teeth in children. It found that water fluoridation resulted in fewer teeth affected by cavities (about 2 primary teeth and 1 permanent tooth), compared to communities that did not have water fluoridation. These differences indicated that initiation of water fluoridation could result in decreases of up to 35 percent in cavities in children. In addition, water fluoridation resulted in higher percentages of children without any cavities (caries-free).

Cochrane's restrictive methodology for including studies in their analyses excluded the majority of studies done after 1975. Although valid, peer-reviewed studies clearly document the effectiveness of community water fluoridation in children and adults even after the use of fluoride toothpaste became widespread, these studies were not considered by Cochrane. As a result, Cochrane found insufficient information available to determine if water fluoridation had an impact in an environment where fluoride products such as toothpaste are now widely used.

Another factor that impacted Cochrane's assessment of the evidence is that their methodology favors randomized controlled trials (RCTs). While RCTs are a preferred study design for studies comparing different clinical treatments among individual patients, this research design is often not feasible for interventions that occur on a community level, like community water fluoridation.

Private Wells

My Home Gets Its Water from a Private Well. What Do I Need to Know about Fluoride and Groundwater from a Well?

Fluoride is present in virtually all waters at some level and it is important to know the fluoride content of your water, particularly if you have children. To find out the fluoride concentration in your well water, it would need to be analyzed by a laboratory. Your public health department should be able to advise how to have your home well water tested.

What Should I Do If the Water from My Well Has Less than the Recommended Level of Fluoride for Preventing Tooth Decay?

The recommended fluoride level in drinking water for good oral health is 0.7 mg/L (milligrams per liter). If fluoride levels in your drinking water are lower than 0.7 mg/L, your child's dentist or pediatrician should evaluate whether your child could benefit from daily fluoride supplements. Their recommendation will depend on your child's risk of developing tooth decay, as well as exposure to other sources of fluoride, such as drinking water at school or daycare, and fluoride toothpaste. It is not currently feasible to add fluoride to an individual resident's well.

What Should I Do If the Water from My Well Has Fluoride Levels That Are Higher than the Recommended Level for Preventing Tooth Decay?

In some regions in the United States, community drinking water and home wells can contain levels of naturally occurring fluoride that are greater than the level recommended by the U.S. Public Health Service (USPHS) for preventing tooth decay. The EPA currently has a nonenforceable recommended guideline for fluoride of 2.0 mg/L that is set to protect against dental fluorosis. If your home is served by a water system that has fluoride levels exceeding this recommended guideline, EPA recommends that children 8 years and younger be provided with alternative sources of drinking water.

What Should I Do If My Well Water Was Measured As Having Too Much Fluoride (Level Greater than 4 mg/L)?

It is unusual to have the fluoride content of water be 4 mg/L or higher. If a laboratory report indicates that you have such a high fluoride content, it's recommended that you retest the water. You should collect at least four samples over four weeks (one sample each week), and compare the results. If one sample is above 4 mg/L and the other samples are less than 4 mg/L, then the high value may have been an error. If the results for all the samples show levels greater than 4 mg/L, you may want to consider alternate sources of water for drinking and cooking, or installing a device to remove the fluoride from your home water source. Physical contact with water with a high fluoride content, such as through bathing or washing dishes, is safe since fluoride does not pass through the skin.

Bottled Water

Consumers drink bottled water for various reasons, including as a taste preference or as a convenient means of hydration. Bottled water may not have a sufficient amount of fluoride, which is important for preventing tooth decay and promoting oral health.

Some bottled waters contain fluoride, and some do not. Fluoride can occur naturally in source waters used for bottling or it can be added.

Does Bottled Water Contain Fluoride?

Bottled water products may contain fluoride, depending on the source of the water. Fluoride can be naturally present in the original source of the water, and many public water systems add fluoride to their water. The U.S. Food and Drug Administration (FDA) sets limits for fluoride in bottled water, based on several factors, including the source of the water. Bottled water products labeled as de-ionized, purified, demineralized, or distilled have been treated in such a way that they contain no or only trace amounts of fluoride, unless they specifically list fluoride as an added ingredient.

How Can I Find Out the Level of Fluoride in Bottled Water?

The FDA does not require bottled water manufacturers to list the amount of fluoride on the label unless the manufacturer has added fluoride within set limits. Contact the bottled water manufacturer to ask about the fluoride content of a particular brand.

Who Regulates Fluoride in Bottled Water?

The EPA regulates public drinking water (tap water), and the FDA regulates bottled water products under the authority of the Federal Food, Drug, and Cosmetic Act (FFDCA).

The FDA has established standards for the maximum amount of naturally occurring fluoride or added fluoride allowed in bottled drinking water. If bottled water meets specific standards of identity and quality set forth by the FDA, and provisions of the authorized health claim, manufacturers may include the following health claim: "Drinking fluoridated water may reduce the risk of [dental caries or tooth decay]."

Section 17.6

Chlorination and Water Disinfection By-Products

This section includes text excerpted from "Safe Water System—Chlorination," Centers for Disease Control and Prevention (CDC), April 23, 2014. Reviewed April 2018.

The Safe Water System (SWS) was developed in the 1990's in response to epidemic cholera in South America by the Centers for Disease Control and Prevention (CDC) and the Pan American Health Organization (PAHO). The treatment method for the SWS is point-of-use chlorination by consumers with a locally-manufactured dilute sodium hypochlorite (chlorine bleach) solution. The SWS also incorporates an emphasis on safe storage of treated water and behavior change communications to improve water and food handling, sanitation, and hygiene practices in the home and in the community. To use the chlorination method, families add one full bottle cap of the sodium hypochlorite solution to clear water (or 2 caps to turbid water) in a standard sized container, agitate, and wait 30 minutes before drinking.

Lab Effectiveness, Field Effectiveness, and Health Impact

At concentrations that are used for household water treatment programs, the hypochlorite solution is effective at inactivating most bacteria and viruses that cause diarrheal disease. However, it is not effective at inactivating some protozoa, such as *Cryptosporidium*. Numerous studies have shown complete removal of bacterial pathogens in SWS treated water in developing countries. In seven randomized, controlled trials, the SWS has resulted in reductions in diarrheal disease incidence in users ranging from 22–84 percent. These studies have been conducted in rural and urban areas, and include adults and children that are poor, living with human immunodeficiency virus (HIV), or using highly turbid water.

Benefits, Drawbacks, and Appropriateness

The benefits of chlorination are:

- Proven reduction of most bacteria and viruses in water
- Residual protection against recontamination
- Ease-of-use and acceptability
- Proven reduction of diarrheal disease incidence
- Scalability and low cost

The drawbacks of chlorination are:

- Relatively low protection against protozoa
- Lower disinfection effectiveness in turbid waters
- Potential taste and odor objections
- Must ensure quality control of the solution
- Potential long-term effects of chlorination by-products

The SWS and chlorination are most appropriate in areas with a consistent supply chain for hypochlorite solution with relatively lower turbidity water, and in urban, rural, and emergency situations where educational messages can reach users to encourage the correct and consistent use of the hypochlorite solution.

Economics and Scalability

A bottle of hypochlorite solution that treats 1,000 liters of water costs about 10 U.S. cents using refillable bottles and 11–50 U.S. cents using disposable bottles, for a cost of 0.01–0.05 cents per liter treated. Education and community motivation add to program costs. SWS programs can achieve full cost recovery (charging the user the full cost of the product, marketing, distribution, and education), partial cost recovery (charging the user only for the product, and subsidizing program costs with donor funds), or can be fully subsidized such as in emergency situations.

Section 17.7

Bottled Water

This section includes text excerpted from "Bottled
Water Everywhere: Keeping It Safe," U.S. Food and Drug
Administration (FDA), December 13, 2017.

The U.S. Food and Drug Administration (FDA) regulates bottled
water products, working to ensure that they're safe to drink.

FDA protects consumers of bottled water through the Federal
Food, Drug, and Cosmetic Act (FFDCA), which makes manufacturers
responsible for producing safe, wholesome, and truthfully labeled food
products.

There are regulations that focus specifically on bottled water,
including:

- "standard of identity" regulations that define different types of
  bottled water

- "standard of quality" regulations that set maximum levels of
  contaminants—including chemical, physical, microbial, and
  radiological contaminants—allowed in bottled water

- "current good manufacturing practice" (CGMP) regulations that
  require bottled water to be safe and produced under sanitary
  conditions

Types of Bottled Water

The FDA describes bottled water as water that's intended for human
consumption and sealed in bottles or other containers with no added
ingredients, except that it may contain a safe and suitable antimicrobial agent. (Fluoride may also be added within the limits set by FDA.)

The agency classifies some bottled water by its origin. Here are four
of those classifications:

- **Artesian well water.** This water is collected from a well that
  taps an aquifer—layers of porous rock, sand, and earth that contain water—which is under pressure from surrounding upper

layers of rock or clay. When tapped, the pressure in the aquifer, commonly called artesian pressure, pushes the water above the level of the aquifer, sometimes to the surface. Other means may be used to help bring the water to the surface.

- **Mineral water.** This water comes from an underground source and contains at least 250 parts per million total dissolved solids. Minerals and trace elements must come from the source of the underground water. They cannot be added later.

- **Spring water.** Derived from an underground formation from which water flows naturally to the surface, this water must be collected only at the spring or through a borehole that taps the underground formation feeding the spring. If some external force is used to collect the water through a borehole, the water must have the same composition and quality as the water that naturally flows to the surface.

- **Well, water.** This is water from a hole bored or drilled into the ground, which taps into an aquifer.

Bottled water may be used as an ingredient in beverages, such as diluted juices or flavored bottled waters. However, beverages labeled as containing "sparkling water," "seltzer water," "soda water," "tonic water," or "club soda," aren't included as bottled water under The FDA's regulations. These beverages are instead considered to be soft drinks.

It May Be Tap Water

Some bottled water also comes from municipal sources—in other words, the tap. Municipal water is usually treated before it is bottled. Examples of water treatments include:

- **Distillation.** Water is turned into a vapor, leaving minerals behind. Vapors are then condensed into water again.

- **Reverse osmosis.** Water is forced through membranes to remove minerals.

- **Absolute 1-micron filtration.** Water flows through filters that remove particles larger than one micron—.00004 inches—in size. These particles include *Cryptosporidium*, a parasitic pathogen that can cause gastrointestinal illness.

- **Ozonation.** Bottlers of all types of waters typically use ozone gas, an antimicrobial agent, instead of chlorine to disinfect the water. (Chlorine can add residual taste and odor to the water.)

Bottled water that has been treated by distillation, reverse osmosis, or another suitable process may meet standards that allow it to be labeled as "purified water."

Ensuring Quality and Safety

Federal quality standards for bottled water were first adopted in 1973. They were based on U.S. Public Health Service (USPHS) standards for drinking water set in 1962.

The 1974 Safe Drinking Water Act (SDWA) gave regulatory oversight of public drinking water (tap water) to the U.S. Environmental Protection Agency (EPA). The FDA subsequently took responsibility, under the FFDCA, for ensuring that the quality standards for bottled water are compatible with EPA standards for tap water.

Each time EPA establishes a standard for a contaminant, the FDA either adopts it for bottled water or finds that the standard isn't necessary for bottled water.

In some cases, standards for bottled water and tap water differ. For example, because lead can leach from pipes as water travels from water utilities to home faucets, EPA has set its limit for lead in tap water at 15 parts per billion (ppb). For bottled water, for which lead pipes aren't used, the lead limit is set at 5 ppb.

For bottled water production, bottlers must follow the Current Good Manufacturing Practice (CGMP) regulations put in place and enforced by FDA. Water must be sampled, analyzed, and found to be safe and sanitary. These regulations also require proper plant and equipment design, bottling procedures, and record keeping.

In addition, FDA oversees inspections of bottling plants. The agency inspects bottled water plants under its general food safety program and has states perform some plant inspections under contract. (Some states also require bottled water firms to be licensed annually.)

Chapter 18

Recreational Water Illnesses

Chapter Contents

Section 18.1

Understanding Recreational Water Illnesses

This section includes text excerpted from "Healthy Swimming—Recreational Water Illnesses," Centers for Disease Control and Prevention (CDC), January 25, 2017.

Recreational water illnesses (RWIs) are caused by germs and chemicals found in the water we swim in. They are spread by swallowing, breathing in mists or aerosols of, or having contact with contaminated water in swimming pools, hot tubs, water parks, water play areas, interactive fountains, lakes, rivers, or oceans. RWIs can also be caused by chemicals in the water or chemicals that turn into gas in the air and cause air quality problems at indoor aquatic facilities.

Knowing the basic facts about RWIs can make the difference between an enjoyable time at the pool, beach, or waterpark, and getting a rash, having diarrhea, or developing other, potentially serious illnesses.

Facts about Recreational Water Illnesses (RWIs)

What Are Recreational Water Illnesses (RWIs)?

Recreational water illnesses (RWIs) are caused by germs spread by swallowing, breathing in mists or aerosols of, or having contact with contaminated water in swimming pools, hot tubs, water parks, water play areas, interactive fountains, lakes, rivers, or oceans. RWIs can also be caused by chemicals in the water or chemicals that evaporate from the water and cause indoor air quality problems. RWIs can be a wide variety of infections, including gastrointestinal, skin, ear, respiratory, eye, neurologic, and wound infections. The most commonly reported RWI is diarrhea. Diarrheal illnesses can be caused by germs such as Crypto (short for *Cryptosporidium*), *Giardia, Shigella*, norovirus, and *E. coli* O157: H7.

Where Are RWIs Found?

RWIs are caused by germs spread through contaminated water in swimming pools, water parks, water play areas, hot tubs, decorative water fountains, oceans, lakes, and rivers.

Swimming Pools, Water Parks, Water Play Areas

The most common RWI is diarrhea. Swallowing even a small amount of water that has been contaminated with feces containing germs can cause diarrheal illness.

To ensure that most germs are killed, check chlorine or other disinfectant levels and pH (potential of hydrogen) regularly as part of good pool operation.

Hot Tubs

Skin infections like "hot tub rash" are a common RWI spread through hot tubs and spas. Respiratory illnesses are also associated with the use of improperly maintained hot tubs.

The high water temperatures in most hot tubs make it hard to maintain the disinfectant levels needed to kill germs. That's why it's important to check disinfectant levels in hot tubs even more regularly than in swimming pools.

The germs that cause "hot tub rash" can also be spread in pools that do not have proper disinfectant levels and in natural bodies of water such as oceans, lakes, or rivers.

Decorative Water Fountains

Not all decorative fountains are chlorinated or filtered. Therefore, when people, especially diaper-aged children, play in the water, they can contaminate the water with fecal matter. Swallowing this contaminated water can then cause diarrheal illness.

Oceans, Lakes, and Rivers

Oceans, lakes, and rivers can be contaminated with germs from sewage spills, animal waste, water runoff following rainfall, fecal incidents, and germs rinsed off the bottoms of swimmers. It is important to avoid swallowing the water because natural recreational water is not disinfected. Avoid swimming after rainfalls or in areas identified as unsafe by health departments.

Why Doesn't Chlorine Kill RWI Germs?

Chlorine (in swimming pools and hot tubs) kills the germs that cause RWIs, but the time it takes to kill each germ varies.

In pools and hot tubs with the correct pH and disinfectant levels, chlorine will kill most germs that cause RWIs in less than an hour.

However, chlorine takes longer to kill some germs, such as Crypto. Crypto can survive for days even in a properly disinfected pool. This is why it is so important for swimmers to keep germs out of the water in the first place.

To protect yourself, your family, and other swimmers from RWIs, it is essential to learn and practice the steps of healthy swimming.

Who Is Most Likely to Get Ill from an RWI?

Children, pregnant women, and people with weakened immune systems (for example, people living with acquired immune deficiency syndrome (AIDS), individuals who have received an organ transplant, or people receiving certain types of chemotherapy) can suffer from more severe illness if infected. People with weakened immune systems should be aware that recreational water might be contaminated with human or animal feces containing Crypto. Crypto can cause a life-threatening infection in persons with weakened immune systems.

People with a weakened immune system should consult their healthcare provider before participating in activities that place them at risk for illness.

How Can We Prevent RWIs?

There are a few easy and effective healthy swimming steps all swimmers can take each time we swim to help protect ourselves, our families, and our friends from RWIs.

Section 18.2

Infections due to Recreational Water Illnesses

This section includes text excerpted from "Healthy Swimming—
Recreational Water Illnesses," Centers for Disease Control and
Prevention (CDC), January 25, 2017. ·

Recreational water illnesses (RWIs) include a wide variety of infections. It includes:

- Diarrheal illness

- Rashes

- Ear infections

- Respiratory infections

- Chemical irritation of the eyes and lungs

- Infections unlikely to be spread through swimming pools

Diarrheal Illness

Diarrhea and swimming don't mix! Diarrhea is the most common recreational water illness (RWI). Swimmers who are sick with diarrhea—or who have been sick in the last two weeks—risk contaminating pool water with germs.

Diarrheal illnesses are caused by germs such as Crypto (short for *Cryptosporidium*), *Giardia, Shigella*, norovirus, and *E. coli* O157: H7. These germs can live from minutes to days in pools, even if the pool is well-maintained. Some germs are very tolerant to chlorine and were not known to cause human disease. Once the pool has been contaminated, all it takes is for someone to swallow a small amount of pool water to become infected.

Crypto has become the leading cause of swimming pool-related outbreaks of diarrheal illness. It can stay alive for days even in well-maintained pools and can cause prolonged diarrhea (for 2–3 weeks).

Giardia is another germ that often causes swimming pool-related outbreaks of diarrheal illness. It has a tough outer shell that allows it to survive for up to 45 minutes even in properly chlorinated pools.

How Is Diarrhea Spread at Recreational Water Venues?

Infectious diarrhea can contain anywhere from hundreds of millions to one billion germs per bowel movement. Swallowing even a small amount of water that has been contaminated with these germs can make you sick. Tiny amounts of fecal matter are rinsed off all swimmers' bottoms as they swim through the water. That is why it is so important to stay out of the pool if you are sick with diarrhea, shower before swimming, and avoid swallowing pool water.

At public swimming facilities, continuous filtration and disinfection of water should reduce the risk of spreading germs. However, swimmers may still be exposed to germs during the time it takes for chlorine to kill germs (certain germs take longer to kill than others) or for water to be recycled through filters. Many pool facilities use one filtration system for several pools. This causes water from various pools to mix and potentially spreads germs throughout connected pools in a very short amount of time. This means that a single diarrheal incident from one person could contaminate water throughout a large pool system or waterpark.

What Should I Do If I Have Diarrhea?

To help protect the health of others, do not swim when you have diarrhea. Microscopic amounts of infected fecal matter can contaminate an entire pool or hot tub and make others sick if they swallow the water.

If you have diarrhea, the most important thing you can do is to drink plenty of fluids to prevent dehydration. This is especially important for young children, pregnant women, and persons with weakened immune systems (such as those living with human immunodeficiency virus (HIV)/acquired immunodeficiency syndrome (AIDS)), those who have received an organ transplant, or those receiving certain types of chemotherapy).

Seek medical care immediately if you experience any of the following symptoms:

- your diarrhea is bloody

- your diarrhea does not resolve within 5 days

- your diarrhea is accompanied by fever or chills

- you are dehydrated (Signs of dehydration include: dry or "cottony" mouth, cracked lips, dry flushed skin, headache, irritability, not urinating at least four times a day, no tears when crying, not sweating, or confusion)

A healthcare provider may prescribe medicine to help replace the fluids your body has lost because of diarrhea. In some cases, over-the-counter (OTC) medications can slow diarrhea.

How Do I Protect Myself and My Family?

Take action! We all share the water we swim in, so each of us plays an essential role in helping to protect ourselves, our families, and our friends from germs that can cause RWIs.

All swimmers should take the following easy and effective healthy swimming steps:

- Keep the pee, poop, sweat, and dirt out of the water!
  - Stay out of the water if you have diarrhea.
  - Shower before you get in the water.
  - Don't pee or poop in the water.
  - Don't swallow the water.
- Every hour—everyone out!
  - Take kids on bathroom breaks.
  - Check diapers, and change them in a bathroom or diaper-changing area—not poolside—to keep germs away from the pool.
  - Reapply sunscreen.
  - Drink plenty of fluids.

"Hot Tub Rash" (Pseudomonas Dermatitis/Folliculitis)

If contaminated water comes in contact with a person's skin for a long period of time, it can cause a rash called hot tub rash, or dermatitis. Hot tub rash is often caused by infection with the germ Pseudomonas aeruginosa. This germ is common in the environment (for example, in the water and soil) and is microscopic, so it can't be seen with the naked eye.

What Are the Symptoms of Hot Tub Rash?

Symptoms of hot tub rash include:

- Itchy spots on the skin that become a bumpy red rash
- The rash is worse in areas that were previously covered by a swimsuit
- Pus-filled blisters around hair follicles

Hot tub rash can affect people of all ages. Most rashes clear up in a few days without medical treatment. However, if your rash lasts longer than a few days, consult your healthcare provider.

How Is Hot Tub Rash Spread at Recreational Water Venues?

Hot tub rash can occur if contaminated water comes in contact with the skin for a long period of time. The rash usually appears within a few days of being in a poorly maintained hot tub (or spa), but it can also appear within a few days after swimming in a poorly maintained pool or contaminated lake. Most rashes clear up in a few days without medical treatment. However, if your rash lasts longer than a few days, consult your healthcare provider.

How Do I Protect Myself and My Family?

Because hot tubs have warmer water than pools, chlorine or other disinfectants used to kill germs (like *Pseudomonas aeruginosa*) break down faster. This can increase the risk of hot tub rash infection for swimmers.

To reduce the risk of hot tub rash:

- Remove your swimsuit and shower with soap after getting out of the water.
- Clean your swimsuit after getting out of the water.
- Ask your pool/hot tub operator if disinfectant (for example, chlorine) and pH levels are checked at least twice per day—hot tubs and pools with good disinfectant and pH control are less likely to spread germs.

Use hot tub test strips to check the hot tub yourself for adequate disinfectant (chlorine or bromine) levels. Centers for Disease Control and Prevention (CDC) recommends the following for pools and hot tubs:

- Pools: Free chlorine (1–3 parts per million or ppm)
- Hot tubs: Free chlorine (2–4 ppm) or bromine (4–6 ppm)
- Both hot tubs and pools should have a pH level of 7.2–7.8
- If you find improper chlorine, bromine, and/or pH levels, tell the hot tub/pool operator or owner immediately

What Can I Ask the Hot Tub Operator?

- What was the most recent health inspection score for the hot tub
- Are disinfectant and pH levels checked at least twice per day
- Are disinfectant and pH levels checked more often when the hot tub is being used by a lot of people

- Are the following maintenance activities performed regularly:
  - Removal of the slime or biofilm layer by scrubbing and cleaning?
  - Replacement of the hot tub water filter according to manufacturer's recommendations?
  - Replacement of hot tub water?

Ear Infections

Ear infections can be caused by leaving contaminated water in the ear after swimming. This infection, known as "swimmer's ear" or otitis externa, is not the same as the common childhood middle ear infection. The infection occurs in the outer ear canal and can cause pain and discomfort for swimmers of all ages. In the United States, swimmer's ear results in an estimated 2.4 million healthcare visits every year and nearly half a billion dollars in healthcare costs.

Below are answers to the most common questions regarding ear infections, swimmer's ear, and healthy swimming.

What Are the Symptoms of Swimmer's Ear?

Symptoms of swimmer's ear usually appear within a few days of swimming and include:

- Itchiness inside the ear
- Redness and swelling of the ear
- Pain when the infected ear is tugged or when pressure is placed on the ear
- Pus draining from the infected ear

Although all age groups are affected by swimmer's ear, it is more common in children and can be extremely painful.

How Is Swimmer's Ear Spread at Recreational Water Venues?

Swimmer's ear can occur when water stays in the ear canal for long periods of time, providing the perfect environment for germs to grow and infect the skin. Germs found in pools and at other recreational water venues are one of the most common causes of swimmer's ear.

Swimmer's ear cannot be spread from one person to another.

If you think you have swimmer's ear, consult your healthcare provider. Swimmer's ear can be treated with antibiotic ear drops.

Is There a Difference between a Childhood-Middle Ear Infection and Swimmer's Ear?

Yes. Swimmer's ear is not the same as the common childhood middle ear infection. If you can wiggle the outer ear without pain or discomfort then your ear condition is probably not swimmer's ear.

How Do I Protect Myself and My Family?

To reduce the risk of swimmer's ear:
DO keep your ears as dry as possible.

- Use a bathing cap, ear plugs, or custom-fitted swim molds when swimming.

DO dry your ears thoroughly after swimming or showering.

- Use a towel to dry your ears well.
  - Tilt your head to hold each ear facing down to allow water to escape the ear canal.
  - Pull your earlobe in different directions while your ear is faced down to help water drain out.
  - If you still have water left in your ears, consider using a hair dryer to move air within the ear canal.
  - Put the dryer on the lowest heat and speed/fan setting.
  - Hold the dryer several inches from your ear.
- DON'T put objects in your ear canal (including cotton-tip swabs, pencils, paperclips, or fingers).
- DON'T try to remove ear wax. Ear wax helps protect your ear canal from infection.
- If you think that your ear canal is blocked by earwax, consult your healthcare provider.
- CONSULT your healthcare provider about using ear drops after swimming.
- Drops should not be used by people with ear tubes, damaged ear drums, outer ear infections, or ear drainage (pus or liquid coming from the ear).

- CONSULT your healthcare provider if you have ear pain, discomfort, or drainage from your ears.

- ASK your pool/hot tub operator if disinfectant and pH levels are checked at least twice per day—hot tubs and pools with proper disinfectant and pH levels are less likely to spread germs.

- USE pool test strips to check the pool or hot tub yourself for adequate disinfectant (chlorine or bromine) levels.

Respiratory Infections

Swimmers are at risk for respiratory infections if they breathe in steam or mist from a pool or hot tub that contains harmful germs. A respiratory disease caused by the germ *Legionella* is one of the most frequent waterborne diseases (drinking water and recreational water) among humans in the United States. Below are answers to the most common questions regarding *Legionella* and healthy swimming.

What Is **Legionella?**

Legionella is a germ that can cause a type of pneumonia called legionellosis, more commonly known as Legionnaires' disease. *Legionella* is microscopic, so it can't be seen with the naked eye.

Why Should I Be Concerned about **Legionella?**

Each year, 8,000–18,000 people in the United States are hospitalized with Legionnaires' disease. Legionnaires' disease is usually treated successfully with antibiotics, but can sometimes be fatal.

Certain groups of people are more likely to become seriously ill when infected with *Legionella*:

- Individuals who are 50 years of age or older

- Smokers

- People with chronic lung disease

- Individuals with weakened immune systems

How Is **Legionella** *Spread at Aquatic Facilities?*

Legionella is not spread from one person to another.

Legionella is naturally found in water, especially warm water. Hot tubs that are not cleaned and disinfected enough can become contaminated with *Legionella*. A person can get infected with *Legionella* when they breathe in steam or mist from a contaminated hot tub.

Legionella can also be found in cooling towers, plumbing systems, and decorative pools or fountains.

How Do I Protect Myself and My Family?

Because high water temperatures make it hard to maintain the disinfectant levels needed to kill germs like *Legionella*, making sure that the hot tub has the right disinfectant and pH levels are essential. Here are some things you can do to determine whether a hot tub has been properly maintained:

Three Steps for Testing Hot Tub Water

- Purchase pool test strips at your local home improvement or pool supply store (be sure to check the expiration date)

- Use the test strips to check hot tub water for adequate free chlorine (2–4 parts per million [ppm]) or bromine (4–6 ppm) and pH (7.2–7.8) levels

- If you find improper chlorine, bromine, and/or pH levels, tell the hot tub operator or owner immediately

Four Questions to Ask Your Hot Tub Operator

- What was the most recent health inspection score for the hot tub?

- Are disinfectant and pH levels checked at least twice per day?

- Are disinfectant and pH levels checked more often when the hot tub is being used by a lot of people?

- Are the following maintenance activities performed regularly:

  - Removal of the slime or biofilm layer by scrubbing and cleaning?

  - Replacement of the hot tub water filter according to manufacturer's recommendations?

  - Replacement of hot tub water?

Chemical Irritation of the Eyes and Lungs

Red eyes or irritated nose or throat after swimming? Blame the pee, poop, and sweat!

To help protect swimmers' health, chlorine is commonly added to the water to kill germs and stop them from spreading. But chlorine can also combine with what comes out of or washes off of swimmers' bodies (for example, pee, poop, sweat, dirt, skin cells, and personal care products). This causes two problems:

Free chlorine, the form of chlorine that kills germs, gets used up and is no longer available to kill germs.

Chemical irritants called chloramines (chlor, short for chlorine, and amines, compounds that contain nitrogen) are formed.

Healthy pools and other places where we swim in chlorinated water don't have a strong chemical smell. If you smell "chlorine" at the place you swim, you are probably smelling chloramines. Chloramines in the water can turn into gas in the surrounding air. This is particularly a problem in indoor pools, which often aren't as well-ventilated as outdoor pools. The chloramines that form in the chlorinated water we swim in are different from the chloramine that is sometimes used to treat drinking water.

What Are the Health Effects Associated with Chloramines?

Breathing in or coming into contact with chloramines at the places we swim can lead to negative health effects in swimmers and others in the swimming area including:

- Everyone (swimmers and others in the swimming area)
  - Respiratory symptoms such as nasal irritation, coughing and wheezing. Asthma attacks can be triggered in people who have asthma
- Swimmers
  - Red and stinging eyes
  - Skin irritation and rashes

What Can I Do to Reduce Chloramine Formation?

We all share the chlorinated water we swim in and the surrounding air we breathe. Here are a few easy and effective steps swimmers can take to help protect our health and the health of our family and friends:

- Keep pee, poop, sweat, and dirt out of the water!

- Stay out of the water if you have diarrhea.

- Use the toilet before getting into the water.

- Shower before getting into the water. Rinsing off in the shower for just 1 minute removes most of the dirt or anything else on your body.

- Wear a bathing cap while in the water.

- Don't pee or poop in the water.

Take a break—every hour!

- Take kids on bathroom breaks

- Check diapers, and change them in a bathroom or diaper-changing station to keep pee and poop out of the water

Talk to others

- Tell other swimmers and parents of young swimmers about chloramines and the steps they can take to help prevent them

- Encourage pool operators to take steps known to prevent and get rid of chloramines

- Tell the lifeguard or pool operator immediately if you or your family or friends:

  - See poop in the water.

  - Smell chemical odors in the swimming area.

  - Experience respiratory, eye, or skin irritation that could be linked to the water or the air surrounding the water.

Chapter 19

Harmful Algae Blooms (Red Tides)

Chapter Contents

Section 19.1

Harmful Algae Blooms: Facts

This section includes text excerpted from "Harmful
Algal Blooms," National Institute of Environmental
Health Sciences (NIEHS), March 16, 2018.

Facts about Harmful Algal Blooms (HAB)

What Is a Harmful Algal Blooms (HAB)?

A harmful algal bloom (HAB) occurs when toxin-producing algae
grow excessively in a body of water. Algae are microscopic organisms
that live in aquatic environments and use photosynthesis to produce
energy from sunlight, just like plants. The excessive algal growth, or
algal bloom, becomes visible to the naked eye and can be green, blue-
green, red, or brown, depending on the type of algae.

Algae are always present in natural bodies of water like oceans,
lakes, and rivers, but only a few types can produce toxins. In these
algae, toxin production can be stimulated by environmental factors
such as light, temperature, and nutrient levels. Algal toxins are
released into the surrounding water or air can seriously harm people,
animals, fish, and other parts of the ecosystem.

Why Do HABs Occur?

Scientists know that environmental conditions trigger HABs, such
as warmer water temperatures in the summer and excessive nutrients
from fertilizers or sewage waste brought by runoff, but are still learning more about why HABs occur. As climate change gradually warms
the earth's climate, scientists expect HABs to become more frequent,
wide-ranging, and severe.

How Are People Exposed?

During a HAB, people can get exposed to toxins from fish they catch
and eat, from swimming in or drinking the water, and from the air
they breathe. In recent years, there have been numerous instances

of HABs in lakes that provide drinking water, like Lake Erie. Importantly, cooking contaminated seafood or boiling contaminated water does not destroy the toxins.

People rarely get sick from HAB-related toxins in commercial seafood, however, because state regulators closely monitored fisheries for HABs and close them during blooms.

People can prevent exposure to HABs by following local health advisories regarding the safety of recreationally caught seafood and drinking water sources.

What Are the Health Effects of HAB?

Depending on the type of algae, HABs can cause serious health effects and even death. For example, eating seafood contaminated by toxins from algae called *Alexandrium* can lead to paralytic shellfish poisoning, which can cause paralysis and even death. The algae *Pseudo-nitzschia* produces a toxin called domoic acid that can cause vomiting, diarrhea, confusion, seizures, permanent short-term memory loss, or death when consumed at high levels.

HABs that occur in freshwater, like the Great Lakes and other drinking water sources, are dominated by the cyanobacteria *Microcystis*. This organism produces a liver toxin that can cause gastrointestinal illness as well as liver damage.

As with many environmental exposures, children and the elderly may be especially sensitive to HAB toxins. Populations that rely heavily on seafood are also at risk of long-term health effects from potentially frequent, low-level exposures to HAB toxins.

Other Impacts from HABs

In addition to health concerns, HABs can damage the environment by depleting oxygen in the water, which can cause fish kills, or simply by blocking sunlight from reaching organisms deeper in the water. The economic impacts of HABs to fisheries and recreational areas can also be extensive. Closed fisheries can lose millions of dollars in revenue each week.

Section 19.2

Harmful Algal Bloom-Associated Illnesses

This section includes text excerpted from "Harmful
Algal Bloom-Associated Illnesses," Centers for Disease
Control and Prevention (CDC), December 13, 2017.

Harmful algal blooms (HABs) can produce toxins that cause illness
in people, companion animals (dogs, cats), livestock (sheep, cattle), and
wildlife (including birds and mammals). Exposures to the toxins can
occur when people or animals have direct contact with contaminated
water by:

- Swimming

- Breathing in aerosols (tiny airborne droplets or mist that contain toxins) from recreational activities or wind-blown sea spray

- Swallowing toxins by drinking contaminated water or eating
  contaminated fish or shellfish

- Human and animal illnesses and symptoms can vary depending
  on the how they were exposed, how long they were exposed, and
  the particular HAB toxin involved

Freshwater Environments

In freshwater, a HAB is most commonly caused by small organisms
called phytoplankton. The phytoplankton that commonly causes HABs
are cyanobacteria, which use sunlight to create food. Some cyanobacteria produce toxins called cyanotoxins. Depending on the specific chemical structure, cyanotoxins can be neurotoxins that affect the nervous
system, hepatotoxins that affect the liver, dermatoxins that affect
the skin, or other toxins that affect the stomach or intestines. Some
common cyanotoxins that are known to cause illnesses in humans and
animals are microcystins, cylindrospermopsin, anatoxins, saxitoxins,
nodularins, and lyngbyatoxins.

Human and animal illnesses and symptoms can vary depending
on the how they were exposed, how long they were exposed, and the

particular HAB toxin involved. No human deaths in the United States have been caused by cyanotoxins; however, companion animal, livestock, and wildlife deaths caused by cyanotoxins have been reported throughout the United States and the world.

Humans and Freshwater HAB-Associated Illnesses

Skin Contact and Inhalation

People or animals can be directly exposed to cyanotoxins in freshwater during recreational activities or by breathing in aerosolized toxins (toxins in water turned into tiny airborne droplets or mist). People or animals exposed to cyanotoxins through direct skin contact or inhalation may experience the following symptoms:

- Skin irritation
- Eye irritation
- Nose irritation
- Throat irritation
- Respiratory irritation

Ingestion

People can be exposed to cyanotoxins by eating freshwater fish from cyanotoxin-contaminated lakes or ponds or by drinking cyanotoxin-contaminated water. Additionally, some toxins may be ingested when taking blue-green algae dietary supplements. People who ingest cyanotoxins may experience the following symptoms:

- Abdominal pain
- A headache
- Neurological symptoms
- Vomiting
- Diarrhea
- Liver damage
- Kidney damage

Animals and Freshwater HAB-Associated Illnesses

Pets, Livestock, and Wildlife

Pets, livestock, and wildlife can be poisoned through direct contact by swimming in waters with a HAB or by drinking cyanotoxin-contaminated water. Coyote deaths have been reported after they were believed to have eaten fish that washed up on the beach from a part of the Gulf of Mexico that was experiencing a HAB. Dogs are especially at risk to cyanotoxin poisoning due to their behaviors, which include swimming in contaminated waters, drinking the water, and licking algae or scum from their fur after swimming. Domestic pets may also be poisoned if they eat dietary supplements that contain algae contaminated with cyanotoxins.

A HAB may also make birds sick. Side effects of cyanotoxin poisoning in birds are sometimes confused with or occur at the same time with, avian botulism, a disease that paralyzes birds. Birds can get avian botulism when they eat toxins produced by the bacteria *Clostridium botulinum* directly or eat insects containing the toxins. Avian botulism is becoming more common in the Great Lakes region since it was first reported in 1963, and there is some evidence that *Clostridium botulinum* can grow in the presence of algae commonly found in the Great Lakes region.

Animals who are exposed to cyanotoxins may experience the following symptoms:

- Excessive salivation
- Vomiting
- Fatigue
- Staggered walking
- Difficulty breathing
- Convulsions
- Liver Failure
- Death
- Death in animals can occur within hours to days of exposure

Fish and Aquatic Animals

When a HAB decomposes, it can use up the oxygen in a body of water. When this happens, fish may not have enough oxygen to breathe and may die. Fish and other aquatic animals (vertebrates or invertebrates that live in the water) may also eat cyanobacteria, storing the cyanotoxins in their bodies. When other animals eat these animals (for example, when small fish are eaten by larger fish), the toxins can build up and move up the food web. This process is called bioaccumulation. Some cyanotoxins can also kill fish by affecting their gills and preventing fish from breathing.

Marine Environments

Marine or saltwater HAB toxins can cause a variety of illnesses in humans and animals. Exposure to marine HAB toxins can occur through direct contact with swimming, breathing in aerosolized toxins (toxins in water turned into tiny airborne droplets or mist), or eating toxin-contaminated shellfish or finfish. In marine mammals, fish, and other aquatic marine life, exposure to HAB toxins can cause widespread illness or death. However, most states at risk for marine HABs have excellent monitoring programs in place to close harvesting when toxins are present in shellfish. Birds can also get sick by eating algae, drinking contaminated water, or eating contaminated marine fish or shellfish. For example, pelicans and cormorants have been poisoned by exposure to these toxins, and, in some cases, thousands of birds have died.

Marine HABs have occurred in the Gulf of Mexico and along the Atlantic and Pacific coasts of the United States. Two major groups of marine phytoplankton, diatoms and dinoflagellates, produce HAB toxins. Some common marine HAB toxins include brevetoxins, azaspiracid, ciguatoxins, domoic acid, okadic acid, saxitoxin, and dinophysistoxins.

Humans and Marine Water-Associated Illnesses

Skin Contact and Inhalation

Marine HABs can cause a variety of illnesses in people. Florida red tides, the most well-known marine HABs in the United States, occur frequently in the Gulf of Mexico. Florida red tides are caused by the dinoflagellate *Karenia brevis*, which can produce toxins called brevetoxins. *Karenia brevis* breaks up easily in ocean waves. When this happens, toxins inside the algae can become incorporated into aerosols that winds blow across the water and inland. People can then be exposed by breathing in these aerosols. People can also be exposed to brevetoxins through skin contact. Human exposure to brevetoxins via inhalation or skin contact can cause various symptoms, including the following:

- Respiratory irritation (coughing, sneezing)
- Shortness of breath
- Throat irritation
- Eye irritation
- Skin irritation

Ingestion: Eating Contaminated Seafood and Marine Toxin Poisoning

Marine HAB toxins can build up in seafood when fish or shellfish eat toxin-producing algae. Humans and animals that eat these contaminated fish or shellfish can become poisoned from HAB toxins, making them sick. Most human illnesses from HABs occur when people eat contaminated seafood. Symptoms of HAB toxin poisoning can vary depending on the type of toxin. Marine toxins and toxin poisoning information are listed below.

Note: Most states at risk for marine HABs have excellent monitoring programs in place to close harvesting when toxins are present in shellfish.

Ciguatera Fish Poisoning (CFP)

The most commonly reported illness caused by a HAB toxin in food is ciguatera fish poisoning (CFP). CFP is caused by eating fish with ciguatera toxins or ciguatoxins produced by a dinoflagellate species, *Gambierdiscus toxicus*. The dinoflagellates are eaten by plant-eating fish that are then eaten by fish-eating fish. As the toxins move through the food web, they change and become poisonous. The toxins can build up in both fish- and plant-eating reef fish in tropical and subtropical waters, such as those found around Hawaii, Puerto Rico, South Florida, and the Gulf of Mexico. When these fish are eaten, the ciguatoxins can cause stomach and intestinal symptoms, including the following:

- Diarrhea
- Abdominal pain
- Nausea
- Vomiting

These symptoms often start within 12–24 hours of eating the contaminated fish and might last for up to 4 days. Stomach and intestinal symptoms might be followed by or accompanied by symptoms related to the heart, blood vessels, and nerves, including:

- Numbness and tingling in the extremities
- Dizziness
- Muscle aches
- Decreased heart rate

- Low blood pressure

- Weakness

- Heightened response to hot or cold temperatures

Symptoms have been reported to last anywhere from a few weeks to years. However, newer information suggests that symptoms of CFP typically go away within months and may be confused with symptoms of other chronic conditions.

Neurotoxic Shellfish Poisoning (NSP)

Neurotoxic Shellfish Poisoning (NSP) is caused by eating shellfish contaminated with brevetoxins, a toxin produced by a dinoflagellate species Karenia brevis. These toxins can be spread throughout the marine food web and have been found in shellfish, including oysters, clams, and mussels. This toxin is most commonly found in shellfish from the Gulf of Mexico but has also been found in shellfish from the in Mid-Atlantic waters.

Symptoms of NSP are often related to the stomach, intestines, and nervous system. Symptoms begin 1–3 hours after eating the contaminated shellfish and can include the following:

- Numbness

- Tingling in the mouth, arms, and legs

- Loss of coordination

- Vomiting

- Diarrhea

- Heightened response to hot or cold temperatures

Symptoms usually resolve in 2–3 days. There have been no reports of long-term effects from NSP, but there have been no follow-up studies of patients to confirm this.

Paralytic Shellfish Poisoning (PSP)

Paralytic shellfish poisoning (PSP) is caused by eating shellfish contaminated with saxitoxins, a toxin produced by dinoflagellates of the genus *Alexandrium*. Saxitoxins, also known as PSP toxins, cause symptoms related to the nervous system. PSP toxins can be found in shellfish (such as mussels, cockles, clams, scallops, oysters, crabs, and lobsters) that usually live in the colder coastal waters near the Pacific states and New England. A species of puffer fish found off the east coast of Florida was recently discovered that also contained saxitoxins.

Symptoms usually begin within 2 hours of eating contaminated shellfish but can start anywhere from 15 minutes to 10 hours after the meal. Symptoms are generally mild and can include the following:

- Numbness or tingling of the face, arms, and legs

- A headache

- Dizziness

- Nausea

- Loss of coordination

- A floating sensation

- Muscle paralysis and respiratory failure can occur in severe cases

In cases of severe poisoning, muscle paralysis and respiratory failure can lead to death in 2–25 hours. The risk of death from PSP is reduced if healthcare professionals have access to machines to help people breathe (ventilators) if the ill person becomes paralyzed.

There are no reports of long-term effects, but there have not been any long-term follow-up studies of those affected.

Domoic Acid Poisoning and Amnesiac Shellfish Poisoning (ASP)

Domoic acid poisoning is caused by eating shellfish contaminated with domoic acid, a toxin produced by the diatoms *Pseudo-nitzschia, Nitzschia,* and *Amphora.* These diatoms have been found in the United States along the Pacific coast, northeast coast, and the western coast of Florida.

Domoic acid poisoning has caused a variety of symptoms ranging from memory loss to death. The first reported human domoic acid poisoning event occurred in Canada in 1987 when 143 people became ill and 3 died from eating domoic acid-contaminated mussels. Reported signs of the poisoning were stomach and intestinal symptoms, confusion, disorientation, memory loss, coma, and death. The illness was named Amnesic Shellfish Poisoning (ASP).

Most of what is known about domoic acid poisoning comes from studies of marine mammals, particularly sea lions. Domoic acid-poisoned animals, including marine mammals (seals, walruses, and sea lions), may exhibit neurotoxic effects, and the poisonings can be fatal.

Shellfish, such as mussels, can accumulate these toxins, making people who eat them sick with various symptoms, including the following:

- Vomiting and diarrhea within 24 hours of eating

- Dizziness

- A headache

- Disorientation

- Short-term memory loss

- Seizures, weakness, paralysis, and death can occur in severe cases

Diarrhetic Shellfish Poisoning (DSP)

Diarrhetic Shellfish Poisoning (DSP) is caused by eating shellfish contaminated with okadic acid and dinophysistoxins, toxins produced by the dinoflagellates *Dinophysis* and *Procentrum*. In the United States, these dinoflagellates have recently been found along the Gulf Coast of Texas.

DSP produces stomach and intestinal symptoms that usually begin 30 minutes to a few hours after eating contaminated shellfish and include:

- Vomiting

- Severe diarrhea

- Nausea

- Abdominal cramps

- Chills

Recovery occurs within about 3 days, with or without medical treatment. DSP is generally not life-threatening.

Azaspiracid Shellfish Poisoning (AZP)

Azaspiracid Shellfish Poisoning (AZP) is the most recently discovered human illness related to shellfish contaminated with a HAB toxin. AZP is believed to be caused by a dinoflagellate that produces toxins that have been found in Ireland, the Netherlands, Belgium, Morocco, and eastern Canada.

Eating contaminated shellfish can result in symptoms including:

- Nausea

- Vomiting

- Diarrhea

- Stomach cramps

Section 19.3

Harmful Algal Bloom: Prevention and Control

This section includes text excerpted from "Harmful Algal Bloom-Associated Illnesses," Centers for Disease Control and Prevention (CDC), December 13, 2017.

Harmful algal blooms (HABs) can produce toxins that cause illness in people, companion animals (dogs, cats), livestock (sheep, cattle), and wildlife (including birds and mammals). Exposures to the toxins can occur when people or animals have direct contact with contaminated water by:

- Swimming

- Breathing in aerosols (tiny airborne droplets or mist that contain toxins) from recreational activities or wind-blown sea spray

- Swallowing toxins by drinking contaminated water or eating contaminated fish or shellfish

- Human and animal illnesses and symptoms can vary depending on the how they were exposed, how long they were exposed, and the particular HAB toxin involved

How to Reduce Exposures and Prevent Illness

Preventing Freshwater Exposures

- Do not drink directly from lakes, rivers, or ponds. Even if the water looks "safe," it might contain toxins or germs that can cause other types of illness.

- Check your state or local environmental health website for beach or lake closures in your area before visiting.

- Do not fish, swim, boat, or play water sports in areas that are experiencing a HAB. Do not let pets eat algae, get in the water, or go to the beach or shoreline.

- Rinse pets off with tap water after they have been in a lake, river, or pond; do not let them lick their fur until they have been rinsed.

- Do not fill pools with water directly from lakes, rivers, or ponds, as the water might contain toxins or germs that can cause other types of illness.

Preventing Marine (Salt) Water Exposures

Check your state or local environmental health website for beach closures in your area before visiting.

- Do not fish, swim, boat, or play water sports in marine waters that are experiencing a HAB. Do not let pets eat algae, get in the water, or go on the beach or shoreline during a HAB.

- Rinse pets off with tap water after they have been in the ocean; do not let them lick their fur until they have been rinsed.

- Avoid eating very large reef fish (especially the head, gut, liver, or roe).

- Follow local guidance if you plan to eat any fish or shellfish that you harvest yourself.

Preventing HABs

Many large-scale efforts around the country are underway to reduce the occurrence of HABs, mainly by decreasing the number of nutrients such as nitrogen and phosphorus that flow into our waters.

The Great Lakes Restoration Initiative (GLRI) has made it a priority to reduce phosphorus runoff in three major watersheds across four states: Indiana, Michigan, Ohio, and Wisconsin. In addition, the U.S. Environmental Protection Agency (EPA), along with six other federal agencies, six states, and the District of Columbia, have collaborated to develop strategies to reduce nutrient inputs into the Chesapeake Bay.

To reduce the occurrence of HABs in your neighborhood:

- Use only the recommended amount of fertilizers in your yard. This will reduce extra nutrients from running off into nearby water bodies.

- Maintain your septic system to prevent wastewater from leaking and seeping into nearby lakes and ponds. Wastewater is filled with nutrients that are food for algae.

What Should I Do If I Have Been Exposed?

If you have any questions about symptoms that you are experiencing, call you're local or state poison information center. The specialists might be able to provide information about HAB-associated illnesses.

Consult a healthcare provider for advice on how to relieve your symptoms. If you do consult a healthcare provider, please let them know that you might have been exposed to a HAB or that you have recently consumed fresh or marine water fish or shellfish that might have been contaminated with toxins. There are currently no available tests or special treatments for HAB-associated illnesses, but information about the suspected cause of your illness might help your healthcare provider to manage symptoms.

Contact your local or state health department if you suspect there is a HAB. Some local and state health departments have web forms or hotlines for reporting suspected HAB-associated illnesses directly to the health department.

What Should I Do If My Pet Has Been Exposed?

If your pet has come into contact water that has an algal bloom, rinse them with tap water as soon as possible.

Seek veterinary care immediately if your pet has consumed or licked algae on its fur after swimming or playing in water that has an algal bloom.

While no HAB-associated human deaths have been reported in the United States, many pet deaths (especially dogs) have been reported after the animal swam in or drank from water bodies with ongoing cyanobacteria blooms. Between 2007–2011, thirteen states reported 67 cases of cyanobacteria toxin-related illness in dogs to Centers for Disease Control and Prevention (CDC). Over half (58%) of these cases resulted in death. Also, there were anecdotal reports of dogs becoming ill after eating foam washed up on a beach during a Florida red tide (Karenia brevis bloom).

Chapter 20

Soil Contamination

Chapter Contents

Section 20.1

Pesticides

This section contains text excerpted from the following sources: Text
in this section begins with excerpts from "Pesticide Exposures,"
Centers for Disease Control and Prevention (CDC), January 10, 2017;
Text beginning with the heading "Pesticides and Public Health"
is excerpted from "Pesticides—Pesticides and Public Health," U.S.
Environmental Protection Agency (EPA), December 13, 2017.

The term pesticide applies to insecticides, herbicides, fungicides, disinfectants, and various other substances that are used to kill, repel, or control any plant or animal life considered to be a pest. Pests are living organisms that occur where they are not wanted or that cause damage to crops or humans or other animals.

When used properly, pesticides may offer a variety of benefits. They may increase crop production, preserve produce, combat insect infestations, and control exotic species. However, pesticides also have the potential for causing harm. In the United States, about 1.1 billion pounds of pesticide active ingredient are used each year and over 20,000 pesticide products are on the market. In 2012, pesticides were the tenth leading cause of poisoning exposure reported to poison control centers in the United States.

People may be exposed to pesticides used in homes, schools, hospitals, and workplaces. Many familiar household products are pesticides, e.g., insect repellents, cleaning products, and weed killers. Because of the widespread use of agricultural chemicals in food production, people are exposed to low levels of pesticides through residues in foods and contaminated drinking water. Scientists do not yet have a clear understanding of the chronic health effects of pesticide exposures.

The National Environmental Public Health Tracking Network (Tracking Network) has data for the following types of pesticides:

- Disinfectants

- Fumigants

- Fungicides

- Herbicides

- Insecticides

- Repellents

- Rodenticides

Pesticides and Public Health

This section focuses on public health problems caused by pests and the role that preventive measures and pesticides may play in protecting people from these health problems.

Why be concerned. Pests such as insects, rodents, and microbes can cause and spread a variety of diseases that pose a serious risk to public health.

What YOU can do. There are a variety of ways that you can control pests and the risks they may pose.

Public Health Issues and Pests

Debilitating and deadly diseases that can be caused or spread by pests such as insects, rodents and microbes pose a serious risk to public health. Examples of significant public health problems that are caused by pests include:

- **Vector-borne diseases.** Infectious diseases such as West Nile virus (WNV), Lyme disease, and rabies can be carried and spread by vectors (disease-carrying) species such as mosquitoes, ticks, and rodents. The U.S. Environmental Protection Agency (EPA) registers several pesticide products, including repellents, that may be used to control the vectors that spread these diseases.

  - Controlling mosquitoes

  - Rodents and rodenticides

  - Insect repellents

- **Asthma and allergies.** Indoor household pests such as cockroaches can contribute to asthma and allergies. In addition to registering products to control these pests, the EPA also provides information to the public about safely using these products in homes and schools.

  - Cockroaches

  - Controlling pests at home

  - Controlling pests at school

- **Microbial contamination.** Various microorganisms, including bacteria, viruses, and protozoans, can cause microbial contamination in hospitals, public health clinics, and food processing facilities. The EPA registers antimicrobial products intended to control these microorganisms and help prevent the spread of numerous diseases.

  - Registration of antimicrobial pesticides

  - Antimicrobial products registered for specific uses

  - Efficacy requirements for antimicrobial pesticides

- **Avian flu.** Avian flu, sometimes called bird flu, is an infection that occurs naturally and chiefly in birds. Infections with these viruses can occur in humans, but the risk is generally low for most people. The EPA works to register and make available antimicrobial pesticide products (sanitizers or disinfectants) that may be used to kill avian influenza virus on inanimate surfaces and to help prevent the spread of avian flu viruses. These products are typically used by the poultry industry to disinfect their facilities.

- **Prions.** Certain proteins found in cells of the central nervous system of humans and animals may exist in abnormal, infectious forms called "prions." Prions share many characteristics of viruses and may cause fatal diseases.

- **Anthrax.** Biological agents such as *Bacillus anthracis* spores can cause a threat to public health and national security. EPA has issued emergency exemptions for several pesticides that were used in anthrax spore decontamination efforts, including (but not limited to):

  - bleach

  - chlorine dioxide

  - ethylene oxide

  - hydrogen peroxide and peroxyacetic acid

  - methyl bromide

  - paraformaldehyde

  - vaporized hydrogen peroxide

Safely Control Pests and Protect Your Health

EPA, along with the Centers for Disease Control and Prevention (CDC) and many pest control professionals, believes that prevention is the most effective way to control disease-carrying pests and their associated public health risks. The combination of preventive measures and reduced-risk treatment methods to reduce the reliance on, and therefore, the corresponding risk from, the use of chemical pesticides is generally known as integrated pest management (IPM).

Prevent Pests

Pests such as cockroaches, rodents, and mosquitoes need food, water, and shelter. Often, problems involving these pests can be solved just by removing these key items. Some actions you can take to reduce or prevent pest problems include:

- Making sure food and food scraps are tightly sealed and garbage is regularly removed from the home

- Not leaving pet food and water out overnight. Also, if you apply pesticides, pet food and water should be removed from the area.

- Fixing leaky plumbing and looking for other sources of water, such as trays under houseplants

- Eliminating standing water in rain gutters, buckets, plastic covers, bird baths, fountains, wading pools, potted plant trays, or any other containers where mosquitoes can breed

- Keeping swimming pool water treated and circulating, and draining temporary pools of water or filling them with dirt

- Closing off entryways and hiding places (e.g., caulking cracks and crevices around cabinets or baseboards)

- Making sure window and door screens are "bug tight"

- Replacing your outdoor lights with yellow "bug" lights which tend to attract fewer mosquitoes than ordinary lights. However, the yellow lights are NOT repellents.

Safely Use Pesticide Products

In addition to preventive measures, traps, bait stations, and other pesticide products (including repellents) can be used to control some pests. These can be used with low risk of exposure to the pesticide, as long as they are kept out of the reach of children and pets and used according to label directions. For assistance choosing an appropriate pest control product:

- Consult your local cooperative extension service office.

- Contact the National Pesticide Information Center (NPIC).

- Find insect repellent products.

Pesticides with public health uses are intended to limit the potential for disease, but in order to be effective, they must be properly applied. By their nature, many pesticides may pose some risk to humans, animals, or the environment because they are designed to kill or otherwise adversely affect living organisms. Safely using pesticides depends on using the appropriate pesticide and using it correctly.

The pesticide label is essential to using a pesticide safely and effectively. It contains important information that must be read and followed when using a pesticide product.

Tips for Hiring a Pest Control Professional

If you have a pest issue that you are uncomfortable dealing with yourself, you may wish to hire a pest control professional.

- Choose a pest control company carefully. Firms offering pest control services must be licensed by your state. Ask to see the company's license and, if you have any concerns, call your state pesticide regulatory agency.

- Hire a pest control service.

- EPA's Citizen's *Guide to Pest Control and Pesticide Safety* offers more tips on how to choose a pest control company.

- For additional assistance and tips on locating and hiring a pest control professional in your area, contact: NPIC, Call 1-800-858-7378, send an e-mail to npic@ace.orst.edu.

- The National Pest Management Association (NPMA): Call (703) 352-6762, send an e-mail to info@pestworld.org.

Regulation of Pesticides with Public Health Uses

EPA is responsible under the (FIFRA) and the Food Quality Protection Act (FQPA) for regulating pesticides with public health uses, as well as ensuring that these products do not pose unintended or unreasonable risks to humans, animals, and the environment.

- **Registration.** Through registration, EPA evaluates pesticides to ensure that they can be used effectively without posing unreasonable risks to human health and the environment.

- **Re-registration.** Under reregistration and tolerance reassessment, EPA reviewed older pesticides (those registered before November 1984) to ensure that they meet current scientific and regulatory standards. It completed re-registration in 2008.

- **Registration review.** Through registration review, EPA plans to review all registered pesticides approximately every 15 years to ensure that they meet current scientific and regulatory standards.

- **Emergency exemptions and special local needs.** In cases where unexpected public health issues arise, EPA works to make pesticides available to states or federal agencies for emergency and special local need uses.

Although pesticides with public health users follow the same regulatory process as agricultural chemicals, EPA recognizes that there may be some differences, including:

- **Exposure.** Pesticide use as part of a public health program may lead to increased exposure for large segments of the population, including exposure to sensitive subpopulations. EPA carefully evaluates human and ecological risks from exposure to pesticides, including a bystander and occupational exposure. EPA places special emphasis on children's health in making regulatory decisions about all pesticides, including pesticides with public health uses.

- **Efficacy.** EPA requires scientific evidence that registered products sold to control pests that are known to carry WNV, Lyme disease, and other vector-borne public health threats are effective against the target pest.

- **Benefits.** EPA considers the benefits from public health pesticides when making regulatory decisions. The benefits information is supplied by many different stakeholders, including our federal partners. CDC is an important source of benefits information for public health pesticides EPA and CDC entered into an agreement in 2000 to formalize this relationship.

Section 20.2

Landfills

This section includes text excerpted from "Basic
Information about Landfills," U.S. Environmental
Protection Agency (EPA), February 14, 2018.

Modern landfills are well engineered and managed facilities for the
disposal of solid waste. Landfills are located, designed, operated and
monitored to ensure compliance with federal regulations. They are
also designed to protect the environment from contaminants, which
may be present in the waste stream. Landfills cannot be built in environmentally sensitive areas, and they are placed using on-site environmental monitoring systems. These monitoring systems check for
any sign of groundwater contamination and for landfill gas, as well as
provide additional safeguards. Landfills must meet stringent design,
operation, and closure requirements established under the Resource
Conservation and Recovery Act (RCRA).

Disposing of waste in landfills is one part of an integrated waste
management system. The U.S. Environmental Protection Agency
(EPA) encourages communities to consider the waste management
hierarchy—favoring source reduction to reduce both the volume and
toxicity of waste and to increase the useful life of manufactured products—when designing waste management systems.

Types of Landfills

Landfills are regulated under RCRA Subtitle D (solid waste) and
Subtitle C (hazardous waste) or under the Toxic Substances Control
Act (TSCA).

Subtitle D focuses on state and local governments as the primary
planning, regulating, and implementing entities for the management
of nonhazardous solid waste, such as household garbage and nonhazardous industrial solid waste. Subtitle D landfills include the following:

- **Municipal solid waste landfills (MSWLFs).** Specifically
  designed to receive household waste, as well as other types of
  nonhazardous wastes.

- **Bioreactor Landfills.** A type of MSWLF that operates to rapidly transform and degrade organic waste.

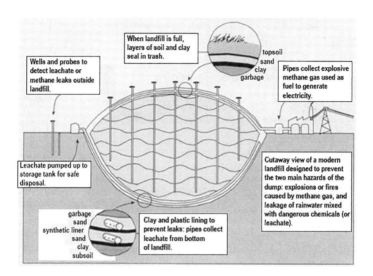

Figure 20.1. *Municipal Solid Waste Landfill* (Source: "Municipal Solid Waste Landfills," U.S. Environmental Protection Agency (EPA).)

- **Industrial waste landfill.** Designed to collect commercial and institutional waste (i.e., industrial waste), which is often a significant portion of solid waste, even in small cities and suburbs.

  - **Construction and demolition (C and D) debris landfill.** A type of industrial waste landfill designed exclusively for construction and demolition materials, which consists of the debris generated during the construction, renovation, and demolition of buildings, roads, and bridges. C and D materials often contain bulky, heavy materials, such as concrete, wood, metals, glass, and salvaged building components.

  - **Coal combustion residual (CCR) landfills.** An industrial waste landfill used to manage and dispose of coal combustion residuals (CCRs or coal ash). EPA established requirements for the disposal of CCR in landfills and published them in the *Federal Register*, April 17, 2015.

- Subtitle C establishes a federal program to manage hazardous wastes from cradle to grave.

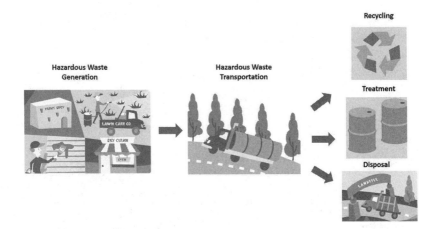

Figure 20.2. *Cradle-to-Grave Hazardous Waste Management System* (Source: "Learn the Basics of Hazardous Waste," U.S. Environmental Protection Agency (EPA).)

The objective of the Subtitle C program is to ensure that hazardous waste is handled in a manner that protects human health and the environment. To this end, there are Subtitle C regulations for the generation, transportation, and treatment, storage or disposal of hazardous wastes. Subtitle C landfills including the following:

- **Hazardous waste landfills.** Facilities used specifically for the disposal of hazardous waste. These landfills are not used for the disposal of solid waste.

- **Polychlorinated Biphenyl (PCB) landfills.** PCBs are regulated by the Toxic Substances Control Act (TSCA). While many PCB decontamination processes do not require EPA approval, some do require approval.

Chapter 21

Bioterrorism and Chemical Emergencies

Bioterrorism: Why It Is a Problem

The word "bioterrorism" refers to biological agents (microbes or toxins) used as weapons to further personal or political agendas. Acts of bioterrorism range from a single exposure directed at an individual by another individual to government sponsored biological warfare resulting in mass casualties. Bioterrorism differs from other methods of terrorism in that the materials needed to make an effective biological agent are readily available, require little specialized knowledge and are inexpensive to produce. Until the aftermath of 9/11, few instances of bioterrorism were documented in the United States.

A bioterrorist attack could be caused by virtually any pathogenic microorganism. The agents of greatest concern are anthrax (a bacterium) and smallpox (a virus). Both can be lethal. Anthrax is not communicable while smallpox is readily transmitted from person to person. In humans, the three forms of anthrax are inhalational, cutaneous

This chapter contains text excerpted from the following sources: Text beginning with the heading "Bioterrorism: Why It Is a Problem" is excerpted from "Bioterrorism," Centers for Disease Control and Prevention (CDC), September 15, 2017; Text beginning with the heading "What Chemical Emergencies Are," is excerpted from "Chemical Emergencies Overview," Centers for Disease Control and Prevention (CDC), November 18, 2015.

and intestinal. Symptoms vary depending upon how the person was exposed but generally occur within 7 days of the exposure. Initial symptoms of inhalational anthrax may resemble the flu. If untreated, symptoms will progress to breathing difficulties and eventual shock. The incubation period for smallpox is 7–17 days following exposure. Symptoms include high fever, fatigue, and head and back pain. A characteristic rash follows in 2–3 days.

Who's at Risk?

In the United States, the risk of contracting anthrax is extremely low. The intentional release of anthrax following the events of 9/11 resulted in only 22 recognized cases of cutaneous and inhalational anthrax. Any risk for inhalational anthrax due to cross-contaminated mail is also very low, even for postal workers. The possibility does exist, however, that if anthrax was dispersed in a public place, a large number of people could be affected. Smallpox has not occurred in the United States since 1949. If the virus was intentionally released, the number of people affected could run to the tens of thousands.

Can It Be Prevented?

Bioterrorism differs from other methods of terrorism in that the effects are not always immediately apparent. An attack may be difficult to distinguish from a naturally occurring infectious disease outbreak. The first evidence of an attack will be in hospital emergency rooms where the proper diagnosis will be essential in treating and preventing the spread of the disease. In the event of intentional anthrax distribution, people at risk should take a 60 day course of prophylactic antibiotics, either doxycycline or ciprofloxacin. Vaccination against smallpox is not recommended to prevent the disease in the general public. In people exposed to smallpox, however, the vaccine can lessen the severity of, or even prevent, illness if given within 4 days of exposure. The United States has a supply of vaccine for emergency use.

The Bottom Line

A story about bioterrorism carries inherent drama but also certain responsibilities. A story can raise concerns and heighten the public's awareness of the topic or it could cause alarm and panic.

And because biological materials are inexpensive and readily available, some thought should be given to whether or not the show will give ideas to potential terrorists. If a person thinks they have been exposed to a biological incident or they suspect a biological threat is planned, they should contact their local health department and/or their local police department. Either of these agencies will promptly notify the Federal Bureau of Investigation (FBI), which is responsible for coordinating interagency investigation of bioterrorism. The symptoms for early inhalational anthrax resemble those of the common cold or flu. Anthrax is diagnosed by isolating B. anthracis from the infected person or through other diagnostic tests. The fatality rate for cutaneous anthrax is about 20 percent; for inhalational anthrax the rate is closer to 75 percent. Smallpox is spread from person to person via airborne saliva droplets. The majority of people infected with smallpox do recover. There is a fatality rate of approximately 30 percent.

Case Examples

- A religious cult has established a base outside town. The cult has applied for a charter to start its own publicly funded school. It's already been voted down once. The charter school is again on the ballot. On election day, hundreds of townspeople become ill and are too sick to get out to vote. In searching the cult headquarters on another matter, a vial of *Salmonella typhimurium* is found. After questioning by the police, one of the cult members reveals that the *salmonella* was used to intentionally contaminate local restaurant salad bars with the aim of limiting the number of people who would vote against the charter school.

- The emergency room (E.R.) is flooded with people experiencing cold and flu symptoms; some people are having difficulty breathing. Police get a phone call from someone claiming they released anthrax in a downtown office building. One of the doctors diagnoses inhalational anthrax. No one on the staff has ever seen a case before. The E.R. is thrown into a panic. Authorities are notified. At shift change, a doctor trained in the Soviet Union comes in and is informed of the case. He has experience with treating anthrax. After viewing a chest X-ray and computed tomography (CT), he's convinced the problem is not anthrax. Cultures come back negative for *B. anthracis,* proving the doctor was correct in his diagnosis.

What Chemical Emergencies Are

A chemical emergency occurs when a hazardous chemical has been released and the release has the potential for harming people's health. Chemical releases can be unintentional, as in the case of an industrial accident, or intentional, as in the case of a terrorist attack.

Where Hazardous Chemicals Come From

Some chemicals that are hazardous have been developed by military organizations for use in warfare. Examples are nerve agents such as sarin and venomous agent X (VX), mustards such as sulfur mustards and nitrogen mustards, and choking agents such as phosgene. It might be possible for terrorists to get these chemical warfare agents and use them to harm people.

Many hazardous chemicals are used in industry (for example, chlorine, ammonia, and benzene). Others are found in nature (for example, poisonous plants). Some could be made from everyday items such as household cleaners. These types of hazardous chemicals also could be obtained and used to harm people, or they could be accidentally released.

Types and Categories of Hazardous Chemicals

Scientists often categorize hazardous chemicals by the type of chemical or by the effects a chemical would have on people exposed to it. The categories/types used by the Centers for Disease Control and Prevention (CDC) are as follows:

- **Biotoxins**—poisons that come from plants or animals

- **Blister agents/vesicants**—chemicals that severely blister the eyes, respiratory tract, and skin on contact

- **Blood agents**—poisons that affect the body by being absorbed into the blood

- **Caustics (acids)**—chemicals that burn or corrode people's skin, eyes, and mucus membranes (lining of the nose, mouth, throat, and lungs) on contact

- **Choking/lung/pulmonary agents**—chemicals that cause severe irritation or swelling of the respiratory tract (lining of the nose and throat, lungs)

- **Incapacitating agents**—drugs that make people unable to think clearly or that cause an altered state of consciousness (possibly unconsciousness)

- **Long-acting anticoagulants**—poisons that prevent blood from clotting properly, which can lead to uncontrolled bleeding

- **Metals**—agents that consist of metallic poisons

- **Nerve agents**—highly poisonous chemicals that work by preventing the nervous system from working properly

- **Organic solvents**—agents that damage the tissues of living things by dissolving fats and oils

- **Riot control agents/tear gas**—highly irritating agents normally used by law enforcement for crowd control or by individuals for protection (for example, mace)

- **Toxic alcohols**—poisonous alcohols that can damage the heart, kidneys, and nervous system

- **Vomiting agents**—chemicals that cause nausea and vomiting

Protecting Yourself If You Don't Know What the Chemical Is

You could protect yourself during a chemical emergency, even if you didn't know yet what chemical had been released.

Chemical Agents: Facts about Evacuation

Some kinds of chemical accidents or attacks, such as a train derailment or a terrorist incident, may make staying put dangerous. In such cases, it may be safer for you to evacuate, or leave the immediate area. You may need to go to an emergency shelter after you leave the immediate area.

How to Know If You Need to Evacuate

You will hear from the local police, emergency coordinators, or government on the radio and/or television emergency broadcast system if you need to evacuate.

If there is a "code red" or "severe" terror alert, you should pay attention to radio and/or television broadcasts so you will know right away if an evacuation order is made for your area.

Every emergency is different and during any emergency people may have to evacuate or to shelter in place depending on where they live.

What to Do

Act quickly and follow the instructions of local emergency coordinators, such as law enforcement personnel, fire departments, or local elected leaders. Every situation can be different, so local coordinators could give you special instructions to follow for a particular situation.

Local emergency coordinators may direct people to evacuate homes or offices and go to an emergency shelter. If so, emergency coordinators will tell you how to get to the shelter. If you have children in school, they may be sheltered at the school. You should not try to get to the school if the children are being sheltered there. Transporting them from the school will put them, and you, at increased risk.

The emergency shelter will have most supplies that people need. The emergency coordinators will tell you which supplies to bring with you, but you may also want to prepare a portable supply kit. Be sure to bring any medications you are taking.

If you have time, call a friend or relative in another state to tell them where you are going and that you are safe. Local telephone lines may be jammed in an emergency, so you should plan ahead to have an out-of-state contact with whom to leave messages. If you do not have private transportation, make plans in advance of an emergency to identify people who can give you a ride.

Evacuating and sheltering in this way should keep you safer than if you stayed at home or at your workplace. You will most likely not be in the shelter for more than a few hours. Emergency coordinators will let you know when it is safe to leave the shelter and anything you may need to do to make sure it is safe to re-enter your home.

Chemical Agents: Facts about Sheltering in Place

What "Sheltering in Place" Means

Some kinds of chemical accidents or attacks may make going outdoors dangerous. Leaving the area might take too long or put you in harm's way. In such a case it may be safer for you to stay indoors than to go outside.

"Shelter in place" means to make a shelter out of the place you are in. It is a way for you to make the building as safe as possible to protect yourself until help arrives. You should not try to shelter in a vehicle unless you have no other choice. Vehicles are not airtight enough to give you adequate protection from chemicals.

Every emergency is different and during any emergency people may have to evacuate or to shelter in place depending on where they live.

How to Prepare to Shelter in Place

Choose a room in your house or apartment for the shelter. The best room to use for the shelter is a room with as few windows and doors as possible. A large room with a water supply is best—something like a master bedroom that is connected to a bathroom. For most chemical events, this room should be as high in the structure as possible to avoid vapors (gases) that sink. This guideline is different from the sheltering in place technique used in tornadoes and other severe weather and for nuclear or radiological events, when the shelter should be low in the home.

You might not be at home if the need to shelter in place ever arises, but if you are at home, the following items, many of which you may already have, would be good to have in your shelter room:

- First aid kit
- Flashlight, battery-powered radio, and extra batteries for both
- A working telephone
- Food and bottled water. Store 1 gallon of water per person in plastic bottles as well as ready to eat foods that will keep without refrigeration in the shelter in place room. If you do not have bottled water, or if you run out, you can drink water from a toilet tank (not from a toilet bowl). Do not drink water from the tap.
- Duct tape and scissors
- Towels and plastic sheeting. You may wish to cut your plastic sheeting to fit your windows and doors before any emergency occurs.

How to Know If You Need to Shelter in Place

Most likely you will only need to shelter for a few hours.

- If there is a "code red" or "severe" terror alert, you should pay attention to radio and television broadcasts to know right away whether a shelter in place alert is announced for your area

- You will hear from the local police, emergency coordinators, or government on the radio and on television emergency broadcast system if you need to shelter in place

What to Do

Act quickly and follow the instructions of your local emergency coordinators such as law enforcement personnel, fire departments, or local elected leaders. Every situation can be different, so local emergency coordinators might have special instructions for you to follow. In general, do the following:

- Go inside as quickly as possible. Bring any outdoor pets indoors.

- If there is time, shut and lock all outside doors and windows. Locking them may pull the door or window tighter and make a better seal against the chemical. Turn off the air conditioner or heater. Turn off all fans, too. Close the fireplace damper and any other place that air can come in from outside.

- Go in the shelter in place room and shut the door.

- Turn on the radio. Keep a telephone close at hand, but don't use it unless there is a serious emergency.

- Sink and toilet drain traps should have water in them (you can use the sink and toilet as you normally would). If it is necessary to drink water, drink stored water, not water from the tap.

- Tape plastic over any windows in the room. Use duct tape around the windows and doors and make an unbroken seal. Use the tape over any vents into the room and seal any electrical outlets or other openings.

- If you are away from your shelter in place location when a chemical event occurs, follow the instructions of emergency coordinators to find the nearest shelter. If your children are at school, they will be sheltered there. Unless you are instructed to do so, do not try to get to the school to bring your children home. Transporting them from the school will put them, and you, at increased risk.

- Listen to the radio for an announcement indicating that it is safe to leave the shelter.

- When you leave the shelter, follow instructions from local emergency coordinators to avoid any contaminants outside. After you come out of the shelter, emergency coordinators may have additional instructions on how to make the rest of the building safe again.

Chemical Agents: Facts About Personal Cleaning and Disposal of Contaminated Clothing

Some kinds of chemical accidents or attacks may cause you to come in contact with dangerous chemicals. Coming in contact with a dangerous chemical may make it necessary for you to remove and dispose of your clothing right away and then wash yourself. Removing your clothing and washing your body will reduce or remove the chemical so that it is no longer a hazard. This process is called decontamination.

People are decontaminated for two primary reasons:

1. to prevent the chemical from being further absorbed by their body or from spreading on their body, and

2. to prevent the chemical from spreading to other people, including medical personnel, who must handle or who might come in contact with the person who is contaminated with the chemical.

Most chemical agents can penetrate clothing and are absorbed rapidly through the skin. Therefore, the most important and most effective decontamination for any chemical exposure is decontamination done within the first minute or two after exposure.

How to Know If You Need to Wash Yourself and Dispose of Your Clothing

In most cases, emergency coordinators will let you know if a dangerous chemical has been released and will tell you what to do.

In general, contact exposure to a chemical in its liquid or solid form may require you to remove your clothing and then thoroughly wash your exposed skin. Exposure to a chemical in its vapor (gas) form generally requires you only to remove your clothing and the source of the toxic vapor.

If you think you have been exposed to a chemical release, but you have not heard from emergency coordinators, you can follow the washing and clothing disposal advice in the next section.

What to Do

Act quickly and follow the instructions of local emergency coordinators. Every situation can be different, so local emergency coordinators might have special instructions for you to follow. The three most important things to do if you think you may have been exposed to a dangerous chemical are to:

1. quickly remove your clothing

2. wash yourself

3. dispose of your clothing

Here's how:

- Quickly take off clothing that has a chemical on it. Any clothing that has to be pulled over your head should be cut off instead of being pulled over your head.

- If you are helping other people remove their clothing, try to avoid touching any contaminated areas of clothing, and remove the clothing as quickly as possible.

- As quickly as possible, wash any chemicals from your skin with large amounts of soap and water. Washing with soap and water will help protect you from any chemicals on your body.

- If your eyes are burning or your vision is blurred, rinse your eyes with plain water for 10–15 minutes. If you wear contacts, remove them and put them with the contaminated clothing. Do not put the contacts back in your eyes (even if they are not disposable contacts). If you wear eyeglasses, wash them with soap and water. You can put your eyeglasses back on after you wash them.

- After you have washed yourself, place your clothing inside a plastic bag. Avoid touching contaminated areas of the clothing. If you can't avoid touching contaminated areas, or you aren't sure where the contaminated areas are, wear rubber gloves or put the clothing in the bag using tongs, tool handles, sticks, or similar objects. Anything that touches the contaminated clothing should also be placed in the bag. If you wear contacts, put them in the plastic bag, too.

- Seal the bag, and then seal that bag inside another plastic bag. Disposing of your clothing in this way will help protect you and other people from any chemicals that might be on your clothes.

- When the local or state health department or emergency personnel arrive, tell them what you did with your clothes. The health department or emergency personnel will arrange for further disposal. Do not handle the plastic bags yourself.

After you have removed your clothing, washed yourself, and disposed of your clothing, you should dress in clothing that is not contaminated. Clothing that has been stored in drawers or closets is unlikely to be contaminated, so it would be a good choice for you to wear.

You should avoid coming in contact with other people who may have been exposed but who have not yet changed their clothes or washed. Move away from the area where the chemical was released when emergency coordinators tell you to do so.

Part Four

Household and Indoor Hazards

Chapter 22

Indoor Air Quality

Chapter Contents

Section 22.1

Importance of Indoor Air Quality

This section includes text excerpted from "Indoor Air Quality (IAQ)—
Introduction to Indoor Air Quality," U.S. Environmental Protection
Agency (EPA), January 29, 2018.

Indoor air quality (IAQ) refers to the air quality within and around
buildings and structures, especially as it relates to the health and
comfort of building occupants. Understanding and controlling common
pollutants indoors can help reduce your risk of indoor health concerns.
Health effects from indoor air pollutants may be experienced soon after
exposure or, possibly, years later.

Indoor Air Pollution and Health

Immediate Effects

Some health effects may show up shortly after a single exposure or
repeated exposures to a pollutant. These include irritation of the eyes,
nose, and throat, headaches, dizziness, and fatigue. Such immediate
effects are usually short term and treatable. Sometimes the treatment
is simply eliminating the person's exposure to the source of the pollution, if it can be identified. Soon after exposure to some indoor air
pollutants, symptoms of some diseases such as asthma may show up,
be aggravated or worsened.

The likelihood of immediate reactions to indoor air pollutants
depends on several factors including age and preexisting medical conditions. In some cases, whether a person reacts to a pollutant depends
on individual sensitivity, which varies tremendously from person to
person. Some people can become sensitized to biological or chemical
pollutants after repeated or high-level exposures.

Certain immediate effects are similar to those from colds or other
viral diseases, so it is often difficult to determine if the symptoms
are a result of exposure to indoor air pollution. For this reason, it is
important to pay attention to the time and place symptoms occur. If
the symptoms fade or go away when a person is away from the area,
for example, an effort should be made to identify indoor air sources

that may be possible causes. Some effects may be made worse by an inadequate supply of outdoor air coming indoors or from the heating, cooling or humidity conditions prevalent indoors.

Long-Term Effects

Other health effects may show up either years after exposure has occurred or only after long or repeated periods of exposure. These effects, which include some respiratory diseases, heart disease and cancer, can be severely debilitating or fatal. It is prudent to try to improve the IAQ in your home even if symptoms are not noticeable.

While pollutants commonly found in indoor air can cause many harmful effects, there is considerable uncertainty about what concentrations or periods of exposure are necessary to produce specific health problems. People also react very differently to exposure to indoor air pollutants. Further research is needed to better understand which health effects occur after exposure to the average pollutant concentrations found in homes and which occurs from the higher concentrations that occur for short periods of time.

Section 22.2

Identifying Problems and Improving the Indoor Air Quality

This section contains text excerpted from the following sources: Text in this section begins with excerpts from "Identifying Problems in the Indoor Environments," U.S. Environmental Protection Agency (EPA), December 1, 2017; Text under the heading "Improving Indoor Air Quality" is excerpted from "Improving Indoor Air Quality," U.S. Environmental Protection Agency (EPA), October 14, 2016.

Some health effects can be useful indicators of an indoor air quality (IAQ) problem, especially if they appear after a person moves to a new residence, remodels or refurnishes a home, or treats a home with pesticides. If you think that you have symptoms that may be related to your home environment, discuss them with your doctor or your local health department to see if they could be caused by indoor air pollution. You may also want to consult a board-certified allergist or an occupational medicine specialist for answers to your questions.

Another way to judge whether your home has or could develop indoor air problems is to identify potential sources of indoor air pollution. Although the presence of such sources does not necessarily mean that you have an IAQ problem, being aware of the type and number of potential sources is an important step toward assessing the air quality in your home.

A third way to decide whether your home may have poor IAQ is to look at your lifestyle and activities. Human activities can be significant sources of indoor air pollution. Finally, look for signs of problems with the ventilation in your home. Signs that can indicate your home may not have enough ventilation include:

- moisture condensation on windows or walls

- smelly or stuffy air

- dirty central heating and air cooling equipment

- areas where books, shoes, or other items become moldy

To detect odors in your home, step outside for a few minutes, and then upon re-entering your home, note whether odors are noticeable.

Measuring Radon Levels

The federal government recommends that you measure the level of radon in your home. Without measurements, there is no way to tell whether radon is present because it is a colorless, odorless, radioactive gas. Inexpensive devices are available for measuring radon. There are specific mitigation techniques that have proven effective in reducing levels of radon in the home.

For pollutants other than radon, measurements are most appropriate when there are either health symptoms or signs of poor ventilation and specific sources for pollutants have been identified as possible causes of IAQ problems. Testing for many pollutants can be expensive. Before monitoring your home for pollutants besides radon, consult your state or local health department or professionals who have experience in solving IAQ problems in nonindustrial buildings.

Weatherizing Your Home

The federal government recommends that homes be weatherized in order to reduce the amount of energy needed for heating and cooling. While weatherization is underway, however, steps should also be taken to minimize pollution from sources inside the home. In addition, residents should be alert to the emergence of signs of inadequate ventilation, such as stuffy air, moisture condensation on cold surfaces, or mold and mildew growth. Additional weatherization measures should not be undertaken until these problems have been corrected.

Weatherization generally does not cause indoor air problems by adding new pollutants to the air. (There are a few exceptions, such as caulking, that can sometimes emit pollutants.) However, measures such as installing storm windows, weather stripping, caulking, and blown-in wall insulation can reduce the amount of outdoor air infiltrating into a home. Consequently, after weatherization, concentrations of indoor air pollutants from sources inside the home can increase.

Improving Indoor Air Quality

Source Control

Usually the most effective way to improve IAQ is to eliminate individual sources of pollution or to reduce their emissions.

Some sources, like those that contain asbestos, can be sealed or enclosed; others, like gas stoves, can be adjusted to decrease the amount of emissions. In many cases, source control is also a more cost-efficient approach to protecting IAQ than increasing ventilation because increasing ventilation can increase energy costs.

Ventilation Improvements

Another approach to lowering the concentrations of indoor air pollutants in your home is to increase the amount of outdoor air coming indoors.

Most home heating and cooling systems, including forced air heating systems, do not mechanically bring fresh air into the house. Opening windows and doors, operating window or attic fans, when the weather permits, or running a window air conditioner with the vent control open increases the outdoor ventilation rate. Local bathroom or kitchen fans that exhaust outdoors remove contaminants directly from the room where the fan is located and also increase the outdoor air ventilation rate.

It is particularly important to take as many of these steps as possible while you are involved in short-term activities that can generate high levels of pollutants—for example, painting, paint stripping, heating with kerosene heaters, cooking, or engaging in maintenance and hobby activities such as welding, soldering, or sanding. You might also choose to do some of these activities outdoors, if you can and if weather permits.

Advanced designs of new homes are starting to feature mechanical systems that bring outdoor air into the home. Some of these designs include energy-efficient heat recovery ventilators (also known as air-to-air heat exchangers).

Ventilation and shading can help control indoor temperatures. Ventilation also helps remove or dilute indoor airborne pollutants coming from indoor sources. This reduces the level of contaminants and improves IAQ. Carefully evaluate using ventilation to reduce indoor air pollutants where there may be outdoor sources of pollutants, such as smoke or refuse, nearby.

The introduction of outdoor air is one important factor in promoting good air quality. Air may enter a home in several different ways, including:

- through natural ventilation, such as through windows and doors

- through mechanical means, such as through outdoor air intakes associated with the heating, ventilation, and air conditioning (HVAC) system

- through infiltration, a process by which outdoor air flows into the house through openings, joints and cracks in walls, floors and ceilings, and around windows and doors

Infiltration occurs in all homes to some extent.

Natural ventilation describes air movement through open windows and doors. If used properly natural ventilation can at times help moderate the indoor air temperature, which may become too hot in homes without air-conditioning systems or when power outages or brownouts limit or make the use of air conditioning impossible.

Natural ventilation can also improve IAQ by reducing pollutants that are indoors. Examples of natural ventilation are:

- opening windows and doors

- window shading such as closing the blinds

Most residential forced air-heating systems and air-conditioning systems do not bring outdoor air into the house mechanically, and infiltration and natural ventilation are relied upon to bring outdoor air into the home. Advanced designs for new homes are starting to add a mechanical feature that brings outdoor air into the home through the HVAC system. Some of these designs include energy efficient heat recovery ventilators to mitigate the cost of cooling and heating this air during the summer and winter.

Air Cleaners

There are many types and sizes of air cleaners on the market, ranging from relatively inexpensive table-top models to sophisticated and expensive whole-house systems. Some air cleaners are highly effective at particle removal, while others, including most tabletop models, are much less so. Air cleaners are generally not designed to remove gaseous pollutants.

The effectiveness of an air cleaner depends on how well it collects pollutants from indoor air (expressed as a percentage efficiency rate) and how much air it draws through the cleaning or filtering element (expressed in cubic feet per minute (CFM)).

A very efficient collector with a low air-circulation rate will not be effective, nor will a cleaner with a high air-circulation rate but a less efficient collector. The long-term performance of any air cleaner depends on maintaining it according to the manufacturer's directions.

Another important factor in determining the effectiveness of an air cleaner is the strength of the pollutant source. Table-top air cleaners, in particular, may not remove satisfactory amounts of pollutants from strong nearby sources. People with a sensitivity to particular sources may find that air cleaners are helpful only in conjunction with con- certed efforts to remove the source.

Over the past few years, there has been some publicity suggesting that houseplants have been shown to reduce levels of some chemicals in laboratory experiments. There is currently no evidence, however, that a reasonable number of houseplants remove significant quantities of pollutants in homes and offices. Indoor houseplants should not be over-watered because overly damp soil may promote the growth of microorganisms which can affect allergic individuals.

At present, U.S. Environmental Protection Agency (EPA) does not recommend using air cleaners to reduce levels of radon and its decay products. The effectiveness of these devices is uncertain because they only partially remove the radon decay products and do not diminish the amount of radon entering the home. EPA plans to do additional research on whether air cleaners are, or could become, a reliable means of reducing the health risk from radon.

Chapter 23

Harmful Agents in Indoor Air

Chapter Contents

Section 23.1

Biological Contaminants

This section includes text excerpted from "Indoor Air Quality (IAQ)—Biological Pollutants' Impact on Indoor Air Quality," U.S. Environmental Protection Agency (EPA), November 6, 2017.

Biological contaminants include bacteria, viruses, animal dander and cat saliva, house dust, mites, cockroaches, and pollen. There are many sources of these pollutants. By controlling the relative humidity level in a home, the growth of some sources of biologicals can be minimized. A relative humidity of 30–50 percent is generally recommended for homes. Standing water, water-damaged materials or wet surfaces also serve as a breeding ground for molds, mildews, bacteria, and insects. House dust mites, the source of one of the most powerful biological allergens, grow in damp, warm environments. Other sources are as follows:

- Pollens, which originate from plants

- Viruses, which are transmitted by people and animals

- Mold

- Bacteria, which are carried by people, animals, and soil and plant debris

- Household pets, which are sources of saliva and animal dander (skin flakes)

- Droppings and body parts from cockroaches, rodents, and other pests or insects

- Viruses and bacteria

- The protein in urine from rats and mice is a potent allergen. When it dries, it can become airborne.

- Contaminated central air handling systems can become breeding grounds for mold, mildew, and other sources of biological contaminants and can then distribute these contaminants through the home.

Many of these biological contaminants are small enough to be inhaled. Biological contaminants produced by living things. Biological contaminants are often found in areas that provide food and moisture or water. For example:

- Damp or wet areas such as cooling coils, humidifiers, condensate pans or unvented bathrooms can be moldy

- Draperies, bedding, carpet, and other areas where dust collects may accumulate biological contaminants

Health Effects from Biological Contaminants

Some biological contaminants trigger allergic reactions, including:

- hypersensitivity pneumonitis
- allergic rhinitis
- some types of asthma

Infectious illnesses, such as influenza, measles, and chickenpox are transmitted through the air. Molds and mildews release disease-causing toxins. Symptoms of health problems caused by biological pollutants include:

- sneezing
- watery eyes
- coughing
- shortness of breath
- dizziness
- lethargy
- fever
- digestive problems

Allergic reactions occur only after repeated exposure to a specific biological allergen. However, that reaction may occur immediately upon re-exposure or after multiple exposures over time. As a result, people who have noticed only mild allergic reactions, or no reactions at all, may suddenly find themselves very sensitive to particular allergens.

Some diseases, like humidifier fever, are associated with exposure to toxins from microorganisms that can grow in large building ventilation systems. However, these diseases can also be traced to microorganisms that grow in home heating and cooling systems and humidifiers.

Children, elderly people and people with breathing problems, allergies, and lung diseases are particularly susceptible to disease-causing biological agents in the indoor air.

Mold, dust mites, pet dander, and pest droppings or body parts can trigger asthma. Biological contaminants, including molds and pollens, can cause allergic reactions for a significant portion of the population. Tuberculosis (TB), measles, *staphylococcus* infections, *Legionella*, and influenza are known to be transmitted by air.

Reducing Exposure to Biological Contaminants

General good housekeeping, and maintenance of heating and air conditioning equipment, are very important. Adequate ventilation and good air distribution also help. The key to mold control is moisture control. If mold is a problem, clean up the mold and get rid of excess water or moisture. Maintaining the relative humidity between 30–60 percent will help control mold, dust mites and cockroaches. Employ integrated pest management to control insect and animal allergens. Cooling tower treatment procedures exist to reduce levels of *Legionella* and other organisms.

- **Install and use exhaust fans that are vented to the outdoors in kitchens and bathrooms and vent clothes dryers outdoors.** These actions can eliminate much of the moisture that builds up from everyday activities. There are exhaust fans on the market that produce little noise, an important consideration for some people. Another benefit to using kitchen and bathroom exhaust fans is that they can reduce levels of organic pollutants that vaporize from hot water used in showers and dishwashers.

- **Ventilate the attic and crawl spaces to prevent moisture buildup.** Keeping humidity levels in these areas below 50 percent can prevent water condensation on building materials.

- **If using cool mist or ultrasonic humidifiers, clean appliances according to manufacturer's instructions and refill with fresh water daily.** Because these humidifiers can become breeding grounds for biological contaminants, they have the potential for causing diseases such as hypersensitivity pneumonitis and humidifier fever. Evaporation trays in air conditioners, dehumidifiers, and refrigerators should also be cleaned frequently.

• **Thoroughly clean and dry water-damaged carpets and building materials (within 24 hours if possible) or consider removal and replacement.** Water-damaged carpets and building materials can harbor mold and bacteria. It is very difficult to completely rid such materials of biological contaminants.

• **Keep the house clean. House dust mites, pollens, animal dander and other allergy-causing agents can be reduced, although not eliminated, through regular cleaning.** People who are allergic to these pollutants should use allergen-proof mattress encasements, wash bedding in hot (130°F) water and avoid room furnishings that accumulate dust, especially if they cannot be washed in hot water. Allergic individuals should also leave the house while it is being vacuumed because vacuuming can actually increase airborne levels of mite allergens and other biological contaminants. Using central vacuum systems that are vented to the outdoors or vacuums with high-efficiency filters may also be of help.

• **Take steps to minimize biological pollutants in basements.** Clean and disinfect the basement floor drain regularly. Do not finish a basement below ground level unless all water leaks are patched and outdoor ventilation and adequate heat to prevent condensation are provided. Operate a dehumidifier in the basement if needed to keep relative humidity levels 30 and 50 percent.

Section 23.2

Carbon Monoxide

This section includes text excerpted from "Indoor Air Quality (IAQ)—Carbon Monoxide's Impact on Indoor Air Quality," U.S. Environmental Protection Agency (EPA), August 30, 2017.

Carbon monoxide (CO) is an odorless, colorless, and toxic gas. Because it is impossible to see, taste, or smell the toxic fumes, CO can kill you before you are aware it is in your home. The effects of CO exposure can vary greatly from person to person depending on age, overall health, and the concentration and length of exposure.

Sources of Carbon Monoxide (CO)

Sources of CO include:

- unvented kerosene and gas space heaters

- leaking chimneys and furnaces

- back-drafting from furnaces, gas water heaters, wood stoves, and fireplaces

- gas stoves

- generators and other gasoline powered equipment

- automobile exhaust from attached garages

- tobacco smoke

- auto, truck, or bus exhaust from attached garages, nearby roads, or parking areas

- incomplete oxidation during combustion in gas ranges, and unvented gas or kerosene heaters

- worn or poorly adjusted and maintained combustion devices (e.g., boilers, furnaces)

- if the flue is improperly sized, blocked, or disconnected

- if the flue is leaking

Health Effects Associated with CO

At low concentrations:

- fatigue in healthy people
- chest pain in people with heart disease

At moderate concentrations:

- angina
- impaired vision
- reduced brain function

At higher concentrations:

- impaired vision and coordination
- headaches
- dizziness
- confusion
- nausea
- flu-like symptoms that clear up after leaving home
- fatal at very high concentrations

Acute effects are due to the formation of carboxyhemoglobin (COHb) in the blood, which inhibits oxygen intake.

At low concentrations, fatigue in healthy people and chest pain in people with heart disease. At higher concentrations, impaired vision and coordination; headaches; dizziness; confusion; nausea. Can cause flu-like symptoms that clear up after leaving home. Fatal at very high concentrations. Acute effects are due to the formation of COHb in the blood, which inhibits oxygen intake. At moderate concentrations, angina, impaired vision, and reduced brain function may result. At higher concentrations, CO exposure can be fatal.

Levels in Homes

Average levels in homes without gas stoves vary from 0.5–5 parts per million (ppm). Levels near properly adjusted gas stoves are often 5–15 ppm and those near poorly adjusted stoves may be 30 ppm or higher.

287

Steps to Reduce Exposure to CO

It is most important to be sure combustion equipment is maintained and properly adjusted. Vehicular use should be carefully managed adjacent to buildings and in vocational programs. Additional ventilation can be used as a temporary measure when high levels of CO are expected for short periods of time.

- Keep gas appliances properly adjusted. Consider purchasing a vented space heater when replacing an unvented one.
- Use proper fuel in kerosene space heaters.
- Install and use an exhaust fan vented to outdoors over gas stoves.
- Open flues when fireplaces are in use.
- Choose properly sized wood stoves that are certified to meet U.S. Environmental Protection Agency (EPA) emission standards. Make certain that doors on all wood stoves fit tightly.
- Have a trained professional inspect, clean and tune-up central heating system (furnaces, flues, and chimneys) annually.
- Repair any leaks promptly.
- Do not idle the car inside a garage.

Measurement Methods

Some relatively high-cost infrared radiation adsorption and electrochemical instruments do exist. Moderately priced real-time measuring devices are also available. A passive monitor is currently under development.

Exposure Limits

[OSHA PEL]. The current Occupational Safety and Health Administration (OSHA) permissible exposure limit (PEL) for CO is 50 parts per million (ppm) parts of air (55 milligrams per cubic meter ($mg/m^{(3)}$)) as an 8-hour time-weighted average (TWA) concentration.

[NIOSH REL]. The National Institute for Occupational Safety and Health (NIOSH) has established a recommended exposure limit (REL) for CO of 35 ppm (40 $mg/m^{(3)}$) as an 8-hour TWA and 200 ppm (229 $mg/m^{(3)}$) as a ceiling. The NIOSH limit is based on the risk of cardiovascular effects.

[ACGIH TLV]. The American Conference of Governmental Industrial Hygienists (ACGIH) has assigned CO a threshold limit value (TLV) of 25 ppm (29 mg/m[(3)]) as a TWA for a normal 8-hour workday and a 40-hour workweek. The ACGIH limit is based on the risk of elevated carboxyhemoglobin levels.

Section 23.3

Combustion Pollutants

This section includes text excerpted from "Indoor Air
Quality (IAQ)—Sources of Combustion Products: An
Introduction to Indoor Air Quality," U.S. Environmental
Protection Agency (EPA), February 22, 2017.

In addition to environmental tobacco smoke, other sources of combustion products are:

- unvented kerosene and gas space heaters

- wood stoves

- fireplaces

- gas stoves

The major pollutants released are:

- carbon monoxide (CO)

- nitrogen dioxide (NO_2)

- particles

Unvented kerosene heaters may also generate acid aerosols.

Combustion gases and particles also come from chimneys and flues that are improperly installed or maintained and cracked furnace heat exchangers. Pollutants from fireplaces and wood stoves with no dedicated outdoor air supply can be "back-drafted" from the chimney into the living space, particularly in weatherized homes.

Health Effects of Combustion Products

Carbon monoxide (CO) is a colorless, odorless gas that interferes with the delivery of oxygen throughout the body.

At high concentrations can cause a range of symptoms, including:

- headaches
- dizziness
- weakness
- nausea
- confusion

- disorientation
- fatigue in healthy people
- episodes of increased chest pain in people with chronic heart disease

The symptoms of CO poisoning are sometimes confused with the flu or food poisoning.

Fetuses, infants, elderly people and people with anemia or with a history of heart or respiratory disease can be especially sensitive to CO exposures.

Nitrogen dioxide is a reddish brown, irritating odor gas that irritates the mucous membranes of the eye, nose, and throat, and causes shortness of breath after exposure to high concentrations. There is evidence that high concentrations or continued exposure to low levels of nitrogen dioxide:

- increases the risk of respiratory infection

- there is also evidence from animals studies that repeated exposures to elevated NO_2 levels may lead, or contribute, to the development of lung disease such as emphysema

People at particular risk from exposure to NO_2 include children and individuals with asthma and other respiratory diseases.

Particles, released when fuels are incompletely burned, can lodge in the lungs and irritate or damage lung tissue. A number of pollutants, including radon and benzo(a)pyrene, both of which can cause cancer, attach to small particles that are inhaled and then carried deep into the lung.

Reducing Exposure to Combustion Products in Homes

- **Take special precautions when operating fuel-burning unvented space heaters.** Consider potential effects of indoor air pollution if you use an unvented kerosene or gas space heater. Follow the manufacturer's directions, especially instructions on the proper fuel and keeping the heater properly adjusted. A persistent yellow-tipped flame is generally an indication of maladjustment and increased pollutant emissions. While a space heater is in use, open a door from the room where the heater is located to the rest of the house and open a window slightly.

- **Install and use exhaust fans over gas cooking stoves and ranges and keep the burners properly adjusted.** Using a stove hood with a fan vented to the outdoors greatly reduces exposure to pollutants during cooking. Improper adjustment, often indicated by a persistent yellow-tipped flame, causes increased pollutant emissions. Ask your gas company to adjust the burner so that the flame tip is blue. If you purchase a new gas stove or range, consider buying one with pilotless ignition because it does not have a pilot light that burns continuously. Never use a gas stove to heat your home. Always make certain the flue in your gas fireplace is open when the fireplace is in use.

- **Keep wood stoves emissions to a minimum.** Choose properly sized new stoves that are certified as meeting U.S. Environmental Protection Agency (EPA) emission standards. Make certain that doors in old wood stoves are tight-fitting. Use aged or cured (dried) wood only and follow the manufacturer's directions for starting, stoking and putting out the fire in wood stoves. Chemicals are used to pressure-treat wood; such wood should never be burned indoors.

- **Have central air handling systems, including furnaces, flues, and chimneys, inspected annually and properly repair cracks or damaged parts.** Blocked, leaking or damaged chimneys or flues release harmful combustion gases and particles and even fatal concentrations of CO. Strictly follow all service and maintenance procedures recommended by the manufacturer, including those that tell you how frequently to change the filter. If manufacturer's instructions are not readily available. change filters once every month or two during periods of use. Proper maintenance is important even for new furnaces because they can also corrode and leak combustion gases, including carbon monoxide.

Section 23.4

Flame Retardants (Polybrominated Diphenyl Ethers, or PBDEs)

This section includes text excerpted from "Toxic Substances Portal—
Polybrominated Biphenyls (PBBs)," Agency for Toxic Substances
and Disease Registry (ATSDR), Centers for Disease Control and
Prevention (CDC), October 6, 2015.

Polybrominated diphenyl ethers (PBDEs) are flame-retardant chemicals that are added to plastics and foam products to make them difficult to burn. There are different kinds of PBDEs; some have only a few bromine atoms attached, while some have as many as ten bromine attached to the central molecule.

PBDEs exist as mixtures of similar chemicals called congeners. Because they are mixed into plastics and foams rather than bound to them, PBDEs can leave the products that contain them and enter the environment.

What Happens to Polybrominated Diphenyl Ethers (PBDEs) When They Enter the Environment?

- PBDEs enter the air, water, and soil during their manufacture and use in consumer products.

- In the air, PBDEs can be present as particles but eventually settle to soil or water.

- Sunlight can degrade some PBDEs.

- PBDEs do not dissolve easily in water, but stick to particles and settle to the bottom of river or lakes.

- Some PBDEs can accumulate in fish but usually at low concentrations.

How Might I Be Exposed to PBDEs?

- The concentrations of PBDEs in human blood, breast milk, and body fat indicate that most people are exposed to low levels of PBDEs.

- You may be exposed to PBDEs from eating foods or breathing air contaminated with PBDEs.

- Workers involved in the manufacture of PBDEs or products that contain PBDEs may be exposed to higher levels than usual.

- Occupational exposure can also occur in people who work in enclosed spaces where PBDE-containing products are repaired or recycled.

How Can PBDEs Affect My Health?

There is no definite information on health effects of PBDEs in people. Rats and mice that ate food with moderate amounts of PBDEs for a few days had effects on the thyroid gland. Those that ate smaller amounts for weeks or months had effects on the thyroid and the liver. Large differences in effects are seen between highly-brominated and less-brominated PBDEs in animal studies.

Preliminary evidence suggests that high concentrations of PBDEs may cause neurobehavioral alterations and affect the immune system in animals.

How Likely Are PBDEs to Cause Cancer?

It's not known whether PBDEs can cause cancer in humans. Rats and mice that ate food with decabromodiphenyl ether (one type of PBDE) throughout their lives, developed liver tumors. Based on this evidence, the U.S. Environmental Protection Agency (EPA) has classified decabromodiphenyl ether as a possible human carcinogen. PBDEs with fewer bromine atoms than decabromodiphenyl ether are listed by the EPA as not classifiable as to human carcinogenicity due to the lack of human and animal cancer studies.

How Can PBDEs Affect Children?

Children are exposed to PBDEs in generally the same way as adults, mainly by eating contaminated food. Because PBDEs dissolve readily in fat, they can accumulate in breast milk and may be transferred to babies and young children. Exposure to PBDEs in the womb and through nursing has caused thyroid effects and neurobehavioral alterations in newborn animals, but not birth defects. It is not known if PBDEs can cause birth defect in children.

293

How Can Families Reduce the Risk of Exposure to PBDEs?

- Children living near hazardous waste sites should be discouraged from playing in the dirt near these sites. Children should also be discouraged from eating dirt and should wash their hands frequently.

- People who are exposed to PBDEs at work should shower and change clothes before going home each day. Work clothes should be stored and laundered separately from the rest of your family's clothes.

Is There a Medical Test to Show Whether I've Been Exposed to PBDEs?

There are tests that can detect PBDEs in blood, body fat, and breast milk. These tests can tell whether you have been exposed to high levels of the chemicals, but cannot tell the exact amount or type of PBDE you were exposed to, or whether harmful effects will occur. Blood tests are the easiest and safest for detecting recent exposures to large amounts of PBDEs. These tests are not routinely available at the doctor's office, but samples can be sent to laboratories that have the appropriate equipment.

Section 23.5

Formaldehyde

This section includes text excerpted from "Toxic Substances Portal—Formaldehyde," Agency for Toxic Substances and Disease Registry (ATSDR), Centers for Disease Control and Prevention (CDC), May 12, 2015.

At room temperature, formaldehyde is a colorless, flammable gas that has a distinct, pungent smell. Small amounts of formaldehyde are naturally produced by plants, animals, and humans. It is used in the production of fertilizer, paper, plywood, and urea-formaldehyde (UF) resins. It is also used as a preservative in some foods and in many household products, such as antiseptics, medicines, and cosmetics.

What Happens to Formaldehyde When It Enters the Environment?

- Once formaldehyde is in the air, it is quickly broken down, usually within hours.

- Formaldehyde dissolves easily but does not last a long time in the water.

- Formaldehyde evaporates from shallow soils.

- Formaldehyde does not build up in plants and animals.

How Might I Be Exposed to Formaldehyde?

- The primary way you can be exposed to formaldehyde is by breathing air containing it.

- Releases of formaldehyde into the air occur from industries using or manufacturing formaldehyde, wood products (such as particle-board, plywood, and furniture), automobile exhaust, cigarette smoke, paints and varnishes, and carpets and permanent press fabrics.

- Indoor air contains higher levels of formaldehyde than outdoor air. Levels of formaldehyde measured in indoor air range from 0.02–4 parts per million (ppm). Formaldehyde levels in outdoor air range from 0.0002–0.006 ppm in rural and suburban areas and 0.001–0.02 ppm in urban areas.

- Breathing contaminated workplace air. The highest potential exposure occurs in the formaldehyde-based resins industry.

How Can Formaldehyde Affect the Health?

Nasal and eye irritation, neurological effects, and increased risk of asthma and/or allergy have been observed in humans breathing 0.1–0.5 ppm. Eczema and changes in lung function have been observed at 0.6–1.9 ppm. Decreased body weight, gastrointestinal ulcers, liver and kidney damage were observed in animals orally exposed to 50–100 milligrams/kilogram/day (mg/kg/day) formaldehyde.

How Likely Is Formaldehyde to Cause Cancer?

The U.S. Department of Health and Human Services (HHS) has determined that formaldehyde is a known human carcinogen-based on sufficient human and animal inhalation studies.

How Can Formaldehyde Affect Children?

A small number of studies have looked at the health effects of formaldehyde in children. It is very likely that breathing formaldehyde will result in nose and eye irritation. It's not known if the irritation would occur at lower concentrations in children than in adults. There is some evidence of asthma or asthma-like symptoms for children exposed to formaldehyde in homes. Animal studies have suggested that formaldehyde will not cause birth defects in humans.

How Can Families Reduce the Risk of Exposure to Formaldehyde?

Formaldehyde is usually found in the air, and levels are usually higher indoors than outdoors. Opening windows and using fans to bring fresh air indoors are the easiest ways to lower levels in the house. Not smoking and not using unvented heaters indoors can lower the formaldehyde levels. Formaldehyde is given off from a number of products used in the home. Removing formaldehyde sources in the home can reduce exposure. Providing fresh air, sealing unfinished manufactured wood surfaces, and washing new permanent press clothing before wearing can help lower exposure.

Is There a Medical Test to Show Whether I've Been Exposed to Formaldehyde?

Formaldehyde cannot be reliably measured in blood, urine, or body tissues following exposure. Formaldehyde is produced in the body and would be present as a normal constituent in body tissues and fluids.

Section 23.6

Household Chemicals

This section includes text excerpted from "Hazardous
Waste—Household Hazardous Waste (HHW)," U.S. Environmental
Protection Agency (EPA), February 26, 2018.

Household Hazardous Waste (HHW)

The U.S. Environmental Protection Agency (EPA) considers some
leftover household products that can catch fire, react, or explode under
certain circumstances, or that are corrosive or toxic as household hazardous waste. Products, such as paints, cleaners, oils, batteries, and
pesticides can contain hazardous ingredients and require special care
when you dispose of them.

Safe Management of HHW

To avoid the potential risks associated with HHWs, it is important
that people always monitor the use, storage, and disposal of products with potentially hazardous substances in their homes. Improper
disposal of HHW can include pouring them down the drain, on the
ground, into storm sewers, or in some cases putting them out with
the regular trash.

The dangers of such disposal methods might not be immediately
obvious, but improper disposal of these wastes can pollute the environment and pose a threat to human health. Certain types of HHW have
the potential to cause physical injury to sanitation workers, contaminate septic tanks or wastewater treatment systems if poured down
drains or toilets. They can also present hazards to children and pets
if left around the house.

Some quick tips for the safe handling of HHWs include:

- Follow any instructions for use and storage provided on product
  labels carefully to prevent any accidents at home.

- Be sure to read product labels for disposal directions to reduce
  the risk of products exploding, igniting, leaking, mixing with

297

other chemicals, or posing other hazards on the way to a disposal facility.

- Never store hazardous products in food containers; keep them in their original containers and never remove labels. Corroding containers, however, require special handling. Call your local hazardous materials official or fire department for instructions.

- When leftovers remain, never mix HHW with other products. Incompatible products might react, ignite, or explode, and contaminated HHW might become unrecyclable.

- Check with your local environmental, health or solid waste agency for more information on HHW management options in your area.

  - If your community doesn't have a year-round collection system for HHW, see if there are any designated days in your area for collecting HHW at a central location to ensure safe management and disposal.

  - If your community has neither a permanent collection site nor a special collection day, you might be able to drop off certain products at local businesses for recycling or proper disposal. Some local garages, for example, may accept used motor oil for recycling. Check around.

- Remember, even empty containers of HHW can pose hazards because of the residual chemicals that might remain so handle them with care also.

Reducing HHW in Your Home

Consider reducing your purchase of products that contain hazardous ingredients. Learn about the use of alternative methods or products—without hazardous ingredients—for some common household needs. When shopping for items such as multipurpose household cleaners, toilet cleaners, laundry detergent, dish soap, dishwashing machine pods and gels, bug sprays and insect pest control, consider shopping for environmentally friendly, natural products or search online for simple recipes you can use to create your own.

Table 23.1. Hazardous Waste Source Reduction around the Home

Drain Cleaner	Use a plunger or plumber's snake.
Glass Cleaner	Mix one tablespoon of vinegar or lemon juice in one quart of water. Spray on and use newspaper to dry.
Furniture Polish	Mix one teaspoon of lemon juice in one pint of mineral or vegetable oil and wipe furniture
Rug Deodorizer	Liberally sprinkles carpets with baking soda. Wait at least 15 minutes and vacuum. Repeat if necessary.
Silver Polish	Boil two to three inches of water in a shallow pan with one teaspoon of salt, one teaspoon of baking soda and a sheet of aluminum foil. Totally submerge silver and boil for two to three more minutes. Wipe away tarnish and repeat if necessary.
Mothballs	Use cedar chips, lavender flowers, rosemary, mints or white peppercorns.

Regulating HHW

While most hazardous wastes that are ignitable, reactive, corrosive or toxic in America are regulated in America under Subtitle C of the Resource Conservation and Recovery Act (RCRA), Congress developed an exclusion for household waste. Under this exclusion, found in Title 40 of the Code of Federal Regulations Part 261.4, wastes generated by normal household activities (e.g., routine house and yard maintenance) are excluded from the definition of hazardous waste. Specifically, wastes covered by the household hazardous waste exclusion must satisfy two criteria:

1. The waste must be generated by individuals on the premise of a temporary or permanent residence, and

2. The waste stream must be composed primarily of materials found in wastes generated by consumers in their homes.

EPA interprets this exclusion to include household-like areas, such as bunkhouses, ranger stations, crew quarters, campgrounds, picnic grounds, and day-use recreation areas.

Although household hazardous waste is excluded from Subtitle C of RCRA, it is regulated under Subtitle D of this law as a solid waste. In other words, household hazardous waste is regulated on the state and local level.

Section 23.7

Pesticides

This section includes text excerpted from "Indoor Air
Quality (IAQ)—Pesticides' Impact on Indoor Air Quality," U.S.
Environmental Protection Agency (EPA), May 10, 2017.

Pesticides are chemicals that are used to kill or control pests which include bacteria, fungi and other organisms, in addition to insects and rodents. Pesticides are inherently toxic.

According to a survey, 75 percent of U.S. households used at least one pesticide product indoors during the past year. Products used most often are insecticides and disinfectants. Another study suggests that 80 percent of most people's exposure to pesticides occurs indoors and that measurable levels of up to a dozen pesticides have been found in the air inside homes.

The amount of pesticides found in homes appears to be greater than can be explained by recent pesticide use in those households; other possible sources include:

- contaminated soil or dust that floats or is tracked in from outside
- stored pesticide containers
- household surfaces that collect and then release the pesticides

Pesticides used in and around the home include products to control:

- insects (insecticides)
- termites (termiticides)
- rodents (rodenticides)
- fungi (fungicides)
- microbes (disinfectants)

They are sold as sprays, liquids, sticks, powders, crystals, balls, and foggers.

In households with children under five years old, almost one-half stored at least one pesticide product within reach of children. The U.S. Environmental Protection Agency (EPA) registers pesticides for use and requires manufacturers to put information on the label about when and how to use the pesticide. It is important to remember that the "-cide" in pesticides means "to kill." These products can be dangerous if not used properly.

In addition to the active ingredient, pesticides are also made up of ingredients that are used to carry the active agent. These carrier agents are called "inerts" in pesticides because they are not toxic to the targeted pest; nevertheless, some inerts are capable of causing health problems.

Sources of Pesticides

- Products used to kill household pests (insecticides, termiticides, and disinfectants)

- Products used on lawns and gardens that drift or are tracked inside the house

Pesticides are classed as semi-volatile organic compounds and include a variety of chemicals in various forms.

Health Effects

Exposure to pesticides may result in:

- Irritation to eye, nose and throat

- damage to central nervous system and kidney

- increased risk of cancer

Symptoms may include:

- headache

- dizziness

- muscular weakness

- nausea

Chronic exposure to some pesticides can result in damage to the:

- liver

- kidneys

- endocrine and nervous systems

Both the active and inert ingredients in pesticides can be organic compounds; therefore, both could add to the levels of airborne organics inside homes. Both types of ingredients can cause the type of effects discussed in Household Chemicals/Products. However, as with other household products, there is insufficient understanding at present about what pesticide concentrations are necessary to produce these effects.

Exposure to high levels of cyclodiene pesticides, commonly associated with misapplication, has produced various symptoms, including:

- headaches

- dizziness

- muscle twitching

- weakness

- tingling sensations

- nausea

In addition, EPA is concerned that cyclodienes might cause long-term damage to the liver and the central nervous system, as well as an increased risk of cancer.

There is no further sale or commercial use permitted for the following cyclodiene or related pesticides: chlordane, aldrin, dieldrin and heptachlor. The only exception is the use of heptachlor by utility companies to control fire ants in underground cable boxes.

Levels in Homes

Preliminary research shows widespread presence of pesticide residues in homes.

Steps to Reduce Exposure

- Use strictly according to manufacturer's directions.

- Mix or dilute outdoors.

- Apply only in recommended quantities.

- Increase ventilation when using indoors. Take plants or pets outdoors when applying pesticides/flea and tick treatments.

- Use nonchemical methods of pest control where possible.

- If you use a pest control company, select it carefully.

- Do not store unneeded pesticides inside the home; dispose of unwanted containers safely.

- Store clothes with moth repellents in separately ventilated areas, if possible.

- Keep indoor spaces clean, dry, and well ventilated to avoid pest and odor problems.

Read the label and follow the directions. It is illegal to use any pesticide in any manner inconsistent with the directions on its label.

Unless you have had special training and are certified, never use a pesticide that is restricted to use by state-certified pest control operators. Such pesticides are simply too dangerous for application by a noncertified person. Use only the pesticides approved for use by the general public and then only in recommended amounts; increasing the amount does not offer more protection against pests and can be harmful to you and your plants and pets.

Ventilate the area well after pesticide use. Mix or dilute pesticides outdoors or in a well-ventilated area and only in the amounts that will be immediately needed. If possible, take plants and pets outside when applying pesticides/flea and tick treatments.

Use nonchemical methods of pest control when possible. Since pesticides can be found far from the site of their original application, it is prudent to reduce the use of chemical pesticides outdoors as well as indoors. Depending on the site and pest to be controlled, one or more of the following steps can be effective:

- use of biological pesticides, such as Bacillus thuringiensis (Bt), for the control of gypsy moths

- selection of disease-resistant plants

- frequent washing of indoor plants and pets

Termite damage can be reduced or prevented by making certain that wooden building materials do not come into direct contact with the soil and by storing firewood away from the home. By appropriately fertilizing, watering and aerating lawns, the need for chemical pesticide treatments of lawns can be dramatically reduced.

If you decide to use a pest control company, choose one carefully. Ask for an inspection of your home and get a written control program for evaluation before you sign a contract. The control program should list specific names of pests to be controlled and chemicals to be used; it should also reflect any of your safety concerns. Insist on a proven record of competence and customer satisfaction.

Dispose of unwanted pesticides safely. If you have unused or partially used pesticide containers you want to get rid of, dispose of them according to the directions on the label or on special household hazardous waste collection days. If there are no such collection days in your community, work with others to organize them.

Keep exposure to moth repellents to a minimum. One pesticide often found in the home is paradichlorobenzene, a commonly used active ingredient in moth repellents. This chemical is known to cause cancer in animals, but substantial scientific uncertainty exists over the effects, if any, of long-term human exposure to paradichlorobenzene. EPA requires that products containing paradichlorobenzene bear warnings such as "avoid breathing vapors" to warn users of potential short-term toxic effects. Where possible, paradichlorobenzene and items to be protected against moths, should be placed in trunks or other containers that can be stored in areas that are separately ventilated from the home, such as attics and detached garages. Paradichlorobenzene is also the key active ingredient in many air fresheners (in fact, some labels for moth repellents recommend that these same products be used as air fresheners or deodorants). Proper ventilation and basic household cleanliness will go a long way toward preventing unpleasant odors.

Integrated Pest Management

If chemicals must be used, use only the recommended amounts, mix or dilute pesticides outdoors or in an isolated well-ventilated area, apply to unoccupied areas, and dispose of unwanted pesticides safely to minimize exposure.

Standards or Guidelines

No air concentration standards for pesticides have been set, however, EPA recommends integrated pest management, which minimizes the use of chemical pesticides. Pesticide products must be used according to application and ventilation instructions provided by the manufacturer.

Section 23.8

Radon

This section contains text excerpted from the following sources: Text in this section begins with excerpts from "A Citizen's Guide to Radon," U.S. Environmental Protection Agency (EPA), 2016; Text under the heading "Health Risk of Radon" is excerpted from "Radon—Health Risk of Radon," U.S. Environmental Protection Agency (EPA), February 23, 2018.

Radon is a radioactive gas. It comes from the natural decay of uranium that is found in nearly all soils. It typically moves up through the ground to the air above and into your home through cracks and other holes in the foundation. Your home traps radon inside, where it can build up. Any home may have a radon problem. This means new and old homes, well-sealed and drafty homes, and homes with or without basements. Radon from soil gas is the main cause of radon problems. Sometimes radon enters the home through well water. In a small number of homes, the building materials can give off radon, too. However, building materials rarely cause radon problems by themselves. Nearly 1 out of every 15 homes in the United States is estimated to have elevated radon levels. Elevated levels of radon gas have been found in homes in your state. Contact your state radon office for general information about radon in your area. While radon problems may be more common in some areas, any home may have a problem. The only way to know about your home is to test. Radon can also be a problem in schools and workplaces. Ask your state radon office (www.epa.gov/radon/whereyoulive.html) about radon problems in schools, daycare and child care facilities, and workplaces in your area (also visit www.epa.gov/radon).

Health Risk of Radon

Exposure to radon causes lung cancer in nonsmokers and smokers alike.

- **Lung cancer** kills thousands of Americans every year. Smoking, radon, and secondhand smoke are the leading causes of lung cancer. Although lung cancer can be treated, the survival rate is one of the lowest for those with cancer. From the time of diagnosis, between 11–15 percent of those afflicted will live beyond five years, depending upon demographic factors. In many cases lung cancer can be prevented.

- **Smoking** is the leading cause of lung cancer. Smoking causes an estimated 160,000 cancer deaths in the United States every year. And the rate among women is rising. On January 11, 1964, Dr. Luther L. Terry, then U.S. Surgeon General, issued the first warning on the link between smoking and lung cancer. Lung cancer now surpasses breast cancer as the number one cause of death among women. A smoker who is also exposed to radon has a much higher risk of lung cancer.

- **Radon** is the number one cause of lung cancer among nonsmokers, according to U.S. Environmental Protection Agency (EPA) estimates. Overall, radon is the second leading cause of lung cancer. Radon is responsible for about 21,000 lung cancer deaths every year. About 2,900 of these deaths occur among people who have never smoked.

- **Secondhand smoke** is the third leading cause of lung cancer and responsible for an estimated 3,000 lung cancer deaths every year. Smoking affects nonsmokers by exposing them to secondhand smoke. Exposure to secondhand smoke can have serious consequences for children's health, including asthma attacks, affecting the respiratory tract (bronchitis, pneumonia), and may cause ear infections.

- For smokers the risk of lung cancer is significant due to the synergistic effects of radon and smoking. For this population about 62 people in a 1,000 will die of lung-cancer, compared to 7.3 people in a 1,000 for never smokers. Put another way, a person who never smoked (never smoker) who is exposed to 1.3 pCi/L has a 2 in 1,000 chance of lung cancer; while a smoker has a 20 in 1,000 chance of dying from lung cancer.

Section 23.9

Secondhand Smoke

This section includes text excerpted from "Indoor Air Quality
(IAQ)—Secondhand Tobacco Smoke and Smoke-Free Homes," U.S.
Environmental Protection Agency (EPA), January 29, 2018.

Secondhand smoke is a mixture of the smoke given off by the burning of tobacco products, such as cigarettes, cigars or pipes and the smoke exhaled by smokers. Secondhand smoke is also called environmental tobacco smoke (ETS) and exposure to secondhand smoke is sometimes called involuntary or passive smoking. Secondhand smoke contains more than 7,000 substances, several of which are known to cause cancer in humans or animals.

- The U.S. Environmental Protection Agency (EPA) has concluded that exposure to secondhand smoke can cause lung cancer in adults who do not smoke. EPA estimates that exposure to secondhand smoke causes approximately 3,000 lung cancer deaths per year in nonsmokers.

- Exposure to secondhand smoke has also been shown in a number of studies to increase the risk of heart disease and stroke.

The Science behind the Risks

Surgeon General Warning: Secondhand Smoke Puts Children at Risk

On June 27, 2006, the Surgeon General released a major report on involuntary exposure to secondhand smoke, concluding that secondhand smoke causes disease and death in children and nonsmoking adults. The report finds a causal relationship between secondhand smoke exposure and sudden infant death syndrome (SIDS), and declares that the home is becoming the predominant location for exposure of children and adults to secondhand smoke.

EPA published a major assessment of the respiratory health risks of passive smoking in 1992 titled *Respiratory Health Effects of Passive Smoking: Lung Cancer and Other Disorders.* The report concluded that exposure to environmental tobacco smoke (ETS)—commonly known as secondhand smoke—is responsible for approximately 3,000 lung cancer deaths each year in nonsmoking adults and impairs the respiratory health of thousands of children.

Key Findings

In adults:

- ETS is a human lung carcinogen, responsible for approximately 3,000 lung cancer deaths annually in U.S. nonsmokers.

- ETS has been classified as a Group A carcinogen under EPA's carcinogen assessment guidelines. This classification is reserved for those compounds or mixtures which have been shown to cause cancer in humans, based on studies in human populations.

In children:

- ETS exposure increases the risk of lower respiratory tract infections such as bronchitis and pneumonia. EPA estimates that between 150,000–300,000 of these cases annually in infants and young children up to 18 months of age are attributable to exposure to ETS. Of these, between 7,500–15,000 will result in hospitalization.

- ETS exposure increases the risk of ear infections in children.

- ETS exposure in children irritates the upper respiratory tract and is associated with a small but significant reduction in lung function.

- ETS exposure increases the frequency of episodes and severity of symptoms in asthmatic children. The report estimates that up to 1,000,000 asthmatic children have their condition worsened by exposure to environmental tobacco smoke.

- ETS exposure is a risk factor for new cases of asthma in children who have not previously displayed symptoms.

Health Risks to Children with Asthma

- Asthma is a chronic disease that affects the airways of the lungs and can lead to coughing, trouble breathing, wheezing and tightness in the chest.

- Asthma is the most common chronic childhood disease affecting 1 in 13 school aged children on average.

- Secondhand smoke is a universal asthma trigger and can elicit an asthma attack or make asthma symptoms more severe.

- Exposure to secondhand smoke may cause new cases of asthma in children who have not previously shown symptoms.

- More than half of U.S. children with asthma are exposed to secondhand smoke.

What You Can Do

- Do not smoke in the house and enforce a smoke-free rule in your home to ensure that all guests smoke outdoors.

- Encourage your multi-unit housing building to implement a smoke-free policy to eliminate infiltration of secondhand smoke from other units and/or common areas.

- Find a community asthma programs near you.

Section 23.10

Multiple Chemical Sensitivity (MCS)

This section contains text excerpted from the following sources: Text in this section begins with excerpts from "Fundamentals of Indoor Air Quality in Buildings," U.S. Environmental Protection Agency (EPA), September 6, 2017; Text under the heading "Evaluation and Management" is excerpted from "Multiple Chemical Sensitivities," U.S. Department of Labor (DOL), December 14, 2010. Reviewed April 2018.

It is generally recognized that some persons can be sensitive to particular agents at levels which do not have an observable affect in the general population. In addition, it is recognized that certain chemicals can be sensitizers in that exposure to the chemical at high levels can result in sensitivity to that chemical at much lower levels.

Some evidence suggests that a subset of the population may be especially sensitive to low levels of a broad range of chemicals at levels common in today's home and working environments. This apparent condition has come to be known as multiple chemical sensitivity (MCS).

Persons reported to have MCS apparently have difficulty being in most buildings. There is significant professional disagreement concerning whether MCS actually exists and what the underlying mechanism might be. Building managers may encounter occupants who have been diagnosed with MCS. Resolution of complaints in such circumstances may or may not be possible with the guidance provided in I-BEAM. Responsibility to accommodate such individuals is subject to negotiation and may involve arrangements to work at home or in a different location.

Evaluation and Management

Limited information is available on effective control measures, exposure assessments, and regulations dealing with multiple chemical sensitivities (MCS). However, OSHA does regulate exposures to specific chemical hazards.

Many physicians are uncertain how to approach the evaluation and care of persons who have multiple symptoms attributed to low-level chemical exposure. The identification of MCS is based largely on the patient's description of the symptoms and the relationship of these symptoms to environmental exposures.

Chapter 24

Molds

Frequently Asked Questions on Molds

What Are Molds?

Molds are fungi that can be found both indoors and outdoors. No one knows how many species of fungi exist but estimates range from tens of thousands to perhaps three hundred thousand or more. Molds grow best in warm, damp, and humid conditions, and spread and reproduce by making spores. Mold spores can survive harsh environmental conditions, such as dry conditions, that do not support normal mold growth.

What Are Some of the Common Indoor Molds?

- Cladosporium
- Penicillium
- Alternaria
- Aspergillus

How Do Molds Affect People?

Some people are sensitive to molds. For these people, exposure to molds can lead to symptoms such as stuffy nose, wheezing, and red or

This chapter includes text excerpted from "Molds in the Environment," Centers for Disease Control and Prevention (CDC), December 20, 2017.

itchy eyes, or skin. Some people, such as those with allergies to molds or with asthma, may have more intense reactions. Severe reactions may occur among workers exposed to large amounts of molds in occupational settings, such as farmers working around moldy hay. Severe reactions may include fever and shortness of breath.

People with a weakened immune system, such as people receiving treatment for cancer, people who have had an organ or stem cell transplant, and people taking medicines that suppress the immune system, are more likely to get mold infections.

Exposure to mold or dampness may also lead to the development of asthma in some individuals. Interventions that improve housing conditions can reduce morbidity from asthma and respiratory allergies.

Where Are Molds Found?

Molds are found in virtually every environment and can be detected, both indoors and outdoors, year round. Mold growth is encouraged by warm and humid conditions. Outdoors they can be found in shady, damp areas, or places where leaves or other vegetation is decomposing. Indoors they can be found where humidity levels are high, such as basements or showers.

How Can People Decrease Mold Exposure?

Sensitive individuals should avoid areas that are likely to have molds, such as compost piles, cut grass, and wooded areas. Inside homes, mold growth can be slowed by controlling humidity levels and ventilating showers and cooking areas. If there is mold growth in your home, you should clean up the mold and fix the water problem. Mold growth can be removed from hard surfaces with commercial products, soap, and water, or a bleach solution of no more than 1 cup of household laundry bleach in 1 gallon of water. Follow the manufacturer's instructions for use (see product label).

If you choose to use bleach to clean up mold:

- Never mix bleach with ammonia or other household cleaners. Mixing bleach with ammonia or other cleaning products will produce dangerous, toxic fumes.

- Open windows and doors to provide fresh air.

- Wear rubber boots, rubber gloves, and goggles during cleanup of affected area.

- Always follow the manufacturer's instructions when using bleach or any other cleaning product.

  Specific recommendations:

- Keep humidity levels as low as you can—no higher than 50 percent–all day long. An air conditioner or dehumidifier will help you keep the level low. Bear in mind that humidity levels change over the course of a day with changes in the moisture in the air and the air temperature, so you will need to check the humidity levels more than once a day.

- Use an air conditioner or a dehumidifier during humid months.

- Be sure the home has adequate ventilation, including exhaust fans.

- Add mold inhibitors to paints before application.

- Clean bathrooms with mold killing products.

- Do not carpet bathrooms and basements.

- Remove or replace previously soaked carpets and upholstery.

What Areas Have High Mold Exposures?

- Antique shops
- Greenhouses
- Saunas
- Farms
- Mills
- Construction areas
- Flower shops
- Summer cottages

If I Found Mold Growing in My Home, How Do I Test the Mold?

Generally, it is not necessary to identify the species of mold growing in a residence, and Centers for Disease Control and Prevention (CDC) does not recommend routine sampling for molds. Current evidence indicates that allergies are the type of diseases most often associated with molds. Since the susceptibility of individuals can vary greatly either because of the amount or type of mold, sampling and culturing are not reliable in determining your health risk. If you are susceptible to mold and mold is seen or smelled, there is a potential health risk; therefore, no matter what type of mold is present, you should arrange for its removal. Furthermore, reliable sampling for mold can be expensive, and standards for judging what is and what is not an acceptable or tolerable quantity of mold have not been established.

A Qualified Environmental Lab Took Samples of the Mold in My Home and Gave Me the Results. Can Centers for Disease Control and Prevention (CDC) Interpret These Results?

Standards for judging what is an acceptable, tolerable, or normal quantity of mold have not been established. If you do decide to pay for environmental sampling for molds, before the work starts, you should ask the consultants who will do the work to establish criteria for interpreting the test results. They should tell you in advance what they will do or what recommendations they will make based on the sampling results. The results of samples taken in your unique situation cannot be interpreted without a physical inspection of the contaminated area or without considering the building's characteristics and the factors that led to the present condition.

What Type of Doctor Should I See Concerning Mold Exposure?

You should first consult a family or general healthcare provider who will decide whether you need a referral to a specialist. Such specialists might include an allergist who treats patients with mold allergies or an infectious disease physician who treats mold infections. If an infection is in the lungs, a pulmonary physician might be recommended. Patients who have been exposed to molds in their workplace may be referred to an occupational physician.

My Landlord or Builder Will Not Take Any Responsibility for Cleaning up the Mold in My Home. Where Can I Go for Help?

If you feel your property owner, landlord, or builder has not been responsive to concerns you've expressed regarding mold exposure, you can contact your local board of health or housing authority. Applicable codes, insurance, inspection, legal, and similar issues about mold generally fall under state and local (not federal) jurisdiction. You could also review your lease or building contract and contact local or state government authorities, your insurance company, or an attorney to learn more about local codes and regulations and your legal rights. You can contact your county or state health department about mold issues in your area to learn about what mold assessment and remediation services they may offer.

I'm Sure That Mold in My Workplace Is Making Me Sick

If you believe you are ill because of exposure to mold in the building where you work, you should first consult your healthcare provider to determine the appropriate action to take to protect your health. Notify your employer and, if applicable, your union representative about your concern so that your employer can take action to clean up and prevent mold growth. To find out more about mold, remediation of mold, or workplace safety, health guidelines, and regulations, you may also want to contact your local (city, county, or state) health department.

I Am Very Concerned about Mold in My Children's School and How It Affects Their Health

If you believe your children are ill because of exposure to mold in their school, first consult their healthcare provider to determine the appropriate medical action to take. Contact the school's administration to express your concern and to ask that they remove the mold and prevent future mold growth. If needed, you could also contact the local school board. Your local health department may also have information on mold, and you may want to get in touch with your state Indoor Air Quality (IAQ) office.

Chapter 25

Asbestos

About Asbestos

Asbestos is a commercial and legal term referring to a class of minerals that naturally form long, thin, very strong fibers. Asbestos has been mined and used in many products worldwide, mostly during the 20th century. In the United States, mining asbestos has ended, but asbestos is still present in older homes and buildings, and some products still contain it. Asbestos occurs in the environment, both naturally and from the breakdown or disposal of old asbestos products.

Asbestos Hazards

Disturbing asbestos minerals or other asbestos-containing materials can release tiny asbestos fibers, too small to see, into the air. Workers and others who breathed asbestos fibers over many years have developed asbestos-related diseases, including asbestosis, pleural disease, lung cancer, and mesothelioma. Some of these diseases can be serious or even fatal.

Asbestos Properties

Asbestos occurs naturally in certain types of rock. Large amounts of asbestos in rocks can look like long fibers, but each asbestos fiber

This chapter includes text excerpted from "Asbestos and Your Health," Centers for Disease Control and Prevention (CDC), November 3, 2016.

is too small to see with the naked eye. Asbestos fibers do not dissolve in water or evaporate. They resist heat and fire and cannot be broken down easily by chemicals or bacteria. Certain areas of the country have natural deposits of asbestos near the ground surface.

Asbestos in Products

Because of its sturdy properties, asbestos was mined and used in making many products, including insulation, fireproofing and acoustic materials, wallboard, plaster, cement, floor tiles, brake linings, and roofing shingles. Beginning in the 1970s, the United States banned many uses of asbestos, but asbestos is still present in old materials and is still used in products such as automobile brakes and roofing materials. Asbestos may also be present in other commercial products, such as vermiculite (especially vermiculite from Libby, Montana) and talc.

Types of Asbestos

The legal definition of asbestos applies to six fibrous minerals in two general classes:

1. **Serpentine class.** Chrysotile (also known as white asbestos)

2. **Amphibole class.** Amosite (brown asbestos), crocidolite (blue asbestos), anthophyllite, tremolite, and actinolite

Exposure to either chrysotile or amphibole asbestos increases the risk of disease. However, amphiboles remain in the lung for a longer period of time. Exposure to amphiboles may result in a higher risk of developing mesothelioma than exposure to chrysotile. Some studies have suggested that other durable, fibrous silicate minerals ("asbestiform" minerals) such as winchite or richterite can have health effects similar to asbestos.

Health Effects of Asbestos

Asbestos is a dangerous substance and should be avoided. But people who have contact with asbestos do not always develop health problems. The risk of disease depends on many factors:

- How much asbestos is in the air

- How often and for how long exposure occurs

- How much time has passed since exposure began

- Whether the person already has lung or breathing conditions

- Whether the person smokes tobacco

Asbestos-Related Diseases

Breathing asbestos can cause tiny asbestos fibers to get stuck in the lungs and irritate lung tissues. Scientific studies have shown that the following noncancer diseases can be caused by breathing asbestos:

- **Asbestosis** is scarring in the lungs caused by breathing asbestos fibers. Oxygen and carbon dioxide do not pass in and out of scarred lungs easily, so breathing becomes harder. Asbestosis usually occurs in people who have had very high exposures over a long time, but years may pass before any symptoms appear.

- **Pleural disease** is a noncancerous lung condition that causes changes in the membrane surrounding the lungs and chest cavity (pleura). The membrane may become thicker throughout (diffuse pleural thickening) or in isolated areas (pleural plaques), or fluid may build up around the lungs (known as a pleural effusion). Not everyone with pleural changes will have problems breathing, but some may have less efficient lung function.

Asbestos exposure also increases the risk of developing certain cancers:

- **Lung cancer** is a malignant tumor that invades and blocks the lungs' air passages. Smoking tobacco combined with asbestos exposure greatly increases the chance of developing lung cancer.

- **Mesothelioma** is a rare cancer of the membrane that covers the lungs and chest cavity (pleura), the membrane lining the abdominal cavity (peritoneum), or membranes surrounding other internal organs. Signs of mesothelioma may not appear until 30–40 years after exposure to asbestos.

In addition to lung cancer and mesothelioma, asbestos exposure can also cause cancer of the larynx and ovary. Evidence also suggests asbestos exposure may cause cancer of the pharynx, stomach, and colorectum.

Advice for People Concerned about Asbestos Exposure

People concerned about asbestos exposure should visit their doctor or another medical provider. Based on the person's detailed exposure and medical history and a physical exam, the doctor will decide if additional testing is needed.

After exposure occurs, asbestos can't be removed from the lungs. Preventing further harm to the respiratory system can lower the chances of the disease developing or slow down the progress of an existing disease. Preventive care guidelines related to asbestos exposure include:

- Having regular medical exams

- Getting regular vaccinations against flu and pneumococcal pneumonia

- Quitting smoking

- Avoiding further asbestos exposure

Asbestos Exposure and Reducing Exposure

Asbestos Exposure

People may be exposed to asbestos by breathing tiny asbestos fibers in the air. The asbestos gets into the air from natural deposits of asbestos in the earth or from past or current commercial products that contain the minerals. Asbestos fibers usually get into the air when something disturbs them in soil, rock, or older products, such as:

- Weathering or erosion of natural deposits of asbestos at the ground surface or old asbestos-containing products

- Crushing rock with natural deposits of asbestos

- Handling, cutting, or crushing old asbestos-containing products, for example, during building renovation or demolition projects

- Disturbing soil contaminated by natural surface deposits or old asbestos-containing products during recreational or other outdoor activities

- Handling or disturbing consumer products contaminated with asbestos (such as vermiculite or talc)

- Gardening in soil contaminated by asbestos from natural deposits or commercial products

- Cleaning or other household activities that might stir up dust containing asbestos from natural deposits or products

The amount of asbestos that gets into the air people breathe depends on many factors, including:

- the location
- the type of material or soil the asbestos is in
- the age and characteristics of that material
- weather conditions and moisture
- the intensity of the activity disturbing the asbestos

Once the asbestos fibers get into the air, they will act the same no matter where they came from. A fiber of chrysotile will cause the same risk of disease whether it came directly from a natural deposit or from a commercial product.

People may also be exposed to asbestos by accidentally swallowing fibers or getting them on their skin. However, these types of contact only cause health effects after large amounts of exposure. Also, the effects of swallowing or touching asbestos are less serious than the health effects of breathing asbestos.

Reducing Asbestos Exposure

People who work around asbestos, or materials that contain it, should:

- Get proper training for handling asbestos.
- Wear the right personal protective equipment.

People who live in older homes should:

- Avoid disturbing materials that might contain asbestos, including:
    - pipe and furnace insulation, siding, flooring, and popcorn ceilings installed from the 1950s to the 1970s
    - vermiculite attic insulation
- Talk to their local or state environmental agency or a certified asbestos contractor if the materials are breaking down or need to be replaced
- Hire contractors who know and follow laws for safe asbestos removal and disposal to avoid contaminating the rest of the home or the environment

People who live in areas with natural asbestos deposits or near areas contaminated by old asbestos-containing products should:

- To keep asbestos levels low in the home:
  - Use wet cleaning methods and high-efficiency particulate air (HEPA) vacuums
  - Use doormats and removing shoes before entering
  - Keep windows closed on windy days to keep asbestos out
  - Avoid breathing dust outside by
  - Use water to wet soil before gardening or playing
  - Spray off patios with water instead of sweeping them
  - Stay on pavement or ground covered with grass or mulch

Chapter 26

Exposures to Lead

Sources of Lead at Home

Older Homes and Buildings

If your home was built before 1978, there is a good chance it has lead-based paint. In 1978, the federal government banned consumer uses of lead-containing paint, but some states banned it even earlier. Lead from paint, including lead-contaminated dust, is one of the most common causes of lead poisoning.

- Lead paint is still present in millions of homes, sometimes under layers of newer paint. If the paint is in good shape, the lead paint is usually not a problem. Deteriorating lead-based paint (peeling, chipping, chalking, cracking, damaged, or damp) is a hazard and needs immediate attention.

- It may also be a hazard when found on surfaces that children can chew or that get a lot of wear-and-tear, such as:

  - Windows and window sills

  - Doors and door frames

  - Stairs, railings, banisters, and porches

- Be sure to keep all paint in excellent shape and clean up dust frequently.

This chapter includes text excerpted from "Protect Your Family from Exposures to Lead," U.S. Environmental Protection Agency (EPA), August 30, 2017.

- Lead in household dust results from indoor sources such as deteriorating lead-based paint.

- Lead dust can also be tracked into the home from soil outside that is contaminated by deteriorated exterior lead-based paint and other lead sources, such as industrial pollution and past use of leaded gasoline.

- Renovation, repair, or painting activities can create toxic lead dust when painted surfaces are disturbed or demolished.

- Pipes and solder. Lead is used in some water service lines and household plumbing materials. It can leach, or enter the water, as water flows through the plumbing. Lead pipes and lead solder were commonly used until 1986.

Dust

Lead in household dust results from indoor sources such as old lead paint on surfaces that are frequently in motion or bump or rub together (such as window frames), deteriorating old lead paint on any surface, home repair activities, tracking lead-contaminated soil from the outdoors into the indoor environment, or even from lead dust on clothing worn at a job site.

Even in well-maintained homes, lead dust can form when lead-based paint is scraped, sanded or heated during home repair activities. Lead paint chips and dust can get on surfaces and objects that people touch. Settled lead dust can re-enter the air when the home is vacuumed or swept, or people walk through it. To reduce exposure to lead dust, it is especially important to maintain all painted surfaces in good condition, and to clean frequently, to reduce the likelihood of chips and dust forming. Using a lead-safe certified renovator to perform renovation, repair and painting jobs is a good way to reduce the likelihood of contaminating your home with lead-based paint dust.

Products

Lead can be found in many products:

- **Painted toys, furniture, and toy jewelry.** That favorite dump truck or rocking chair handed down in the family, antique doll furniture, or toy jewelry could contain lead-based paint or contain lead in the material it is made from. Biting or swallowing toys or toy jewelry that contain lead can cause a child to suffer from lead poisoning.

- **Cosmetics**
- **Food or liquid containers.** Food and liquids stored or served in lead crystal or lead-glazed pottery or porcelain can become contaminated because lead can leach from these containers into the food or liquid.
- **Plumbing products.** Materials, like pipes and fixtures, that contain lead can corrode over time.

Drinking Water

Lead can enter drinking water through corrosion of plumbing materials, especially where the water has high acidity or low mineral content that corrodes pipes and fixtures. Homes built before 1986 are more likely to have lead pipes, fixtures, and solder. However, new homes are also at risk: even legally "lead-free" plumbing may contain up to 8 percent lead.

Beginning January 2014, changes to the Safe Drinking Water Act (SDWA) further reduced the maximum allowable lead content of pipes, pipe fittings, plumbing fittings, and fixtures to 0.25 percent. The most common problem is with brass or chrome-plated brass faucets and fixtures with lead solder, from which significant amounts of lead can enter into the water, especially hot water.

Corrosion is a dissolving or wearing away of metal caused by a chemical reaction between water and your plumbing. A number of factors are involved in the extent to which lead enters the water including the chemistry of the water (acidity and alkalinity), the amount of lead it comes into contact with, how long the water stays in the plumbing materials, and the presence of protective scales or coatings inside the plumbing materials.

To address corrosion of lead and copper into drinking water, EPA issued the Lead and Copper Rule (LCR) under the authority of the SDWA. The LCR requires corrosion control treatment to prevent lead and copper from contaminating drinking water. Corrosion control treatment means systems must make drinking water less corrosive to the materials it comes into contact with on its way to consumers' taps.

Jobs and Hobbies

You could bring lead home on your hands or clothes, or contaminate your home directly if you:

- Work with lead and/or lead-based paint (for example, renovation and painting, mining, smelting, battery recycling, refinishing old furniture, auto body, shooting ranges); or

- Have a hobby that uses lead (for example, hunting, fishing, stained glass, stock cars, making pottery).

  - Lead can be found in shot, fishing sinkers, and jigs; came and solder used in stained glass; weights used in stock cars; dyes and glazes used in pottery; and many other places.

If you have a job or hobby where you may come into contact with lead:

- Never put leaded materials (for example, fishing sinkers, lead came or solder for stained glass or leaded pottery clay or glaze) in your mouth.

- Avoid handling food or touching your mouth or face while engaged in working with lead materials and wash hands before eating or drinking following such activities.

- Shower and change clothes before entering your vehicle or coming home.

- Launder your work and hobby clothes separately from the rest of your family's clothes.

- Keep all work and hobby materials away from living areas.

If someone in your family is a renovator or contractor working in older housing, find out more about lead-safe work practices. If you are an owner or operator of outdoor rifle, pistol, trap, skeet or sporting clay ranges, find out more about lead management at ranges.

Folk Remedies

Some folk remedies that contain lead, such as "greta" and "azarcon," are used to treat an upset stomach. Some folk remedies for morning sickness, including "nzu," "poto," and "calabash chalk," contain dangerous levels of lead and other chemicals. Consuming even small amounts of lead can be harmful. Lead poisoning from folk remedies can cause serious and irreversible illness.

Chapter 27

Volatile Organic Compounds (VOCs)

Volatile organic compounds (VOCs) are emitted as gases from certain solids or liquids. VOCs include a variety of chemicals, some of which may have short- and long-term adverse health effects. Concentrations of many VOCs are consistently higher indoors (up to ten times higher) than outdoors. VOCs are emitted by a wide array of products numbering in the thousands.

Organic chemicals are widely used as ingredients in household products. Paints, varnishes, and wax all contain organic solvents, as do many cleaning, disinfecting, cosmetic, degreasing, and hobby products. Fuels are made up of organic chemicals. All of these products can release organic compounds while you are using them, and, to some degree, when they are stored.

U.S. Environmental Protection Agency (EPA) Office of Research and Development's (ORD) "Total Exposure Assessment Methodology (TEAM) Study" found levels of about a dozen common organic pollutants to be 2–5 times higher inside homes than outside, regardless of whether the homes were located in rural or highly industrial areas. TEAM studies indicated that while people are using products containing organic chemicals, they can expose themselves and others to very

This chapter includes text excerpted from "Volatile Organic Compounds' Impact on Indoor Air Quality," U.S. Environmental Protection Agency (EPA), November 6, 2017.

high pollutant levels, and elevated concentrations can persist in the air long after the activity is completed.

Sources of VOCs

Household products, including:

- paints, paint strippers, and other solvents
- wood preservatives
- aerosol sprays
- cleansers and disinfectants
- moth repellents and air fresheners
- stored fuels and automotive products
- hobby supplies
- dry-cleaned clothing
- pesticide

Other products, including:

- building materials and furnishings
- office equipment such as copiers and printers, correction fluids, and carbonless copy paper
- graphics and craft materials including glues and adhesives, permanent markers, and photographic solutions

Health Effects

Health effects may include:

- Eye, nose, and throat irritation
- Headaches, loss of coordination, and nausea
- Damage to liver, kidney, and central nervous system (CNS)
- Some organics can cause cancer in animals, some are suspected or known to cause cancer in humans

Key signs or symptoms associated with exposure to VOCs include:

- conjunctival irritation
- nose and throat discomfort

- a headache
- allergic skin reaction
- dyspnea
- declines in serum cholinesterase levels
- nausea
- emesis
- epistaxis
- fatigue
- dizziness

The ability of organic chemicals to cause health effects varies greatly from those that are highly toxic to those with no known health effect.

As with other pollutants, the extent and nature of the health effect will depend on many factors including level of exposure and length of time exposed. Among the immediate symptoms that some people have experienced soon after exposure to some organics include:

- eye and respiratory tract irritation
- headaches
- dizziness
- visual disorders and memory impairment

At present, not much is known about what health effects occur from the levels of organics usually found in homes.

Levels in Homes

Studies have found that levels of several organics average 2–5 times higher indoors than outdoors. During and for several hours immediately after certain activities, such as paint stripping, levels may be 1,000 times background outdoor levels.

Steps to Reduce Exposure

- Increase ventilation when using products that emit VOCs.
- Meet or exceed any label precautions.
- Do not store opened containers of unused paints and similar materials within the school.

- Formaldehyde, one of the best known VOCs, is one of the few indoor air pollutants that can be readily measured.

- Identify, and if possible, remove the source.

- If not possible to remove, reduce exposure by using a sealant on all exposed surfaces of paneling and other furnishings.

- Use integrated pest management techniques to reduce the need for pesticides.

- Use household products according to manufacturer's directions.

- Make sure you provide plenty of fresh air when using these products.

- Throw away unused or little-used containers safely; buy in quantities that you will use soon.

- Keep out of reach of children and pets.

- Never mix household care products unless directed on the label.

Follow Label Instructions Carefully

Potentially hazardous products often have warnings aimed at reducing exposure of the user. For example, if a label says to use the product in a well-ventilated area, go outdoors or in areas equipped with an exhaust fan to use it. Otherwise, open up windows to provide the maximum amount of outdoor air possible.

Throw Away Partially Full Containers of Old or Unneeded Chemicals Safely

Because gases can leak even from closed containers, this single step could help lower concentrations of organic chemicals in your home. (Be sure that materials you decide to keep are stored not only in a well-ventilated area but are also safely out of reach of children.) Do not simply toss these unwanted products in the garbage can. Find out if your local government or any organization in your community sponsors special days for the collection of toxic household wastes. If such days are available, use them to dispose of the unwanted containers safely. If no such collection days are available, think about organizing one.

Buy Limited Quantities

If you use products only occasionally or seasonally, such as paints, paint strippers and kerosene for space heaters or gasoline for lawn mowers, but only as much as you will use right away.

Keep Exposure to Emissions from Products Containing Methylene Chloride to a Minimum

Consumer products that contain methylene chloride include paint strippers, adhesive removers and aerosol spray paints. Methylene chloride is known to cause cancer in animals. Also, methylene chloride is converted to carbon monoxide in the body and can cause symptoms associated with exposure to carbon monoxide. Carefully read the labels containing health hazard information and cautions on the proper use of these products. Use products that contain methylene chloride outdoors when possible; use indoors only if the area is well ventilated.

Keep Exposure to Benzene to a Minimum

Benzene is a known human carcinogen. The main indoor sources of this chemical are:

- environmental tobacco smoke
- stored fuels
- paint supplies
- automobile emissions in attached garages

Actions that will reduce benzene exposure include:

- eliminating smoking within the home
- providing for maximum ventilation during painting
- discarding paint supplies and special fuels that will not be used immediately

Keep Exposure to Perchloroethylene Emissions from Newly Dry-Cleaned Materials to a Minimum

Perchloroethylene is the chemical most widely used in dry cleaning. In laboratory studies, it has been shown to cause cancer in animals. Studies indicate that people breathe low levels of this chemical both in homes where dry-cleaned goods are stored and as they wear dry-cleaned clothing. Dry cleaners recapture the perchloroethylene during the dry-cleaning process so they can save money by re-using it, and they remove more of the chemical during the pressing and finishing processes. Some dry cleaners, however, do not remove as much perchloroethylene as possible all of the time.

331

Taking steps to minimize your exposure to this chemical is prudent.

- If dry-cleaned goods have a strong chemical odor when you pick them up, do not accept them until they have been properly dried.

- If goods with a chemical odor are returned to you on subsequent visits, try a different dry cleaner.

Chapter 28

Radiation Exposure Risks

Chapter Contents

Section 28.1

Microwave Oven Radiation

This section includes text excerpted from "Microwave Oven Radiation," U.S. Food and Drug Administration (FDA), December 12, 2017.

The U.S. Food and Drug Administration (FDA) has regulated the manufacture of microwave ovens since 1971. Microwave oven manufacturers are required to certify their products and meet safety performance standards created and enforced by the FDA to protect the public health. On the basis of current knowledge about microwave radiation, the Agency believes that ovens that meet the FDA standard and are used according to the manufacturer's instructions are safe for use.

What Is Microwave Radiation?

Microwaves are a form of electromagnetic (EM) radiation; that is, they are waves of electrical and magnetic energy moving together through space. EM radiation spans a broad spectrum from very long radio waves to very short gamma rays. The human eye can only detect a small portion of this spectrum called visible light. A radio detects a different portion of the spectrum, and an X-ray machine uses yet another portion.

Visible light, microwaves, and radio frequency (RF) radiation are forms of nonionizing radiation. Nonionizing radiation does not have enough energy to knock electrons out of atoms. X-rays are a form of ionizing radiation. Exposure to ionizing radiation can alter atoms and molecules and cause damage to cells in organic matter.

Microwaves are used to detect speeding cars and to send telephone and television (TV) communications. Industry uses microwaves to dry and cure plywood, to cure rubber and resins, to raise bread and doughnuts, and to cook potato chips. But the most common consumer use of microwave energy is in microwave ovens. Microwaves have three characteristics that allow them to be used in cooking: they are reflected by metal; they pass through glass, paper, plastic, and similar materials; and they are absorbed by foods.

Cooking with Microwaves

Microwaves are produced inside the oven by an electron tube called a magnetron. The microwaves are reflected in the metal interior of the oven where they are absorbed by food. Microwaves cause water molecules in food to vibrate, producing heat that cooks the food. That's why foods that are high in water content, like fresh vegetables, can be cooked more quickly than other foods. The microwave energy is changed to heat as it is absorbed by food, and does not make food "radioactive" or "contaminated."

Although heat is produced directly in the food, microwave ovens do not cook food from the "inside out." When thick foods are cooked, the outer layers are heated and cooked primarily by microwaves while the inside is cooked mainly by the conduction of heat from the hot outer layers.

Microwave cooking can be more energy efficient than conventional cooking because foods cook faster and the energy heats only the food, not the whole oven compartment. Microwave cooking does not reduce the nutritional value of foods any more than conventional cooking. In fact, foods cooked in a microwave oven may keep more of their vitamins and minerals, because microwave ovens can cook more quickly and without adding water.

Glass, paper, ceramic, or plastic containers are used in microwave cooking because microwaves pass through these materials. Although such containers cannot be heated by microwaves, they can become hot from the heat of the food cooking inside. Some plastic containers should not be used in a microwave oven because they can be melted by the heat of the food inside. Generally, metal pans or aluminum foil should also not be used in a microwave oven, as the microwaves are reflected off these materials causing the food to cook unevenly and possibly damaging the oven. The instructions that come with each microwave oven indicate the kinds of containers to use. They also cover how to test containers to see whether or not they can be used in microwave ovens.

Avoiding Injuries from Super-Heated Water in Microwave Ovens

The FDA received reports in the past of serious skin burns or scalding injuries around people's hands and faces as a result of hot water erupting out of a cup after it had been overheated in a microwave oven. Super-heated water (water heated past its boiling temperature) does not appear to be boiling and occurs when water is heated by itself in a clean cup. If super-heating has occurred, a slight disturbance or movement such as picking up the cup, or pouring in a spoon full of instant coffee, may result in a violent eruption with the boiling water exploding out of the cup. Adding substances such as instant coffee or sugar before heating greatly reduces this risk.

Users should closely follow the precautions and recommendations provided in the microwave oven instruction manuals, specifically regarding heating times. Users should make sure that they do not exceed the recommended heating times when determining the best time settings to heat water to the desired temperature.

Microwave Oven Safety Standard

Through its Center for Devices and Radiological Health (CDRH), the FDA sets and enforces standards of performance for electronic products to assure that radiation emissions do not pose a hazard to public health.

A federal standard (21 CFR 1030.10) limits the number of microwaves that can leak from an oven throughout its lifetime to 5 milliwatts (mW) of microwave radiation per square centimeter at approximately 2 inches from the oven surface. This limit is far below the level known to harm people. Microwave energy also decreases dramatically as you move away from the source of radiation. A measurement made 20 inches from an oven would be approximately 1/100th of the value measured at 2 inches from the oven.

The standard also requires all ovens to have two independent interlock systems that stop the production of microwaves the moment the latch is released or the door is opened. In addition, a monitoring system stops oven operation in case one or both of the interlock systems fail.

All ovens must have a label stating that they meet the safety standard. In addition, the FDA requires that all ovens have a label explaining precautions for use. This requirement may be dropped if the manufacturer has proven that the oven will not exceed the allowable leakage limit even if used under the conditions cautioned against on the label.

To make sure the standard is met, the FDA tests microwave ovens in its own laboratory. The FDA also evaluates manufacturers' radiation testing and quality control programs at their factories.

Microwave Ovens and Health

Microwave radiation can heat body tissue the same way it heats food. Exposure to high levels of microwaves can cause a painful burn.

Two areas of the body, the eyes, and the testes are particularly vulnerable to RF heating because there is relatively little blood flow in them to carry away excess heat. Additionally, the lens of the eye is particularly sensitive to intense heat, and exposure to high levels of microwaves can cause cataracts. But these types of injuries—burns and cataracts—can only be caused by exposure to large amounts of microwave radiation.

Consumers should take common-sense precautions regarding the handling of hot foods and beverages.

Have Radiation Injuries Resulted from Microwave Ovens?

Most injuries related to microwave ovens are the result of heat-related burns from hot containers, overheated foods, or exploding liquids. Most injuries are not radiation-related. That said, there have been very rare instances of radiation injury due to unusual circumstances or improper servicing. In general, microwave oven radiation injuries are caused by exposure to large amounts of microwave radiation leaking through openings such as gaps in the microwave oven seals. However, the FDA regulations require that microwave ovens are designed to prevent these high-level radiation leaks.

Microwave Ovens and Pacemakers

At one time, there was concern that radiation leakage from microwave ovens could interfere with certain electronic cardiac pacemakers. Similar concerns were raised about pacemaker interference from electric shavers, auto ignition systems, and other electronic products. While the FDA does not specifically require microwave ovens to carry warnings for people with pacemakers, this problem has largely been resolved as pacemakers are designed to shield against such electrical interference. However, patients with pacemakers are encouraged to consult their physicians if they have concerns.

Checking Ovens for Leakage and Other Radiation Safety Problems

There is little cause for concern about excess microwaves leaking from ovens unless the door hinges, latch, or seals are damaged. The FDA recommends looking at your oven carefully, and not using an oven if the door doesn't close firmly or is bent, warped, or otherwise damaged.

The FDA also monitors appliances for radiation safety issues and has received reports of microwave ovens that appear to stay on—and operate—while the door is open. When operating as intended, microwave ovens have safety features to prevent them from continuing to generate microwaves if the door is open. However, if an oven does continue to operate with the door open, consumers cannot be 100 percent sure that microwave radiation is not being emitted. Thus, if this occurs, the FDA recommends immediately discontinuing use of the oven.

How to Report Microwave Oven Radiation Safety Problems

If you suspect a radiation safety problem with your microwave oven, you may contact the microwave oven manufacturer. Manufacturers who discover that any microwave ovens produced, assembled, or imported by them have a defect or failure to comply with an applicable federal standard are required to immediately notify the FDA. In addition, manufacturers/importers are required to report all accidental radiation occurrences to the FDA, unless the incident is associated with a defect or noncompliance that has previously been reported (21 CFR 1002.20).

Tips on Safe Microwave Oven Operation

- Follow the manufacturer's instruction manual for recommended operating procedures and safety precautions for your oven model.

- Use microwave safe cookware specially manufactured for use in the microwave oven.

- Don't operate a microwave oven if the door does not close firmly or is bent, warped, or otherwise damaged.

- Stop using a microwave oven if it continues to operate with the door open.

- As an added safety precaution, don't stand directly against an oven (and don't allow children to do this) for long periods of time while it is operating.

- Do not heat water or liquids in the microwave oven longer than recommended in the manufacturer's instructions.

- Some ovens should not be operated when empty. Refer to the instruction manual for your oven.

- Regularly clean the oven cavity, the outer edge of the cavity, and the door with water and a mild detergent. A special microwave oven cleaner is not necessary. Be sure to not use scouring pads, steel wool, or other abrasives.

Section 28.2

Cell Phone Radiation

This section contains text excerpted from the following sources: Text in this section begins with excerpts from "Cell Phones," National Institute of Environmental Health Sciences (NIEHS), April 10, 2018; Text under the heading "Why Is There Concern That Cell Phones May Cause Cancer or Other Health Problems?" is excerpted from "Cell Phones and Cancer Risk," National Cancer Institute (NCI), February 16, 2018.

Personal (cellular) telecommunications is a rapidly evolving technology that uses radio frequency energy or radiation for mobile communication. Most Americans use cell phones. Given this large number of users, if adverse health effects are shown to be associated with cell phone use, this could potentially be a widespread public health concern. Current scientific evidence has not conclusively linked cell phone use with any adverse health problems in humans, but more research is needed.

Why Is There Concern That Cell Phones May Cause Cancer or Other Health Problems?

There are three main reasons why people are concerned that cell phones (also known as "mobile" or "wireless" telephones) might have the potential to cause certain types of cancer or other health problems:

1. Cell phones emit radiofrequency (RF) energy (radio waves), a form of nonionizing radiation, from their antennas. Tissues nearest to the antenna can absorb this energy.

2. The number of cell phone users has increased rapidly. As of December 2014, there were more than 327.5 million cell phone

subscribers in the United States, according to the Cellular Telecommunications and Internet Association (CTIA). This is a nearly threefold increase from the 110 million users in 2000. Globally, the number of subscriptions is estimated by the International Telecommunications Union (ITU) to be 5 billion.

3. Over time, the number of cell phone calls per day, the length of each call, and the amount of time people use cell phones have increased. However, improvements in cell phone technology have resulted in devices that have lower power outputs than earlier models.

What Is Radiofrequency (RF) Energy and How Does It Affect the Body?

RF energy is a form of electromagnetic (EM) radiation. EM radiation can be categorized into two types: ionizing (e.g., X-rays, radon, and cosmic rays) and nonionizing (e.g., RF and extremely low frequency, or power frequency). EM radiation is defined according to its wavelength and frequency, which is the number of cycles of a wave that pass a reference point per second. EM frequencies are described in units called hertz (Hz).

The energy of EM radiation is determined by its frequency; ionizing radiation is high frequency, and therefore, high energy, whereas nonionizing radiation is low frequency, and therefore, low energy.

The frequency of RF-EM radiation ranges from 30 kilohertz (30 kHz, or 30,000 Hz) to 300 gigahertz (300 GHz, or 300 billion Hz). EM fields in the RF range are used for telecommunications applications, including cell phones, televisions, and radio transmissions. The human body absorbs energy from devices that emit RF-EM radiation. The dose of the absorbed energy is estimated using a measure called the specific absorption rate (SAR), which is expressed in watts per kilogram of body weight.

Exposure to ionizing radiation, such as from X-rays, is known to increase the risk of cancer. However, although many studies have examined the potential health effects of nonionizing radiation from radar, microwave ovens, cell phones, and other sources, there is currently no consistent evidence that nonionizing radiation increases cancer risk.

The only consistently recognized biological effect of RF energy is heating. The ability of microwave ovens to heat food is one example of this effect of RF energy. RF exposure from cell phone use does cause heating to the area of the body where a cell phone or other device is held (ear, head, etc.). However, it is not sufficient to measurably increase body temperature, and there are no other clearly established effects on the body from RF energy.

It has been suggested that RF energy might affect glucose metabolism, but two small studies that examined brain glucose metabolism after use of a cell phone showed inconsistent results. Whereas one study showed increased glucose metabolism in the region of the brain close to the antenna compared with tissues on the opposite side of the brain, the other study found reduced glucose metabolism on the side of the brain where the phone was used.

Another study investigated whether exposure to the RF energy from cell phones affects the flow of blood in the brain and found no evidence of such an effect.

The authors of these studies noted that the results are preliminary and that possible health outcome from changes in glucose metabolism are still unknown. Such inconsistent findings are not uncommon in experimental studies of the biological effects of RF-EM radiation. Some contributing factors include assumptions used to estimate doses, failure to consider temperature effects, and lack of blinding of investigators to exposure status.

How Is RF Energy Exposure Measured in Epidemiologic Studies?

Epidemiologic studies use information from several sources, including questionnaires and data from cell phone service providers. Direct measurements are not yet possible outside of a laboratory setting. Estimates take into account the following:

- How "regularly" study participants use cell phones (the number of calls per week or month)

- The age and the year when study participants first used a cell phone and the age and the year of last use (allows calculation of the duration of use and time since the start of use)

- The average number of cell phone calls per day, week, or month (frequency)

- The average length of a typical cell phone call

- The total hours of lifetime use, calculated from the length of typical call times, the frequency of use, and the duration of use

341

What Has Research Shown about the Possible Cancer-Causing Effects of RF Energy?

RF energy, unlike ionizing radiation, does not cause deoxyribonucleic acid (DNA) damage that can lead to cancer. It's only consistently observed the biological effect in humans is tissue heating. In animal studies, it has not been found to cause cancer or to enhance the cancer-causing effects of known chemical carcinogens. The National Toxicology Program (NTP), a federal interagency program headquartered at the National Institute of Environmental Health Sciences (NIEHS), which is part of the National Institutes of Health (NIH), completed a series of large-scale studies in rodents of exposure to RF energy (the type used in cell phones). This investigation was conducted in highly specialized labs that can specify and control sources of radiation and measure their effects.

In February 2018, two draft technical reports summarizing the findings were made available in advance of the formal peer-review process in March 2018. Peer review is a critical component of the scientific process to ensure that research findings are meaningful, accurate, and appropriately interpreted.

The U.S. Food and Drug Administration (FDA) issued a statement on the NTP reports stating they "believe the current safety limits for cell phones are acceptable for protecting the public health." the FDA and Federal Communications Commission (FCC) share responsibility for regulating cell phone technologies and the FDA originally nominated this topic for study by NTP.

Researchers have carried out several types of epidemiologic studies in humans to investigate the possibility of a relationship between cell phone use and the risk of malignant (cancerous) brain tumors, such as gliomas, as well as benign (noncancerous) tumors, such as acoustic neuromas (tumors in the cells of the nerve responsible for hearing), most meningiomas (tumors in the meninges, membranes that cover and protect the brain and spinal cord), and parotid gland tumors (tumors in the salivary glands).

In one type of study, called a case-control study, cell phone use is compared between people with these types of tumors and people without them. In another type of study, called a cohort study, a large group of people who do not have cancer at study entry is followed over time and the rate of these tumors in people who did and didn't use cell phones is compared. Cancer incidence data can also be analyzed over time to see if the rates of cancer changed in large populations during the time that cell phone use increased dramatically. These studies have not shown clear evidence of a relationship between cell phone use and cancer. However, researchers have reported some statistically significant associations for certain subgroups of people.

Three large epidemiologic studies have examined the possible association between cell phone use and cancer: Interphone, a case-control study; the Danish Study, a cohort study; and the Million Women Study, another cohort study.

Interphone

How the study was done. This is the largest health-related case-control study of cell phone use and the risk of head and neck tumors. It was conducted by a consortium of researchers from 13 countries. The data came from questionnaires that were completed by study participants.

What the study showed. Most published analyses from this study have shown no statistically significant increases in the brain or central nervous system cancers related to higher amounts of cell phone use. One analysis showed a statistically significant, although modest, increase in the risk of glioma among the small proportion of study participants who spent the total time on cell phone calls. However, the researchers considered this finding inconclusive because they felt that the amount of use reported by some respondents was unlikely and because the participants who reported lower levels of use appeared to have a slightly reduced risk of brain cancer compared with people who did not use cell phones regularly. Another analysis from this study found no relationship between brain tumor locations and regions of the brain that were exposed to the highest level of RF energy from cell phones.

Danish Study

How the study was done. This cohort study, conducted in Denmark, linked billing information from more than 358,000 cell phone subscribers with brain tumor incidence data from the Danish Cancer Registry.

What the study showed. No association was observed between cell phone use and the incidence of glioma, meningioma, or acoustic neuroma, even among people who had been cell phone subscribers for 13 or more years.

Million Women Study

How the study was done. This prospective cohort study conducted in the United Kingdom used data obtained from questionnaires that were completed by study participants.

What the study showed. Self-reported cell phone use was not associated with an increased risk of glioma, meningioma, or noncentral nervous system tumors. Although the original published findings reported an association with an increased risk of acoustic neuroma, this association disappeared after an additional follow-up of the cohort.

Why Are the Findings from Different Studies of Cell Phone Use and Cancer Risk Inconsistent?

A limited number of studies have shown some evidence of statistical association between cell phone use and brain tumor risks, but most studies have found no association. Reasons for these discrepancies include the following:

- **Recall bias,** which can occur when data about prior habits and exposures are collected from study participants using questionnaires administered after diagnosis of a disease in some of the participants. It is possible that study participants who have brain tumors may remember their cell phone use differently from individuals without brain tumors. Many epidemiologic studies of cell phone use and brain cancer risk lack verifiable data about the total amount of cell phone use over time. In addition, people who develop a brain tumor may have a tendency to recall cell phone use mostly on the same side of the head where their tumor was found, regardless of whether they actually used their phone on that side of the head a lot or only a little.

- **Inaccurate reporting,** which can happen when people say that something has happened more or less often than it actually did. People may not remember how much they used cell phones in a given time period.

- **Morbidity and mortality** among study participants who have brain cancer. Gliomas are particularly difficult to study, for example, because of their high death rate and the short survival of people who develop these tumors. Patients who survive initial treatment are often impaired, which may affect their responses to questions. Furthermore, for people who have died, next-of-kin are often less familiar with the cell phone use patterns of their deceased family member and may not accurately describe their patterns of use to an interviewer.

- **Participation bias,** which can happen when people who are diagnosed with brain tumors are more likely than healthy people (known as controls) to enroll in a research study. Also, controls who did not or rarely used cell phones were less likely to participate in the Interphone study than controls who used cell phones regularly. For example, the Interphone study reported participation rates of 78 percent for meningioma patients (range 56–92 percent for the individual studies), 64 percent for glioma patients (range 36–92 percent), and 53 percent for control subjects (range 42–74 percent).

- **Changing technology and methods of use.** Older studies evaluated RF energy exposure from analog cell phones. However, most cell phones use digital technology, which operates at a different frequency and a lower power level than analog phones. Digital cell phones have been in use for more than a decade in the United States, and cellular technology continues to change. Texting, for example, has become a popular way of using a cell phone to communicate that does not require bringing the phone close to the head. Furthermore, the use of hands-free technology, such as wired and wireless headsets, is increasing and may decrease RF energy exposure to the head and brain.

What Do Expert Organizations Conclude about the Cancer Risk from Cell Phone Use?

In 2011, the International Agency for Research on Cancer (IARC), a component of the World Health Organization (WHO), appointed an expert Working Group to review all available evidence on the use of cell phones. The Working Group classified cell phone use as "possibly carcinogenic to humans," based on limited evidence from human studies, limited evidence from studies of RF energy and cancer in rodents, and inconsistent evidence from mechanistic studies.

The Working Group indicated that, although the human studies were susceptible to bias, the findings could not be dismissed as reflecting bias alone, and that a causal interpretation could not be excluded. The Working Group noted that any interpretation of the evidence should also consider that the observed associations could reflect chance, bias, or confound rather than an underlying causal effect. In addition, the Working Group stated that the investigation of the risk of cancer of the brain associated with cell phone use poses complex methodologic challenges in the conduct of the research and in the analysis and interpretation of findings.

The American Cancer Society (ACS) states that the IARC classification means that there could be some cancer risk associated with RF energy, but the evidence is not strong enough to be considered causal and needs to be investigated further. Individuals who are concerned about RF energy exposure can limit their exposure, including using an earpiece and limiting cell phone use, particularly among children.

The National Institute of Environmental Health Sciences (NIEHS) states that the weight of the current scientific evidence has not conclusively linked cell phone use with any adverse health problems, but more research is needed.

The U.S. Food and Drug Administration (FDA) notes that studies reporting biological changes associated with RF energy have failed to be replicated and that the majority of human epidemiologic studies have failed to show a relationship between exposure to RF energy from cell phones and health problems.

The Centers for Disease Control and Prevention (CDC) states that no scientific evidence definitively answers whether cell phone use causes cancer.

The Federal Communications Commission (FCC) concludes that no scientific evidence establishes a causal link between wireless device use and cancer or other illnesses.

In 2015 the European Commission Scientific Committee on Emerging and Newly Identified Health Risks (SCENIHR) concluded that, overall, the epidemiologic studies on cell phone RF-EM radiation exposure do not show an increased risk of brain tumors or of other cancers of the head and neck region. The Committee also stated that epidemiologic studies do not indicate an increased risk for other malignant diseases, including childhood cancer.

What Studies Are Underway That Will Help Further Our Understanding of the Possible Health Effects of Cell Phone Use?

A large prospective cohort study of cell phone use and its possible long-term health effects was launched in Europe in March 2010. This study, known as a cohort study of mobile phone use and health (COSMOS), has enrolled approximately 290,000 cell phone users aged 18 years or older to date and will follow them for 20–30 years.

Participants in COSMOS will complete a questionnaire about their health, lifestyle, and current and past cell phone use. This information will be supplemented with information from health records and cell phone records.

The challenge of this ambitious study is to continue following the participants for a range of health effects over many decades. Researchers will need to determine whether participants who leave the study are somehow different from those who remain throughout the follow-up period.

Although recall bias is minimized in studies such as COSMOS that link participants to their cell phone records, such studies face other problems. For example, it is impossible to know who is using the listed cell phone or whether that individual also places calls using other cell phones. To a lesser extent, it is not clear whether multiple users of a single phone will be represented on a single phone company account.

Do Children Have a Higher Risk of Developing Cancer Due to Cell Phone Use than Adults?

There are theoretical considerations as to why the possible risk should be investigated separately in children. Their nervous systems are still developing and, therefore, more vulnerable to factors that may cause cancer. Their heads are smaller than those of adults and consequently, have a greater proportional exposure to the field of radiofrequency radiation that is emitted by cell phones. And, children have the potential of accumulating more years of cell phone exposure than adults do.

Thus far, the data from studies in children with cancer do not support this theory. The first published analysis came from a large case-control study called CEFALO, which was conducted in Denmark, Sweden, Norway, and Switzerland. The study included children who were diagnosed with brain tumors, when their ages ranged from 7–19. Researchers did not find an association between cell phone use and brain tumor risk either by time since initiation of use, amount of use or by the location of the tumor.

Several studies that will provide more information are underway. Researchers from the Centre for Research in Environmental Epidemiology (CREAL) in Spain are conducting another international case-control study—Mobi-Kids—that will include 2000 young people (aged 10–24 years) with newly diagnosed brain tumors and 4000 healthy young people. The goal of the study is to learn more about risk factors for childhood brain tumors.

What Can Cell Phone Users Do to Reduce Their Exposure to RF Energy?

The FDA has suggested some steps that concerned cell phone users can take to reduce their exposure to RF energy:

- Reserve the use of cell phones for shorter conversations or for times when a landline phone is not available.

- Use a device with hands-free technology, such as wired head-sets, which place more distance between the phone and the head of the user.

Hands-free kits reduce the amount of RF energy exposure to the head because the antenna, which is the source of energy, is not placed against the head. Exposures decline dramatically when cell phones are used hands-free.

Where Can I Find More Information about RF Energy from My Cell Phone?

The FCC provides information about the specific absorption rate (SAR) of cell phones produced and marketed within the last 1–2 years. The SAR corresponds to the relative amount of RF energy absorbed by the head of a cell phone user. Consumers can access this information using the phone's FCC ID number, which is usually located in the case of the phone, and the FCC's ID search form.

Chapter 29

Electric and Magnetic Field Exposure

What Are Electric and Magnetic Fields?

Electric and magnetic fields are invisible areas of energy (also called radiation) that are produced by electricity, which is the movement of electrons, or current, through a wire.

An electric field is produced by voltage, which is the pressure used to push the electrons through the wire, much like water being pushed through a pipe. As the voltage increases, the electric field increases in strength. Electric fields are measured in volts per meter (V/m).

A magnetic field results from the flow of current through wires or electrical devices and increases in strength as the current increases. The strength of a magnetic field decreases rapidly with increasing distance from its source. Magnetic fields are measured in microteslas (μT, or millionths of a Tesla).

Electric fields are produced whether or not a device is turned on, whereas magnetic fields are produced only when current is flowing, which usually requires a device to be turned on. Power lines produce magnetic fields continuously because the current is always flowing through them. Electric fields are easily shielded or weakened by walls and other objects, whereas magnetic fields, can pass through buildings, living things, and most other materials.

This chapter includes text excerpted from "Electromagnetic Fields and Cancer," National Cancer Institute (NCI), May 27, 2016.

Electric and magnetic fields together are referred to as electromagnetic (EM) fields or EMFs. The electric and magnetic forces in EMFs are caused by EM radiation. There are two main categories of EMFs:

1. Higher-frequency EMFs, which include X-rays and gamma rays. These EMFs are in the ionizing radiation part of the EM spectrum and can damage deoxyribonucleic acid (DNA) or cells directly.

2. Low-to mid-frequency EMFs, which include static fields (electric or magnetic fields that do not vary with time), magnetic fields from electric power lines and appliances, radio waves, microwaves, infrared radiation, and visible light. These EMFs are in the nonionizing radiation part of the EM spectrum and are not known to damage DNA or cells directly. Low-to mid-frequency EMFs include extremely low frequency (ELF) EMFs (ELF-EMFs) and radiofrequency (RF) EMFs. ELF-EMFs have frequencies of up to 300 cycles per second, or hertz (Hz), and RF EMFs range from 3 kilohertz (3 kHz, or 3,000 Hz) to 300 gigahertz (300 GHz, or 300 billion Hz). RF radiation is measured in watts per meter squared (W/m2).

What Are Common Sources of Nonionizing EMFs?

There are both natural and human-made sources of nonionizing EMFs. The earth's magnetic field, which causes the needle on a compass to point North, is one example of a naturally occurring EMF.

Human-made EMFs fall into both the ELF and RF categories of nonionizing part of the EM spectrum. These EMFs can come from a number of sources.

Extremely Low-Frequency EMFs (ELF-EMFs)

Sources of ELF-EMFs include power lines, electrical wiring, and electrical appliances such as shavers, hair dryers, and electric blankets.

RF Radiation

The most common sources of RF radiation are wireless telecommunication devices and equipment, including cell phones, smart meters, and portable wireless devices, such as tablets and laptop computers. In the United States, cell phones currently operate in a frequency range of about 1.8–2.2 GHz.

Other common sources of RF radiation include:

- **Radio and television signals.** Amplitude-modulated/frequency-modulated (AM/FM) radios and older very high frequency/

ultra high frequency (VHF/UHF) televisions operate at lower RFs than cell phones. Radio signals are AM (amplitude-modulated) or FM (frequency-modulated). AM radio is used for broadcasting over very long distances, whereas FM radio covers more localized areas. AM signals are transmitted from large arrays of antennas that are placed at high elevation on sites that are off-limits to the general public because exposures close to the source can be high. Maintenance workers could receive substantial RF exposures from AM radio antennas, but the general public would not. FM radio antennas and TV broadcasting antennas, which are much smaller than AM antennas, are generally mounted at the top of high towers. RF exposures near the base of these towers are below guideline limits, so exposure of the general population is very low. Sometimes small local radio and television (TV) antennas are mounted on the top of a building; access to the roof of such buildings is usually controlled.

- **Radar, satellite stations, magnetic resonance imaging (MRI) devices, and industrial equipment.** These operate at somewhat higher RFs than cell phones.

- **Microwave ovens** used in homes, which also operate at somewhat higher RFs than cell phones. Microwave ovens are manufactured with effective shielding that has reduced the leakage of RF radiation from these appliances to barely detectable levels.

- **Cordless telephones,** which can operate on an analog or digital enhanced cordless telecommunications (DECT) technology and typically emit RFs similar to those of cell phones. However, because cordless phones have a limited range and require a nearby base, their signal strengths are generally much lower than those of cell phones.

- **Cell phone base stations.** Antenna towers or base stations, including those for mobile phone networks and for broadcasting for radio and for television, emit various types of RF energy. Because the majority of individuals in the general population are exposed only intermittently to base stations and broadcast antennas, it is difficult to estimate exposures for a population. The strength of these exposures varies based on the population density of the region, the average distance from the source, and the time of day or the day of the week (lower exposures on the weekends or at night). In general, exposures decrease with increasing distance from the source. Exposures among maintenance workers have been found to vary depending on their tasks, the type of antenna, and the location of the worker in relation to the source. Cumulative exposures of such workers are very difficult to estimate.

- **Televisions and computer screens** produce electric and magnetic fields at various frequencies, as well as static electric fields. The liquid crystal displays (LCDs) found in some laptop and desktop computers do not produce substantial electric or magnetic fields. Modern computers have conductive screens that reduce static fields produced by the screen to normal background levels.

- **Wireless local area networks,** commonly known as wireless fidelity (Wi-Fi) are specific types of wireless networking systems and an increasingly common source of RF radiation. Wireless networks use radio waves to connect Wi-Fi enabled devices to an access point that is connected to the Internet, either physically or through some form of data connection. Most Wi-Fi devices operate at RFs that are broadly similar to cell phones, typically 2.4–2.5 GHz, although in Wi-Fi devices that operate at somewhat higher frequencies (5, 5.3, or 5.8 GHz) have appeared. RF radiation exposure from Wi-Fi devices is considerably lower than that from cell phones. Both sources emit levels of RF radiation that are far below the guideline of 10 W/m2 as specified by the International Commission on Non-Ionizing Radiation Protection (ICNIRP).

- **Digital electric and gas meters, also known as "smart meters."** These devices, which operate at about the same RFs as cell phones, transmit information on consumption of electricity or gas to utility companies. Smart meters produce very low-level fields that sometimes cannot be distinguished from the total background RF radiation levels inside a home.

For household appliances and other devices used in the home that require electricity, magnetic field levels are highest near the source of the field and decrease rapidly the farther away the user is from the source. Magnetic fields drop precipitously at a distance of about 1 foot from most appliances. For computer screens, at a distance of 12–20 inches from the screen that most persons using computers sit, magnetic fields are similarly dramatically lower.

Why Are Nonionizing EMFs Studied in Relation to Cancer?

Power lines and electrical appliances that emit nonionizing EMFs are present everywhere in homes and workplaces. For example, wireless local networks are nearly always "on" and are increasingly commonplace in homes, schools, and many public places.

No mechanism by which ELF-EMFs or RF radiation could cause cancer has been identified. Unlike high-energy (ionizing) radiation, EMFs in the nonionizing part of the EM spectrum cannot damage DNA or cells directly. Some scientists have speculated that ELF-EMFs could cause cancer through other mechanisms, such as by reducing levels of the hormone melatonin. There is some evidence that melatonin may suppress the development of certain tumors.

Studies of animals have not provided any indications that exposure to ELF-EMFs is associated with cancer. The few high-quality studies in animals have provided no evidence that Wi-Fi is harmful to health. The National Institute of Environmental Health Sciences (NIEHS), which is part of the National Institutes of Health (NIH), is carrying out a large-scale study in rodents of exposure to RF energy (the type used in cell phones). This investigation is being conducted in highly specialized labs that can specify and control sources of radiation and measure their effects.

Although there is no known mechanism by which nonionizing EMFs could damage DNA and cause cancer, even a small increase in risk would be of clinical importance given how widespread exposure to these fields is.

What Have Studies Shown About Possible Associations between Nonionizing EMFs and Cancer in Children?

Numerous epidemiologic studies and comprehensive reviews of the scientific literature have evaluated possible associations between exposure to nonionizing EMFs and risk of cancer in children. (Magnetic fields are the component of nonionizing EMFs that are usually studied in relation to their possible health effects.) Most of the research has focused on leukemia and brain tumors, the two most common cancers in children. Studies have examined associations of these cancers with living near power lines, with magnetic fields in the home, and with exposure of parents to high levels of magnetic fields in the workplace. No consistent evidence for an association between any source of nonionizing EMF and cancer has been found.

353

Exposure from Power Lines

Although a study pointed to a possible association between living near electric power lines and childhood leukemia, more studies have had mixed findings. Most of these studies did not find an association or found one only for those children who lived in homes with very high levels of magnetic fields, which are present in few residences.

Several studies have analyzed the combined data from multiple studies of power line exposure and childhood leukemia:

- A pooled analysis of nine studies reported a twofold increase in the risk of childhood leukemia among children with exposures of 0.4 μT or higher. Less than 1 percent of the children in the studies experienced this level of exposure.

- A meta-analysis of 15 studies observed a 1.7-fold increase in childhood leukemia among children with exposures of 0.3 μT or higher. A little more than 3 percent of children in the studies experienced this level of exposure.

- A pooled analysis of seven studies published after 2000 reported a 1.4-fold increase in childhood leukemia among children with exposures of 0.3 μT or higher. However, less than one half of 1 percent of the children in the studies experienced this level of exposure.

For the two pooled studies and the meta-analysis, the number of highly exposed children was too small to provide stable estimates of the dose-response relationship. This means that the findings could be interpreted to reflect linear increases in risk, a threshold effect at 0.3 or 0.4 μT, or no significant increase.

The interpretation of the finding of increased childhood leukemia risk among children with the highest exposures (at least 0.3 μT) is unclear.

Exposure from Electrical Appliances

Another way that children can be exposed to magnetic fields is from household electrical appliances. Although magnetic fields near many electrical appliances are higher than those near power lines, appliances contribute less to a person's total exposure to magnetic fields because most appliances are used for only short periods of time. And moving even a short distance from most electrical appliances reduces exposure dramatically. Again, studies have not found consistent evidence for an association between the use of household electrical appliances and risk of childhood leukemia.

Exposure to Wi-Fi

In view of the widespread use of Wi-Fi in schools, the U.K. Health Protection Agency (now part of Public Health England) has conducted the largest and most comprehensive measurement studies to assess exposures of children to RF-EM fields from wireless computer networks. This agency concluded that RF exposures were well below recommended maximum levels and that there was "no reason why Wi-Fi should not continue to be used in schools and in other places."

A review of the published literature concluded that the few high-quality studies to date provide no evidence of biological effects from Wi-Fi exposures.

Exposure to Cell Phone Base Stations

Few studies have examined cancer risk in children living close to cell phone base stations or radio or TV transmitters. None of the studies that estimated exposures on an individual level found an increased risk of pediatric tumors.

Parental Exposure and Risk in Offspring

Several studies have examined possible associations between maternal or paternal exposure to high levels of magnetic fields before conception and/or during pregnancy and the risk of cancer in their future children. The results to date have been inconsistent. This question requires further evaluation.

Exposure and Cancer Survival

A few studies have investigated whether magnetic field exposure is associated with prognosis or survival of children with leukemia. Several small retrospective studies of this question have yielded inconsistent results. An analysis that combined prospective data for more than 3,000 children with acute lymphoid leukemia (ALL) from eight countries showed that ELF magnetic field exposure was not associated with their survival or risk of relapse.

What Have Studies Shown about Possible Associations between Nonionizing EMFs and Cancer in Adults?

Many studies have examined the association between nonionizing EMF exposure and cancer in adults, of which few studies have reported evidence of increased risk.

Residential Exposures

The majority of epidemiologic studies have shown no relationship between breast cancer in women and exposure to extremely low-frequency EMFs (ELF-EMFs) in the home, although a few individual studies have suggested an association; the only one reported results that were statistically significant.

Workplace Exposures to ELF Radiation

Several studies conducted have shown that people who worked in some electrical occupations that exposed them to ELF radiation (such as power station operators and telephone line workers) had higher-than-expected rates of some types of cancer, particularly leukemia, brain tumors, and male breast cancer. Most of the results were based on participants' job titles and not on actual measurements of their exposures. More studies, including some that considered exposure measurements as well as job titles, have generally not shown an increased risk of leukemia, brain tumors, or female breast cancer with increasing exposure to magnetic fields at work.

Workplace Exposures to RF Radiation

A limited number of studies have evaluated risks of cancer in workers exposed to RF radiation. A large study of U.S. Navy personnel found no excess of brain tumors among those with a high probability of exposure to radar (including electronics technicians, aviation technicians, and fire control technicians); however, nonlymphocytic leukemia, particularly acute myeloid leukemia (AML), was increased in electronics technicians in aviation squadrons, but not in Navy personnel in the other job categories. A case-control study among U.S. Air Force personnel found the suggestion of an increased risk of brain cancer among personnel who maintained or repaired RF or microwave-emitting equipment. A case-control study found the suggestion of an increased risk of death from brain cancer among men occupationally exposed to microwave and/or RF radiation, with all of the excess risk among workers in electrical and electronics jobs involving design, manufacture, repair, or installation of electrical or electronics equipment. There was no evidence that electrical utility workers who were exposed to pulsed EM fields produced by power lines were more likely to develop brain tumors or leukemia than the general population. Employees of a large manufacturer of wireless communication products were not more likely to die from brain tumors or cancers of the hematopoietic or lymphatic system than the general population.

What Do Expert Organizations Conclude about the Cancer Risk from EMFs?

The International Agency for Research on Cancer (IARC), a component of the World Health Organization (WHO), appointed an expert Working Group to review all available evidence on static and extremely low frequency electric and magnetic fields. The Working Group classified ELF-EMFs as "possibly carcinogenic to humans," based on limited evidence from human studies in relation to childhood leukemia. Static electric and magnetic fields and extremely low-frequency electric fields were determined "not classifiable as to their carcinogenicity to humans."

The European Commission Scientific Committee on Emerging and Newly Identified Health Risks (SCENIHR) reviewed EM fields in general, as well as cell phones in particular. It found that, overall, epidemiologic studies of extremely low-frequency fields show an increased risk of childhood leukemia with estimated daily average exposures above 0.3–0.4 μT, although no mechanisms have been identified and there is no support from experimental studies that explains these findings. It also found that the epidemiologic studies on RF exposure do not show an increased risk of brain tumors or other cancers of the head and neck region, although the possibility of an association with acoustic neuroma remains open.

Part Five

Foodborne Hazards

Chapter 30

Food Safety

Chapter Contents

Section 30.1

Food Safety at Home

This section includes text excerpted from "For Woman—Food Safety at Home," U.S. Food and Drug Administration (FDA), January 19, 2018.

Four Basic Steps for Food Safety

Each year millions of people get sick from food illnesses which can cause you to feel like you have the flu. Food illnesses can also cause serious health problems, even death. Follow these four steps to help keep you and your family safe.

Step1. Clean. Always wash your food, hands, counters, and cooking tools.

- Wash hands in warm soapy water for at least 20 seconds. Do this before and after touching food.

- Wash your cutting boards, dishes, forks, spoons, knives, and countertops with hot soapy water. Do this after working with each food item.

- Rinse fruits and veggies

- Clean the lids on canned goods before opening

Step 2. Separate. Keep raw foods to themselves. Germs can spread from one food to another.

- Keep raw meat, poultry, seafood, and eggs away from other foods.

- Do this in your shopping cart, bags, and refrigerator.

- Do not reuse marinades used on raw foods unless you bring them to a boil first.

- Use a special cutting board or plate for raw foods only.

Step 3. Cook. Foods need to get hot and stay hot. Heat kills germs.

- Cook to safe temperatures:
  - Beef, pork, lamb 145°F.
  - Fish 145°F.
  - Ground beef, pork, lamb 160°F.
  - Turkey, chicken, duck 165°F.
- Use a food thermometer to make sure that food is done. You can't always tell by looking.

  Step 4. Chill. Put food in the refrigerator right away.

- **Two-Hour rule.** Put foods in the refrigerator or freezer within 2 hours after cooking or buying from the store. Do this within 1 hour if it is 90 degrees or hotter outside.
- Never thaw food by simply taking it out of the refrigerator
- Thaw food:
  - In the refrigerator
  - Under cold water
  - In the microwave
- Marinate foods in the refrigerator

Think You Have a Food Illness?

Call your doctor and get medical care right away if you think you have a food illness. Save the food package, can, or carton. Then report the problem.

- Call the U.S. Department of Agriculture (USDA) at 888-674-6854 if you think the illness was caused by meat, poultry, or eggs
- Call the U.S. Food and Drug Administration (FDA) at 866-300-4374 for all other foods
- Call your local health department if you think you got sick from food you ate in a restaurant or another food seller

Anyone can get sick from eating spoiled food. Some people are more likely to get sick from food illnesses.

- Pregnant women
- Older Adults

- People with certain health conditions like cancer, human immunodeficiency virus (HIV)/acquired immunodeficiency syndrome (AIDS), diabetes, and kidney disease

Some foods are more risky for these people. Talk to your doctor or other health provider about which foods are safe for you to eat.

Section 30.2

Food Safety Modernization Act (FSMA)

This section includes text excerpted from "Background on the FDA Food Safety Modernization Act (FSMA)," U.S. Food and Drug Administration (FDA), January 30, 2018.

About 48 million people (1 in 6 Americans) get sick, 128,000 are hospitalized, and 3,000 die each year from foodborne diseases, according to recent data from the Centers for Disease Control and Prevention (CDC). This is a significant public health burden that is largely preventable.

The U.S. Food and Drug Administration (FDA) Food Safety Modernization Act (FSMA), signed into law by President Obama on January 4, enables the FDA to better protect public health by strengthening the food safety system. It enables the FDA to focus more on preventing food safety problems rather than relying primarily on reacting to problems after they occur. The law also provides the FDA with new enforcement authorities designed to achieve higher rates of compliance with prevention- and risk-based food safety standards and to better respond to and contain problems when they do occur. The law also gives the FDA important new tools to hold imported foods to the same standards as domestic foods and directs the FDA to build an integrated national food safety system in partnership with state and local authorities.

Building a new food safety system based on prevention will take time, and the FDA is creating a process for getting this work done. Congress has established specific implementation dates in the legislation. Some authorities will go into effect quickly, such as the FDA's new authority to order companies to recall food, and others require the FDA to prepare and issue regulations and guidance documents. The funding the Agency gets each year, which affects staffing and vital operations, will also affect how quickly the FDA can put this legislation into effect. the FDA is committed to implementing the requirements through an open process with opportunity for input from all stakeholders.

The following are among the FDA's key new authorities and mandates. Specific implementation dates specified in the law are noted in parentheses.

Prevention

For the first time, the FDA will have a legislative mandate to require comprehensive, science-based preventive controls across the food supply. This mandate includes:

- **Mandatory preventive controls for food facilities.** Food facilities are required to implement a written preventive controls plan. This involves: evaluating the hazards that could affect food safety, specifying what preventive steps, or controls, will be put in place to significantly minimize or prevent the hazards, specifying how the facility will monitor these controls to ensure they are working, maintaining routine records of the monitoring, and specifying what actions the facility will take to correct problems that arise.

- **Mandatory produce safety standards.** The FDA must establish science-based, minimum standards for the safe production and harvesting of fruits and vegetables. Those standards must consider naturally occurring hazards, as well as those that may be introduced either unintentionally or intentionally, and must address soil amendments (materials added to the soil such as compost), hygiene, packaging, temperature controls, animals in the growing area and water.

- **Authority to prevent intentional contamination.** The FDA must issue regulations to protect against the intentional adulteration of food, including the establishment of science-based mitigation strategies to prepare and protect the food supply chain at specific vulnerable points.

Inspection and Compliance

The FSMA recognizes that preventive control standards improve food safety only to the extent that producers and processors comply with them. Therefore, it will be necessary for the FDA to provide oversight, ensure compliance with requirements and respond effectively when problems emerge. FSMA provides the FDA with important new tools for inspection and compliance, including:

- **Mandated inspection frequency.** The FSMA establishes a mandated inspection frequency, based on risk, for food facilities and requires the frequency of inspection to increase immediately. All high-risk domestic facilities must be inspected within five years of enactment and no less than every three years thereafter. Within one year of enactment, the law directs the FDA to inspect at least 600 foreign facilities and double those inspections every year for the next five years.

- **Records access.** The FDA will have access to records, including industry food safety plans and the records firms will be required to keep documenting implementation of their plans.

- **Testing by accredited laboratories.** The FSMA requires certain food testing to be carried out by accredited laboratories and directs the FDA to establish a program for laboratory accreditation to ensure that the U.S. food testing laboratories meet high-quality standards.

Response

The FSMA recognizes that the FDA must have the tools to respond effectively when problems emerge despite preventive controls. New authorities include:

- **Mandatory recall.** The FSMA provides the FDA with authority to issue a mandatory recall when a company fails to voluntarily recall unsafe food after being asked to by FDA.

- **Expanded administrative detention.** The FSMA provides the FDA with a more flexible standard for administratively detaining products that are potentially in violation of the law (administrative detention is the procedure the FDA uses to keep suspect food from being moved).

- **Suspension of registration.** The FDA can suspend registration of a facility if it determines that the food poses a reasonable probability of serious adverse health consequences or death. A facility that is under suspension is prohibited from distributing food.

- **Enhanced product tracing abilities.** The FDA is directed to establish a system that will enhance its ability to track and trace both domestic and imported foods. In addition, the FDA is directed to establish pilot projects to explore and evaluate methods to rapidly and effectively identify recipients of food to prevent or control a foodborne illness outbreak.

- **Additional recordkeeping for high-risk foods.** The FDA is directed to issue proposed rulemaking to establish record-keeping requirements for facilities that manufacture, process, pack, or hold foods that the Secretary designates as high-risk foods.

Imports

The FSMA gives the FDA unprecedented authority to better ensure that imported products meet the U.S. standards and are safe for the U.S. consumers. New authorities include:

- **Importer accountability.** For the first time, importers have an explicit responsibility to verify that their foreign suppliers have adequate preventive controls in place to ensure that the food they produce is safe.

- **Third-party certification.** The FSMA establishes a program through which qualified third parties can certify that foreign food facilities comply with the U.S. food safety standards. This certification may be used to facilitate the entry of imports.

- **Certification for high-risk foods.** The FDA has the authority to require that high-risk imported foods be accompanied by a credible third-party certification or other assurance of compliance as a condition of entry into United States.

- **Voluntary qualified importer program.** The FDA must establish a voluntary program for importers that provides for expedited review and entry of foods from participating importers. Eligibility is limited to, among other things, importers offering food from certified facilities.

- **Authority to deny entry.** The FDA can refuse entry into the United States of food from a foreign facility if the FDA is denied access by the facility or the country in which the facility is located.

Enhanced Partnerships

The FSMA builds a formal system of collaboration with other government agencies, both domestic and foreign. In doing so, the statute explicitly recognizes that all food safety agencies need to work together in an integrated way to achieve its public health goals. The following are examples of enhanced collaboration:

- **State and local capacity building.** The FDA must develop and implement strategies to leverage and enhance the food safety and defense capacities of state and local agencies. The FSMA provides the FDA with a new multi-year grant mechanism to facilitate investment in state capacity to more efficiently achieve national food safety goals.

- **Foreign capacity building.** The law directs the FDA to develop a comprehensive plan to expand the capacity of foreign governments and their industries. One component of the plan is to address training of foreign governments and food producers on the U.S. food safety requirements.

- **Reliance on inspections by other agencies.** The FDA is explicitly authorized to rely on inspections of other federal, state, and local agencies to meet its increased inspection mandate for domestic facilities. The FSMA also allows the FDA to enter into interagency agreements to leverage resources with respect to the inspection of seafood facilities, both domestic and foreign, as well as seafood imports.

Additional partnerships are required to develop and implement a national agriculture and food defense strategy, to establish an integrated consortium of laboratory networks, and to improve foodborne illness surveillance.

Section 30.3

New FDA Rules Will Make Your Foods Safer

This section includes text excerpted from "5 Ways New
FDA Rules Will Make Your Foods Safer," U.S. Food and
Drug Administration (FDA), January 4, 2018.

The first two of seven rules proposed to implement the landmark
U.S. Food and Drug Administration (FDA) Food Safety Modernization Act (FSMA) (the preventive controls rules for human and animal
food—meaning food companies will apply greater controls to prevent
hazards) are now final. Here are five ways your life will be touched
by the FSMA rules.

1. **Food companies will apply greater controls to help prevent hazards.** "Rather than just react to outbreaks, we are
   requiring food facilities to take measures to prevent them from
   the get-go," says Jenny Scott, M.S., a senior advisor in the
   FDA's Office of Food Safety. Food facilities will need to think
   upfront about what could be harmful to consumers, and then
   put controls in place to minimize or prevent those hazards.

   For example, Scott says the facilities could take steps to kill
   bacteria that cause foodborne illness or to prevent them from
   growing in food. If allergens (substances that can cause an
   allergic reaction) are a hazard, the facility could pay particular
   attention to how equipment is cleaned when it is used for more
   than one product so that allergens aren't transferred from one
   food to another, and ensure that the product label identifies
   the presence of food allergens. Unidentified food allergens are
   a major cause of food recalls by industry.

2. **You and your pet get protections from tainted animal
   food.** With the Preventive Controls for Animal Food rule, "the
   same upfront thinking now required of human food manufacturing will also apply to manufacturers of animal food, including pet food," says Dan McChesney, Ph.D., director of the
   Office of Surveillance and Compliance (OS&C) in the FDA's
   Center for Veterinary Medicine (CVM).

369

If pet food manufacturers have methods in place to kill harmful bacteria, it will be much safer for both the pet and for anyone handling the food, McChesney says.

With a new prevention-oriented system in place, the FDA expects reductions in the risk of serious illness and death to animals when hazards, such as harmful levels of substances in a product, are controlled, McChesney says.

3. **Eating healthfully and eating safely will go hand in hand.** The final Produce Safety rule safeguards to help prevent illnesses in ways that are appropriate for farms.

"Farms, unlike factories, are open environments," says Samir Assar, Ph.D., director of the FDA's Division of Produce Safety. "There are elements we understand that farms can't necessarily control." However, there are actions that can, and must, be taken to minimize the likelihood of contamination in ways that are practical and feasible for growers.

Farming conditions and methods for growing the same crop can differ widely from state to state and coast to coast, so the new regulations will focus on major conduits of contamination that are common to all or most farming environments, says Assar. For example, standards have been proposed for agricultural water, farm worker hygiene or cleanliness, compost and sanitation conditions affecting buildings, equipment, and tools. These standards will apply to both domestic and imported produce.

The FDA anticipates that the produce rule as proposed would prevent hundreds of thousands of illnesses caused by produce each year.

4. **There will be greater oversight of foods imported from other countries.** We import a lot of food. In 2013, 19 percent of our overall food supply was imported from other countries, including 80 percent of our seafood, nearly 52 percent of our fresh fruit, and 22 percent of our fresh vegetables.

The rules specifically affecting imports—Foreign Supplier Verification Programs (FSVP) and Third-Party Certification—will be enhancing the oversight of imported foods.

"The FSVP rule, when finalized, will require importers to assume greater responsibility to verify that the foods they import into the United States meet the same safety standards required of domestic producers," says senior policy advisor Brian Pendleton, J.D.

5. **Consumers like you will be more confident that their food is safe.** "Up until now, everything has been reactive," says Darin Detwiler, senior policy coordinator for the advocacy group STOP Foodborne Illness. "This is the most sweeping food safety legislation passed within the last 70 years."

FDA is taking a series of steps to move the food safety system from reactive to proactive prevention.

Section 30.4

Irradiated Foods

This section includes text excerpted from "Overview of Irradiation of Food and Packaging," U.S. Food and Drug Administration (FDA), January 4, 2018.

Ionizing radiation can extend shelf life and improve the quality and safety of foods. National and international organizations and regulatory agencies have concluded that irradiated food is safe and wholesome. A brief background of the food irradiation issues leading to these conclusions is given. Despite its limited use in the past, use of food irradiation is increasing as consumers are beginning to appreciate the benefits of irradiated food. Interest in the use of food irradiation increased following the 1997 U.S. Food and Drug Administration (FDA) approval of irradiation for pathogen control in unprocessed red meat and meat products. This approval led to numerous studies on a variety of food irradiation applications. Since food is usually prepackaged prior to irradiation, the possibility of radiolytic products being released from packaging materials into food requires a safety evaluation. Therefore, the use of these packaging materials is subject to regulatory review and approval prior to their use.

Ionizing Radiation

Radiation for the treatment of food is achieved through the application of gamma rays (with Co-60 or Cesium-137 radioisotope), electron beams (high energy of up to 10 MeV), or X-rays (high energy of up to 5 MeV). Radiation principles explain how the gamma rays, e-beams and X-rays interact with matter. These interactions result in the formation of energetic electrons at random throughout the matter, which cause the formation of energetic molecular ions. These ions may be subject to electron capture and dissociation, as well as rapid rearrangement through ion-molecule reactions, or they may dissociate with time depending on the complexity of the molecular ion. Effects of radiation on matter depend on the type of the radiation and its energy level, as well as the composition, physical state, temperature and the atmospheric environment of the absorbing material. The chemical changes in matter can occur via primary radiolysis effects, which occur as a result of the adsorption of the energy by the absorbing matter, or via secondary effects, which occur as a result of the high reactivity of the free radicals and excited ions produced as a result of the primary effects. These highly reactive intermediates can undergo a variety of reactions leading to stable chemical products. In general, it is these chemical products that are detected and referred to as radiolysis products. For living things, these chemical changes can ultimately have biological consequences in the case where the target materials include living organisms.

Irradiation of Food

The use of ionizing radiation for food preservation began in the early 1920s. Later, during the 1950s–1960s, the U.S. Army conducted research into low-dose and high-dose irradiation of military rations. These experiments prompted similar studies in other countries, and the interest in food irradiation has grown ever since. With proper application, irradiation can be an effective means of eliminating and/or reducing microbial and insect infestations along with the foodborne diseases they induce, thereby improving the safety of many foods as well as extending shelf life.

Safety for Consumption of Irradiated Foods

The safety of irradiated foods for human consumption has been questioned because ionizing radiation can lead to chemical changes. The wholesomeness of irradiated foods has, therefore, been the subject of considerable national and international research, which has been reviewed and evaluated by joint expert committees of the International Atomic Energy Agency (IAEA), the World Health Organization (WHO), and the Food and Agricultural Organization (FAO) of the United Nations (UN). These expert groups have uniformly concluded that the food irradiation process does not present any enhanced toxicological, microbiological, or nutritional hazard beyond those brought about by conventional food processing techniques. These organizations, along with the Codex Alimentarius Commission (CAC) and numerous regulatory agencies, have endorsed the safety of food irradiation, providing that Good Manufacturing Practices (GMPs) and Good Irradiation Practices (GIPs) are used. This has resulted in the approval of irradiated foods by many national governments, although not all of these approvals have led to use of irradiation in the marketplace.

Identification and Detection of Irradiated Foods

The ability to reliably differentiate between irradiated and nonirradiated foods or ingredients is in the interest of government agencies, food processors, and consumers. In addition, detection tests can be used to enforce the labeling requirements for identifying irradiated foods. Labeling will enhance consumer confidence by providing assurance of the consumer's right to choose. Furthermore, the knowledge of radiation-induced chemical changes in food provides the scientific basis for the safety evaluation of the consumption of irradiated food.

Several detection methods have been subjected to interlaboratory collaborative studies including electron spin resonance (ESR), luminescence methods, physical methods, chemical methods, and biological methods. ESR measures the concentration of free radicals in irradiated matter. The luminescence methods measure the presence of excited molecules such as light emission upon heating material (thermoluminescence, TL). The physical methods are based on changes in physical properties of matter e.g., viscosity. The chemical methods are based on measurement of radiolytic products, e.g., using gas chromatography (GC) to measure volatile radiolytic products such as alkanes, alkenes, and 2-alkylcyclobutanones in fat-containing food, or to measure nonvolatile compounds such as 6-ketocholesterol and o-tyrosine. The biological methods are based on measurements of changes in viable microorganisms or changes in plant germination as a result of irradiation. The most practical methods are ESR (for foods containing bones, shells, or other particles), TL (for foods containing mineral dust particles), and GC (for fat-containing food). Continuing efforts to

373

develop detection methods are focusing on the deoxyribonucleic acid (DNA) comet assay, and the changes in protein molecular mass distribution measured by discontinuous SDS-polyacrylamide electrophoresis and quantified by laser scanning densitometry.

Labeling

Like other forms of processing, irradiation can affect the characteristics of food. Consumer choice mandates that irradiated food be adequately labeled and under the general labeling requirements, it is necessary that the food processor inform the consumer that food has been irradiated. Labeling of irradiated foods, however, is undergoing reevaluation in the United States. If whole foods have been irradiated, the FDA requires that the label bear the radura symbol and the phrase "treated with radiation" or "treated by irradiation." Yet, if irradiated ingredients are added to foods that have not been irradiated, no special labeling is required on retail packages. Special labeling is required for foods not yet in the retail market that may undergo further processing in order to ensure that foods are not irradiated multiple times. In this regulation, the FDA advises that other truthful statements, such as the reason for irradiating the food, may be included.

Because the words "radiation" and "irradiation" may have negative connotations, the labeling requirement has been viewed as an obstacle to consumer acceptance. Many in the food industry believe that an alternative wording, e.g., "electronically pasteurized," would be helpful. In 1997, Congress attempted to resolve this issues in two ways. First, it mandated that the FDA could not require print size on a label statement to be larger than that required for ingredients and second, it directed the FDA to reconsider the label requirement and to seek public comment on possible changes. The FDA had not in fact mandated a type size but did require a statement that would be "prominent and conspicuous." In response to this congressional directive, the FDA published an Advance Notice of Proposed Rulemaking (ANPR) in 1999 seeking public comment on the labeling of irradiated food, particularly on whether the current label may be misleading by implying a warning and invited suggestions of alternative labeling that would inform consumers without improperly alarming them. Thousands of comments were received, with a large number compiled into a categorical database for further examination by the Center for Food Safety and Applied Nutrition (CFSAN) Office of Nutritional Products, Labeling, and Dietary Supplements (ONPLDS). This leading office for labeling policy has not yet determined whether there will be a change in labeling requirements.

Consumer Acceptance

Consumer advocacy groups have expressed their perception that consumers do not want irradiated food products. Consumer acceptance is based on a complex decision-making process weighing the perceived risks and benefits of food irradiation compared to the existing alternatives. The acceptance is related to the needs, beliefs, and attitudes of the individual consumer and the nature of the economic, political and social environment in which food choices take place. Even though the benefits and safety of food irradiation have been scientifically documented, public awareness of such information has been limited. Consumers consequently reject food irradiation due to consumer confusion over what food irradiation is. Lack of knowledge of food irradiation and how it works generates fear that irradiated food is radioactive. Another concern is that irradiated food contains free radicals and radiolytic products. Food and health professionals could take an instrumental role in educating the consumer about the advantages and limitations of food irradiation and thus facilitate consumer acceptance of irradiated food products. The advantages of food irradiation (process safety, reduction of chemical use, and improved quality and safety of foods) over other food preservation techniques such as canning, freezing, or chemical treatment far outweigh the drawbacks—a slight reduction in nutrients (vitamins).

Though the levels of consumer acceptance vary among countries, consumers in North America are rapidly increasing their acceptance of irradiated foods. Consumer education has resulted in an appreciation of the benefits of irradiated foods. Survey results indicated that consumers develop a positive attitude toward food irradiation after receiving information on product benefits; safety and wholesomeness; environmental safety issues; and endorsement by recognized health authorities. A positive response to irradiated foods can be enhanced if the consumer is allowed to compare irradiated and nonirradiated foods side by side. Increasing numbers of consumers are willing to purchase irradiated food because they prefer the advantages irradiation processing provides. Further promotion of irradiated food has been achieved by marketing tests in various countries.

Food Irradiation Regulations

Governmental regulation of irradiation of food varies considerably from country to country. Where irradiation is permitted, regulations are needed to license the plant, radioactive materials or process; to ensure radiation safety, environmental security, and general health and safety during plant operation; and to provide for safe disposal of any hazardous materials at the end of the operation. Each country has adopted its own unique approach to the introduction, approval, and regulation of the technology for food production. Although there is an agreement among international committee experts that food is safe and wholesome for consumption after irradiation up to a dose of 10 KiloGray (kGy), there is no approval for irradiation of all foods up to this limit in any country. Most countries approve food irradiation on a case-by-case basis.

In the United States, the Food Additives Amendment to the Federal Food, Drug, and Cosmetic Act (FFDCA) of 1958 places food irradiation under the food additive regulations. It is because of this act that the FDA regulates food irradiation as a food additive and not a food process. Congress explicitly defined a source of radiation as a food additive when it stated that "Sources of radiation (including radioactive isotopes, particle accelerators, and X-ray machines) intended for use in processing food are included in the term 'food additive' as defined in this legislation." The Food Additives Amendment states that a food is adulterated (thus it cannot be marketed legally) if it has been intentionally irradiated, unless the irradiation is carried out in conformity with a regulation prescribing safe conditions of use. For clarification, the statute does not define the form of energy or the process as an additive, but rather the equipment used to irradiate the food as it may affect the characteristics of the food.

A food additive regulation, in general, may be established or amended in one of two ways: by the FDA's own initiative to propose a regulation, or in response to petitions filed by proponents of an additive's use. A petition, the more common method of regulatory alteration, is a scientific and legal document that forms the basis for the administrative record under-pinning the Agency's decision. This decision must be based on an explicit, complete, and unassailable record. The record must contain adequate information to demonstrate that the additive is safe under all conditions of use that would be permitted. When authorized, the regulation is granted generically; anyone can use the additive in conformance with the specified conditions of use permitted under the regulation.

The Food Additives Amendment does not exempt the foods that are regulated by other authorities. Meat or meat food products are subject to the Federal Meat Inspection Act (FMIA). Poultry products are subject to the Poultry Products Inspection Act (PPIA). Irradiated meat and poultry are then subject to the requirements of the Acts, which are administered by the Food Safety and Inspection Service (FSIS) of the U.S. Department of Agriculture (USDA). In addition, the USDA's

Animal and Plant Health Inspection Service (APHIS) administers the law that quarantines certain crops from transport into the country. Irradiation is one quarantine treatment method that can be used with some foods to protect U.S. agriculture from the import of exotic pests; therefore, such a use must also meet the requirements of APHIS.

At an international conference on ensuring the safety and quality of food through radiation processing, it was evident that food irradiation regulations in several countries have been or are being harmonized through compliance with the Codex General Standard for Irradiated Foods and the relevant recommendations of the International Consultative Group on Food Irradiation (ICGFI). The participants of the conference agreed that national regulations need not stipulate maximum dose limits from a toxicological and nutritional perspective under good manufacturing and irradiation practices. The regulations should focus on the production of microbiologically safe products that meet the stated technical purposes, should provide appropriate flexibility for processors, and should be in conformity with Codex as well as the World Trade Organization (WTO) agreement on the sanitary and phytosanitary measures. These measures are required to protect human, animal and plant health and must be based on the standards and recommendations of the recognized international authorities including the CAC.

Emerging Food Irradiation Applications

Irradiation is an effective form of food preservation that extends the shelf life of the food and, therefore, reduces the spoilage of food. The process also benefits the consumer by reducing the risk of illnesses caused by foodborne diseases. Food irradiation may be achieved using low-dose, medium-dose, or high-dose levels of radiation. Low-dose irradiation (<2 kGy) is used to delay sprouting of vegetables and aging of fruits; medium dose (between 1 and 10 kGy) is used to reduce the levels of pathogenic organisms, similar to pasteurization; and high dose (>10 kGy) is used to achieve sterility of the product. Ahmed reported that 37 countries have approved one or more items of irradiated food products for human consumption, and 25 countries have commercialized the irradiation process.

Since worldwide foodborne diseases are increasing and attempts to reduce them have been unsuccessful, the WHO considers food irradiation important toward ensuring food safety and reducing food losses. Irradiation can be a useful control measure in the production of several types of raw or minimally processed foods such as poultry, meat and meat products, fish, seafood, and fruits and vegetables. The United States sets an example for the increase in permitted food irradiation uses as exemplified by the 1997 FDA approval of the irradiation of unprocessed red meat and meat products and the 1999 FSIS/USDA approval of plant facilities. The list of FDA-approved, irradiated foods for pathogen control has recently been amended to include fresh shell eggs and seeds for sprouting. There is continued interest in using this technology, as suggested by the pending petition submitted by the Food Irradiation Coalition to amend the permitted use of ionizing radiation to treat a variety of human foods to a maximum irradiation dose of 4.5 kGy for nonfrozen and nondry products, and 10.0 kGy for frozen or dry products.

As the outbreaks of foodborne pathogens continue, an increase of food irradiation research also continues. Irradiation is being considered as a method to ensure the hygienic quality of food, as a legitimate sanitary and phytosanitary treatment of food and agricultural commodities, as a quarantine treatment of fresh horticultural commodities, and as a substitute for fumigants in Asian countries and the United States of America. Low-dose and medium-dose irradiation applications are currently being investigated with food products, but the use of irradiation in combination with other processes, and high-dose food irradiations are beginning to emerge. Strategies for food irradiation continue to evolve and are updated periodically.

Irradiation of Food Packaging

To prevent recontamination, food is usually packaged prior to irradiation. Therefore, the effects of radiation on the food-packaging materials must also be considered when evaluating the safety of irradiated foods. Irradiation can cause changes to the packaging that might affect integrity as a barrier to microbial contamination. Irradiation might also produce radiolysis products that could migrate into food, affecting odor, taste, and possibly the safety of the food.

Many food-packaging materials are made of polymers. Radiation effects on polymers are the result of competing crosslinking or chain scission, i.e., degradation, reactions. Crosslinking is the joining of two polymer chains via a bridge-type chemical bond, leading to an increase in molecular weight. Crosslinking in many plastics and rubber is essentially a curing process that modifies the physical and mechanical properties of the polymer. Radiation-induced crosslinking dominates under vacuum or an inert atmosphere. Chain scission, on the other hand, is the fragmentation of polymer chains, which leads to a decrease in average molecular weight and dominates during irradiation in the presence of oxygen or air. Both reactions are assumed to be random and are generally proportional to dose, as well as dependent on dose rate and the oxygen content of the atmosphere in which the polymer is irradiated. Radiation does not affect all the properties of a polymer to the same degree. Therefore, when selecting a polymer for a particular application, the effect of radiation on the overall stability of the material must be considered.

Regulatory Requirements-Chemistry Considerations

Both crosslinking and chain scission reactions can occur during irradiation of food-packaging materials. If crosslinking dominates, the migration of packaging components is not expected to increase and, in fact, is likely to decrease compared to that observed for unirradiated packaging. In contrast, if chain scission dominates, lower molecular weight molecules are formed, and these potentially mobile molecules may migrate into food. The safety of these compounds must be evaluated because, in the United States all commercial facilities that irradiate food and other bulk materials such as medical supplies are currently irradiating in air. In addition, the migration of low-molecular-weight radiolysis products into food could affect the odor and taste of the irradiated food.

In the United States components of packaging used to hold food during irradiation must undergo premarket approval by the FDA and may be used only if they comply with the regulations in 21 CFR 179.45 or are the subject of an effective food contact notification or Threshold of Regulation exemption. Regardless of the review channel, chemistry data supporting the identity of and human dietary exposure to a new food-contact substance intended to be used during the irradiation of prepackaged food, as well as its radiolysis products, must be submitted to the FDA. If the packaging material is already approved for unirradiated uses, comparisons can be made to an unirradiated control to determine exposures that would result from the new irradiated use.

Evaluation of Irradiated Food-Packaging Materials

Studies of the effects of radiation on polymeric food-packaging materials have been limited compared to those for medical devices and pharmaceutical products. Ionizing radiation for sterilization of medical devices and pharmaceuticals provides advantages over traditional heat and chemical sterilization methods. Radiation sterilization has been successfully applied to medical products and their packaging, which is made of both thermoplastics and thermosets and includes polyesters, polystyrenes, polyethylenes, elastomers, nylon, acrylics and cellulose, and their copolymers. Since several thermoplastics are used with both food and medical devices, similar radiation effects on these polymers are anticipated. However, the typical dose used on medical devices is 25 kGy, whereas a dose less than 10 kGy is usually applied to food. This means that the levels of radiolysis products should be proportionately lower in food-packaging polymers as compared to medical devices. The observation of radiation-induced alterations in medical products focuses mainly on the physical and performance changes of the devices. Therefore, there are limited quantitative chemical data available to aid in the analysis of the migration of radiolysis products from polymers into food. Additional investigations are needed to evaluate the suitability of modern food- packaging materials and adjuvants intended for use during the irradiation of prepackaged food.

Most of the packaging materials listed in 21 CFR 179.45 are films and homogeneous structures that were approved in the 1960s. These materials do not fully meet today's needs, as modern materials are more desirable to the food industry. Many modern materials have not yet been evaluated by the FDA. These materials may contain adjuvants that prevent undesirable reactions from occurring during polymer processing and subsequent irradiation. Adjuvants may be added to minimize the loss of chemical and physical properties, e.g., antioxidants are added to polymers to prevent the polymer from oxidizing, ultraviolet (UV) stabilizers are added to prevent discoloration of polymers when exposed to light, and release agents are added to enable high-speed production. Adjuvants are especially prone to degradation upon irradiation because they degrade preferentially over the polymer. Therefore, the radiation-induced degradation of various polymer adjuvants, including antioxidants, plasticizers, coatings, release agents, and stabilizers must be evaluated as well.

Chapter 31

Food Allergies and Intolerance

Chapter Contents

Section 31.1

All You Need to Know about Food Allergies

This section contains text excerpted from the following
sources: Text in this section begins with excerpts from "Food
Allergies: Reducing the Risks," U.S. Food and Drug Administration
(FDA), December 18, 2017; Text beginning with the heading
"Frequently Asked Questions about Food Allergies" is excerpted from
"Frequently Asked Questions about Food Allergies," U.S. Food and
Drug Administration (FDA), December 18, 2017.

A food allergy is a specific type of adverse food reaction involving
the immune system. The body produces what is called an allergic, or
immunoglobulin E (IgE), antibody to a food. Once a specific food is
ingested and binds with the IgE antibody, an allergic response ensues.

A food allergy should not be confused with a food intolerance or
other nonallergic food reactions. Various epidemiological surveys have
indicated that almost 80 percent of people who are asked if they have
a food allergy respond that they do when, in fact, they do not have a
true IgE-mediated food allergy.

Food intolerance refers to an abnormal response to a food or
additive, but it differs from an allergy in that it does not involve the
immune system. For example, people who have recurring gastrointestinal problems when they drink milk may say they have a milk allergy.
But they really may be lactose intolerant.

The main differences between food allergies and food intolerances
are that food allergies can result in an immediate, life-threatening
response. Thus, compared to food intolerances, food allergic reactions
pose a much greater health risk.

Frequently Asked Questions about Food Allergies

What Are the Most Common Food Allergy Signs and Symptoms?

Symptoms of food allergies typically appear from within a few minutes
to two hours after a person has eaten the food to which he or she is allergic.

Allergic reactions can include:

- Hives
- Flushed skin or rash
- Tingling or itchy sensation in the mouth
- Face, tongue, or lip swelling
- Vomiting and/or diarrhea
- Abdominal cramps
- Coughing or wheezing
- Dizziness and/or lightheadedness
- Swelling of the throat and vocal cords
- Difficulty breathing
- Loss of consciousness

People with food allergies can also experience a severe, life-threatening allergic reaction called anaphylaxis after eating a food allergen(s). Anaphylaxis can lead to:

- Constricted airways in the lungs
- Severe lowering of blood pressure and shock ("anaphylactic shock")
- Suffocation by swelling of the throat

Each year in the United States, it is estimated that anaphylaxis to food results in:

- 30,000 emergency room visits
- 2,000 hospitalizations
- 150 deaths

Prompt administration of epinephrine by autoinjector during early symptoms of anaphylaxis may help prevent these serious consequences.

What to Do If Symptoms Occur?

Severe food allergies can be life-threatening. If you or someone you care for has symptoms of food allergies, avoid these foods and consult your healthcare provider for appropriate testing and evaluation.

- Read food labels and avoid the foods or ingredients that have caused symptoms.

- Recognize the early symptoms of an allergic reaction, especially in the event of accidental ingestion, and be properly educated on—and armed with—appropriate treatment measures, such as an autoinjector.

- Initiate treatment immediately if you have a known food allergy and experience symptoms while or after eating a food. Go to a nearby emergency room if symptoms progress.

For adverse events related to food products, consumers can call U.S. Food and Drug Administration's (FDA) emergency number at 866-300-4374 or 301-796-8240 or report directly to MedWatch. You may also contact the FDA consumer complaint coordinator in your geographic area.

What Are Major Food Allergens?

To help Americans avoid the health risks posed by food allergens, Congress passed the Food Allergen Labeling and Consumer Protection Act of 2004 (FALCPA). The law applies to all foods whose labeling is regulated by the FDA, both domestic and imported. (FDA regulates the labeling of all foods, except for poultry, most meats, certain egg products, and most alcoholic beverages.)

Although more than 160 foods can cause allergic reactions in people with food allergies, the law identifies the eight most common allergenic foods. These foods account for 90 percent of food allergic reactions, and are the food sources from which many other ingredients are derived (such as whey from milk).

The eight foods identified by the law are:

- Milk

- Eggs

- Fish (e.g., bass, flounder, cod)

- Crustacean shellfish (e.g., crab, lobster, shrimp)

- Tree nuts (e.g., almonds, walnuts, pecans)

- Peanuts

- Wheat

- Soybeans

How Are Major Food Allergens Listed?

If you're allergic to a food ingredient, you probably look for it on the food product's label. The law requires that food labels identify the food source names of all major food allergens used to make the food. This requirement is met if the common or usual name of an ingredient (e.g., buttermilk) that is a major food allergen already identifies that allergen's food source name (i.e., milk). Otherwise, the allergen's food source name must be declared at least once on the food label in one of two ways.

Major food allergen names must appear:

1. **In parentheses following the name of the ingredient.** Examples: "lecithin (soy)," "flour (wheat)," and "whey (milk)";

   or

2. **Immediately after or next to the list of ingredients in a "contains" statement.** Example: "Contains Wheat, Milk, and Soy."

What Is Cross-Contact?

In the context of food allergens, "cross-contact" occurs when a residue or trace amount of an allergenic food becomes incorporated into another food not intended to contain it. Because of cross-contact, manufacturers may voluntarily place an advisory or precautionary allergen labeling statement on food products to notify consumers about the possible presence of food allergen(s). The FDA guidance for the food industry states that food allergen advisory statements, e.g., "may contain [allergen,]" "produced in a facility that also uses [allergen,]" etc., should not be used as a substitute for adhering to current good manufacturing practices and must be truthful and not misleading.

What about Gluten?

Gluten is the protein that occurs naturally in wheat, rye, barley, and crossbreeds of these grains. Foods that typically contain gluten include bread, cakes, cereals, pasta, and many other foods. Although gluten can cause allergic reactions in wheat-allergic individuals, for the estimated 3 million Americans suffering from celiac disease, an auto-immune digestive disorder, consuming gluten can have other serious health consequences.

On August 5, 2013, the FDA issued a final rule defining the term "gluten-free" for voluntary use in the labeling of foods. Food products bearing a gluten-free claim labeled on or after August 5, 2014, must meet the rule's requirements. The law requires that food labels list the product's ingredients. When Lupin or gluten is present in a food, it is, therefore, required to be listed on the label.

Section 31.2

Is It Food Allergy or Food Intolerance?

This section includes text excerpted from "Is It Food Allergy or Food Intolerance?" U.S. Department of Veterans Affairs (VA), May 23, 2017.

A food allergy occurs when a food you eat abnormally triggers your body's immune system. Sometimes even a very small amount of a food can trigger such a response. The body may respond to the food allergen with such symptoms as digestive problems, hives or impaired airway. In some cases, the reaction may be as extreme as to be life-threatening, with a reaction called anaphylaxis. Anaphylaxis is a severe whole-body reaction to an allergen.

Food allergies are often seen in children. Children who have food allergies may find that the food item is no longer an offense to their immune system as they grow older. A common food allergy for children is an allergy to soy.

Adult foods often associated with allergic reactions:

• Fish and shellfish

• Peanuts, walnuts

• Eggs

'Food intolerance' is different from a food allergy. Food intolerance is a reaction to a food that does not involve the body's immune system. While the reaction may feel as if it is a food allergy, if the immune system is not responding, it is a food intolerance. Sometimes it is an additive to a food item that may trigger the intolerance symptoms. Some common intolerance in adults are:

- **Monosodium glutamate (MSG)** is a flavor enhancer which, in large amounts, can cause such symptoms as flushing, headache, and chest discomfort. MSG is found in prepared foods such as sauces, dressing, chips, and seasonings.

- **Sulfites** are naturally occurring in some foods, such as some wines, and are used in food to increase crispness. Intolerance to sulfites can cause breathing problems for people with asthma.

"Lactose Intolerance" defines food intolerance as a sugar, lactose, found in milk and milk products. While uncommon in young children, it is more common in adults. The enzyme needed to break down the lactase declines as people age. When lactase is not broken down by the needed enzyme, the gut may respond with symptoms such as abdominal pain, bloating, and diarrhea. Your healthcare provider can run some laboratory tests to determine if you have lactose intolerance.

Chapter 32

Common Chemical Contaminants in the Food Supply

Chapter Contents

Section 32.1

Persistent Organic Pollutants (POPs)

This section includes text excerpted from "Persistent
Organic Pollutants: A Global Issue, A Global Response," U.S.
Environmental Protection Agency (EPA), October 26, 2017.

Persistent organic pollutants (POPs) are toxic chemicals that
adversely affect human health and the environment around the
world. Because they can be transported by wind and water, most
POPs generated in one country can and do affect people and wildlife
far from where they are used and released. They persist for long
periods of time in the environment and can accumulate and pass
from one species to the next through the food chain. To address
this global concern, the United States joined forces with 90 other
countries and the European Community to sign a groundbreaking
United Nations treaty in Stockholm, Sweden, in May 2001. Under
the treaty, known as the Stockholm Convention, countries agreed
to reduce or eliminate the production, use, and/or release of 12 key
POPs, and specified under the Convention a scientific review process that has led to the addition of other POPs chemicals of global
concern.

Many of the POPs included in the Stockholm Convention are no longer produced in this country. However, U.S. citizens and habitats can
still be at risk from POPs that have persisted in the environment from
unintentionally produced POPs that are released in the United States,
from POPs that are released elsewhere and then transported here (by
wind or water, for example), or from both. Although most developed
nations have taken strong action to control POPs, a great number of
developing nations have only fairly recently begun to restrict their
production, use, and release.

The Stockholm Convention adds an important global dimension to
our national and regional efforts to control POPs. Though the United
States is not yet a party to the Stockholm Convention, the Convention
has played a prominent role in the control of harmful chemicals on
both a national and global level. For example, the U.S. Environmental
Protection Agency (EPA) and the states have significantly reduced the

release of dioxins and furans to land, air, and water from U.S. sources. In addition to assessing dioxins, the EPA has also been working diligently on the reduction of dichloro diphenyl trichloroethane (DDT) from global sources.

The United States and Canada signed an agreement for the virtual elimination of persistent toxic substances in the Great Lakes to reduce emissions from toxic substances. The United States has also signed the regional protocol of the United Nations Economic Commission for Europe (UNECE) on POPs under the Convention on Long-Range Transboundary Air Pollution (CLRTAP) which addresses the Stockholm Convention POPs and other chemicals.

In addition to the POPs-related agreements the United States has taken part in signing, the United States has also provided ample financial and technical support to countries across the globe supporting POPs reduction. A few of these initiatives include dioxin and furan release inventories in Asia and Russia, and the reduction of polychlorinated biphenyls (PCB) sources in Russia.

About Persistent Organic Pollutants (POPs)

Many POPs were widely used during the boom in industrial production after World War II when thousands of synthetic chemicals were introduced into commercial use. Many of these chemicals proved beneficial in pest and disease control, crop production, and industry. These same chemicals, however, have had unforeseen effects on human health and the environment.

Many people are familiar with some of the most well-known POPs, such as PCBs, DDT, and dioxins. POPs include a range of substances that include:

- **Intentionally produced chemicals** currently or once used in agriculture, disease control, manufacturing, or industrial processes. Examples include PCBs, which have been useful in a variety of industrial applications (e.g., in electrical transformers and large capacitors, as hydraulic and heat exchange fluids, and as additives to paints and lubricants) and DDT, which is still used to control mosquitoes that carry malaria in some parts of the world.

- **Unintentionally produced chemicals,** such as dioxins, that result from some industrial processes and from combustion (for example, municipal and medical waste incineration and backyard burning of trash).

The Dichlorodiphenyltrichloroethane (DDT) Dilemma

DDT is likely one of the most famous and controversial pesticides ever made. An estimated 4 billion pounds of this inexpensive and historically effective chemical have been produced and applied worldwide since 1940. In the United States, DDT was used extensively on agricultural crops, particularly cotton, from 1945 to 1972. DDT was also used to protect soldiers from insect-borne diseases such as malaria and typhus during World War II, and it remains a valuable public health tool in parts of the tropics. The heavy use of this highly persistent chemical, however, led to widespread environmental contamination and the accumulation of DDT in humans and wildlife—a phenomenon brought to public attention by Rachel Carson in her 1962 book, Silent Spring. A wealth of scientific laboratory and field data have now confirmed research from the 1960s that suggested, among other effects, that high levels of dichlorodiphenyldichloroethylene (DDE), a metabolite of DDT, in certain birds of prey caused their eggshells to thin so dramatically they could not produce live offspring.

One bird species especially sensitive to DDE was the bald eagle. Public concern about the Eagles' decline and the possibility of other long-term harmful effects of DDT exposure to both humans and wildlife prompted the EPA to cancel the registration of DDT in 1972. The bald eagle has since experienced one of the most dramatic species recoveries in our history.

Transboundary Travelers

A major impetus for the Stockholm Convention was the finding of POPs contamination in relatively pristine Arctic regions—thousands of miles from any known source. Much of the evidence for long-range transport of airborne gaseous and particulate substances to the United States focuses on dust or smoke because they are visible in satellite images. Tracing the movement of most POPs in the environment is complex because these compounds can exist in different phases (e.g., as a gas or attached to airborne particles) and can be exchanged among environmental media. For example, some POPs can be carried for many miles when they evaporate from water or land surfaces into the air, or when they adsorb to airborne particles. Then, they can return to Earth on particles or in snow, rain, or mist. POPs also travel through oceans, rivers, lakes, and, to a lesser extent, with the help of animal carriers, such as migratory species.

Domestic Actions Taken to Control POPs

The United States has taken strong domestic action to reduce emissions of POPs. For example, none of the original POPs pesticides listed in the Stockholm Convention is registered for sale and distribution in the United States. In 1978, Congress prohibited the manufacture of PCBs and severely restricted the use of remaining PCB stocks. In addition, since 1987, the EPA and the states have effectively reduced environmental releases of dioxins and furans to land, air, and water from U.S. sources. These regulatory actions, along with voluntary efforts by U.S. industry, resulted in a greater than 85 percent decline in total dioxin and furan releases after 1987 from known industrial sources. To better understand the risks associated with dioxin releases, the EPA has been conducting a comprehensive reassessment of dioxin science and will be evaluating additional actions that might further protect human health and the environment.

Stopping DDT Use

Over the years, the United States has taken a number of steps to restrict the use of DDT:

- **1969.** After studying the persistence of DDT residues in the environment, the U.S. Department of Agriculture (USDA) canceled the registration of certain uses of DDT (on shade trees, on tobacco, in the home, and in aquatic environments).

- **1970.** USDA cancels DDT applications on crops, commercial plants, and wood products, as well as for building purposes.

- **1972.** Under the authority of the EPA, the registrations of the remaining DDT products are canceled.

- **1989.** The remaining exempted uses (public health use for controlling vector-borne diseases, the military use for quarantine, and prescription drug use for controlling body lice) are voluntarily stopped.

  As of date. There is no U.S. registration for DDT, meaning that it cannot legally be sold or distributed in the United States.

Controlling Dioxins

The EPA has pursued regulatory control and management of dioxins and furans releases to air, water, and soil. The Clean Air Act (CAA) requires the application of maximum achievable control technology for hazardous air pollutants, including dioxins and furans. Major sources regulated under this authority include municipal, medical, and hazardous waste incineration; pulp and paper manufacturing; and certain metals production and refining processes. Dioxin releases to water are managed through a combination of risk-based and technology-based tools established under the Clean Water Act (CWA). The cleanup of dioxin-contaminated land is an important part of the EPA Superfund and Resource Conservation and Recovery Act Corrective Action programs. Voluntary actions to control dioxins and furans include the EPA's Persistent, Bioaccumulative, and Toxics (PBTs) program and the Dioxin Exposure Initiative (DEI), both of which gather information to inform future actions and further reduce risks associated with dioxin exposure.

Impact of POPs on People and Wildlife

Studies have linked POPs exposures to declines, diseases, or abnormalities in a number of wildlife species, including certain kinds of fish, birds, and mammals. Wildlife also can act as sentinels for human health: abnormalities or declines detected in wildlife populations can sound an early warning bell for people. Behavioral abnormalities and birth defects in fish, birds, and mammals in and around the Great Lakes, for example, led scientists to investigate POPs exposures in human populations.

In people, reproductive, developmental, behavioral, neurologic, endocrine, and immunologic adverse health effects have been linked to POPs. People are mainly exposed to POPs through contaminated foods. Less common exposure routes include drinking contaminated water and direct contact with the chemicals. In people and other mammals alike, POPs can be transferred through the placenta and breast milk to developing offspring. It should be noted, however, that despite this potential exposure, the known benefits of breastfeeding far outweigh the suspected risks.

A number of populations are at particular risk of POPs exposure, including people whose diets include large amounts of fish, shellfish, or wild foods that are high in fat and locally obtained. For example, indigenous peoples may be particularly at risk because they observe cultural and spiritual traditions related to their diet. To them, fishing and hunting are not sport or recreation but are part of a traditional, subsistence way of life, in which no useful part of the catch is wasted. In remote areas of Alaska and elsewhere, locally obtained subsistence food may be the only readily available option for nutrition.

In addition, sensitive populations, such as children, the elderly, and those with suppressed immune systems, are typically more susceptible to many kinds of pollutants, including POPs. Because POPs have been linked to reproductive impairments, men and women of childbearing age may also be at risk.

POPs and the Food Chain

POPs work their way through the food chain by accumulating in the body fat of living organisms and becoming more concentrated as they move from one creature to another. This process is known as "biomagnification." When contaminants found in small amounts at the bottom of the food chain biomagnify, they can pose a significant hazard to predators that feed at the top of the food chain. This means that even small releases of POPs can have significant impacts.

Biomagnification in Action. A 1997 study by the Arctic Monitoring and Assessment Programme (AMAP), called Arctic Pollution Issues: A State of the Arctic Environment Report, found that caribou in Canada's Northwest Territories had as much as 10 times the levels of PCBs as the lichen on which they grazed; PCB levels in the wolves that fed on the caribou were magnified nearly 60 times as much as the lichen.

The Role of Science

Although scientists have more to learn about POPs chemicals, decades of scientific research have greatly increased our knowledge of POPs' impacts on people and wildlife. For example, laboratory studies have shown that low doses of certain POPs adversely affect some organ systems and aspects of development. Studies also have shown that chronic exposure to low doses of certain POPs can result in reproductive and immune system deficits. Exposure to high levels of certain POPs chemicals—higher than normally encountered by humans and wildlife—can cause serious damage or death. Epidemiological studies of exposed human populations and studies of wildlife might provide more information on health impacts. However, because such studies are less controlled than laboratory studies, other stresses cannot be ruled out as the cause of adverse effects.

The EPA developed a report summarizing the science on POPs.

Reservoirs of POPs

POPs can be deposited in marine and freshwater ecosystems through effluent releases, atmospheric deposition, runoff, and other means. Because POPs have low water solubility, they bond strongly to particulate matter in aquatic sediments. As a result, sediments can serve as reservoirs or "sinks" for POPs. When sequestered in these sediments, POPs can be taken out of circulation for long periods of time. If disturbed, however, they can be reintroduced into the ecosystem and food chain, potentially becoming a source of local, and even global, contamination.

The Great Lakes: A Story of Trials and Triumphs

The Great Lakes—Superior, Michigan, Huron, Erie, and Ontario— and their connecting channels make up the largest system of fresh surface water in the world. A vital resource for the United States and Canada, the Great Lakes are used for fishing, swimming, boating, agriculture, industry, and tourism; they are also a source of drinking water and energy.

Despite their size, however, the Great Lakes are vulnerable to pollution. Until the 1970s, a variety of POPs, heavy metals, and other agricultural and industrial pollutants were routinely discharged into the Great Lakes. Toxic substances also entered the Great Lakes Basin through other avenues, including waste sites, river runoff, and atmospheric deposition. These pollutants existed in large enough quantities to warrant concern regarding the effects on human health and wildlife, including several species of fish and shellfish, bald eagles and other birds of prey, and fish-eating mammals such as mink.

Extensive cleanup and pollution control efforts were subsequently launched, and many contaminant levels have declined dramatically in the Great Lakes as a result, illustrating the positive outcomes that can be achieved when communities, government, and industry work together to reduce pollution. Still, some POPs exist at significant concentrations, indicating their persistence and the possibility of continued contamination from other sources, particularly long-range atmospheric transport of POPs from other areas.

In 1972, the United States and Canada signed the first Great Lakes Water Quality Agreement (GLWQA), calling for the two countries to clean up and control pollution of these waters. In 1978, they signed a new agreement, which added a commitment to work together to rid the Great Lakes of persistent toxic chemicals, some of which are POPs. As part of this agreement, both countries have been monitoring atmospheric loadings of these chemicals to the Great Lakes since 1990.

The Great Lakes Binational Toxics Strategy (GLBTS), signed by the United States and Canada in 1997, was an agreement aimed to reduce several persistent toxic pollutants, including certain POPs, in the Great Lakes Basin over a 10-year period. The strategy provided a guide for governments and stakeholders toward the virtual elimination of 12 identified substances through cost-efficient and expedient pollution prevention and other incentive-based actions.

Over the course of the 10-year period, working closely with state, provincial, tribal, and local governments and stakeholders from industry, academia, environmental and community groups, both governments made significant progress in meeting that goal of virtually eliminating persistent toxic substances such as mercury, PCBs, and dioxin from discharging into the Great Lakes environment. The two governments agreed to continue to extend the agreement in order to work together to identify new challenges that are presented by emerging substance of concern, such as flame retardants.

Great Lakes Research

Much of our knowledge of POPs, populations at risk, and possible health effects comes from research conducted in the Great Lakes region. It's learned, for example, that a major route of exposure is through contaminated food, particularly fish. Studies conducted in the 1970s showed a correlation between fish consumption and elevated POPs levels in the blood, leading researchers to conclude that people can be exposed to POPs by eating contaminated fish.

As a result, extensive fish contaminant monitoring programs have been established in the Great Lakes states, and fish consumption advisories are regularly released to help inform people which fish are safe to eat and how much is safe to eat. It's also learned that currently some POPs primarily enter the Great Lakes from the air and that urban areas are major sources of airborne POPs.

The Stockholm Convention

The Stockholm Convention (Convention) on POPs, which was adopted in 2001 and entered into force in 2004, is a global treaty whose purpose is to safeguard human health and the environment from highly harmful chemicals that persist in the environment and affect the well-being of humans as well as wildlife. The Convention requires parties to eliminate and/or reduce POPs, which have a potential of causing devastating effects such as cancer and diminished intelligence and have the ability to travel over great distances.

The Convention is managed by the United Nations Environment Program (UNEP) and its Secretariat is based in Geneva, Switzerland. UNEP is the leading international environmental entity that supports the agenda and implementation of environmental sustainability for the United Nations. The COP, or the Conference of the Parties of the Convention, governs the POPs Convention, with its members being the Convention's parties (Parties).

The role of Parties is to implement the obligations of the Convention, including eliminating or restricting the production and use of the intentionally produced POPs, prohibiting and eliminating production and use or import of POPs, conducting research, identifying areas contaminated with POPs, and providing financial support and incentives for the Convention. The process of becoming a Party begins with a state or regional economic integration organization submitting a means of ratification, acceptance, approval or accession to the depositary. Official contact points and national focal points are nominated to carry out administrative, communications, and information exchange procedure.

Monitoring Process

The Convention provides for an effectiveness evaluation, based on a POPs monitoring and data collection effort that will use existing monitoring programs and mechanisms to the extent possible.

Table 32.1. The Dirty Dozen

POP	Global Historical Use/Source	Overview of U.S. Status
Aldrin and Dieldrin	Insecticides used on crops such as corn and cotton; also used for termite control.	Under FIFRA: • No U.S. registrations; most use canceled in 1969; all uses by 1987. • All tolerances on food crops revoked in 1986. No production, import, or export.

Table 32.1. Continued

POP	Global Historical Use/Source	Overview of U.S. Status
Chlordane	Insecticide used on crops, including vegetables, small grains, potatoes, sugarcane, sugar beets, fruits, nuts, citrus, and cotton. Used on home lawn and garden pests. Also used extensively to control termites.	Under FIFRA: • No U.S. registrations; most use canceled in 1978; all uses by 1988. • All tolerances on food crops revoked in 1986. No production (stopped in 1997), import, or export. Regulated as a hazardous air pollutant (CAA).
DDT	Insecticide used on agricultural crops, primarily cotton, and insects that carry diseases such as malaria and typhus.	Under FIFRA: No U.S. registrations; most use canceled in • 1972; all uses by 1989. • Tolerances on food crops revoked in 1986. No U.S. production, import, or export. DDE (a metabolite of DDT) regulated as a hazardous air pollutant (CAA). Priority toxic pollutant (CWA).
Endrin	Insecticide used on crops such as cotton and grains; also used to control rodents.	Under FIFRA, no U.S. registrations; most uses canceled in 1979; all uses by 1984. No production, import, or export. Priority toxic pollutant (CWA).
Mirex	Insecticide used to combat fire ants, termites, and mealybugs. Also used as a fire retardant in plastics, rubber, and electrical products.	Under FIFRA, no U.S. registrations; all uses canceled in 1977. No production, import, or export.

Table 32.1. Continued

POP	Global Historical Use/Source	Overview of U.S. Status
Heptachlor	Insecticide used primarily against soil insects and termites. Also used against some crop pests and to combat malaria.	Under FIFRA: • Most uses canceled by 1978; registrant voluntarily canceled use to control fire ants in underground cable boxes in early 2000. • All pesticide tolerances on food crops revoked in 1989. No production, import, or export.
hexachlorobenzene	Fungicide used for seed treatment. Also, an industrial chemical used to make fireworks, ammunition, synthetic rubber, and other substances. Also unintentionally produced during combustion and the manufacture of certain chemicals. Also an impurity in certain pesticides.	Under FIFRA, no U.S. registrations; all uses canceled by 1985. No production, import, or export as a pesticide. Manufacture and use for chemical intermediate (as allowed under the Convention). Regulated as a hazardous air pollutant (CAA). Priority toxic pollutant (CWA).
PCBs	Used for a variety of industrial processes and purposes, including in electrical transformers and capacitors, as heat exchange fluids, as paint additives, in carbonless copy paper, and in plastics. Also unintentionally produced during combustion.	Manufacture and new use prohibited in 1978 (TSCA). Regulated as a hazardous air pollutant (CAA). Priority toxic pollutant (CWA).

Table 32.1. Continued

POP	Global Historical Use/Source	Overview of U.S. Status
Toxaphene	Insecticide used to control pests on crops and livestock, and to kill unwanted fish in lakes.	Under FIFRA: • No U.S. registrations; most use canceled in 1982; all uses by 1990. All tolerances on food crops revoked in 1993. • No production, import, or export. • Regulated as a hazardous air pollutant (CAA).
Dioxins and Furans	Unintentionally produced during most forms of combustion, including the burning of municipal and medical wastes, backyard burning of trash, and industrial processes. Also can be found as trace contaminants in certain herbicides, wood preservatives, and in PCB mixtures.	Regulated as hazardous air pollutants (CAA). Dioxin in the form of 2,3,7,8-TCDD is a priority toxic pollutant (CWA).

FIFRA: Federal Insecticide, Fungicide and Rodenticide Act
TSCA: Toxic Substances Control Act
CAA: Clean Air Act
CWA: Clean Water Act

Section 32.2

Polychlorinated Biphenyls (PCBs)

This section includes text excerpted from "Polychlorinated Biphenyls (PCBs)," U.S. Environmental Protection Agency (EPA), April 13, 2018.

About Polychlorinated Biphenyls (PCBs)

Polychlorinated biphenyls (PCBs) are a group of manufactured organic chemicals consisting of carbon, hydrogen and chlorine atoms.

The number of chlorine atoms and their location in a PCB molecule determines many of its physical and chemical properties. PCBs have no known taste or smell, and range in consistency from an oil to a waxy solid.

PCBs belong to a broad family of manufactured organic chemicals known as chlorinated hydrocarbons. PCBs were domestically manufactured from 1929 until manufacturing was banned in 1979. They have a range of toxicity and vary in consistency from thin, light-colored liquids to yellow or black waxy solids. Due to their nonflammability, chemical stability, high boiling point, and electrical insulating properties, PCBs were used in hundreds of industrial and commercial applications including:

- Electrical, heat transfer, and hydraulic equipment

- Plasticizers in paints, plastics, and rubber products

- Pigments, dyes, and carbonless copy paper

- Other industrial applications

Commercial Uses for PCBs

Although no longer commercially produced in the United States, PCBs may be present in products and materials produced before the 1979 PCB ban. Products that may contain PCBs include:

- Transformers and capacitors

- Electrical equipment including voltage regulators, switches, re-closers, bushings, and electromagnets

- Oil used in motors and hydraulic systems

- Old electrical devices or appliances containing PCB capacitors

- Fluorescent light ballasts

- Cable insulation

- Thermal insulation material including fiberglass, felt, foam, and cork

- Adhesives and tapes

- Oil-based paint

- Caulking

- Plastics

- Carbonless copy paper

- Floor finish

The PCBs used in these products were chemical mixtures made up of a variety of individual chlorinated biphenyl components known as congeners. Most commercial PCB mixtures are known in the United States by their industrial trade names, the most common being Arochlor.

Release and Exposure of PCBs

As of date, PCBs can still be released into the environment from:

- Poorly maintained hazardous waste sites that contain PCBs

- Illegal or improper dumping of PCB wastes

- Leaks or releases from electrical transformers containing PCBs

- Disposal of PCB-containing consumer products into municipal or other landfills not designed to handle hazardous waste

- Burning some wastes in municipal and industrial incinerators

PCBs do not readily break down once in the environment. They can remain for long periods cycling between air, water, and soil. PCBs can be carried long distances and have been found in snow and sea water in areas far from where they were released into the environment. As a consequence, they are found all over the world. In general, the lighter the form of PCB, the further it can be transported from the source of contamination.

PCBs can accumulate in the leaves and above-ground parts of plants and food crops. They are also taken up into the bodies of small organisms and fish. As a result, people who ingest fish may be exposed to PCBs that have bioaccumulated in the fish they are ingesting.

The National Center for Health Statistics (NCHS), a division of the Centers for Disease Control and Prevention (CDC), conducts the National Health and Nutrition Examination Surveys (NHANES). NHANES is a series of U.S. national surveys on the health and nutrition status of the noninstitutionalized civilian population, which includes data collection on selected chemicals. Interviews and physical examinations are conducted with approximately 10,000 people in each two-year survey cycle.

PCB Congeners

A PCB congener is any single, unique well-defined chemical compound in the PCB category. The name of a congener specifies the total number of chlorine substituents and the position of each chlorine. For example 4,4-Dichlorobiphenyl is a congener comprising the biphenyl structure with two chlorine substituents—one on each of the 4 carbons of the two rings. In 1980, a numbering system was developed which assigned a sequential number to each of the 209 PCB congeners.

PCB Homologs

Homologs are subcategories of PCB congeners that have equal numbers of chlorine substituents. For example, the tetrachlorobiphenyls are all PCB congeners with exactly 4 chlorine substituents that can be in any arrangement.

PCB Mixtures and Trade Names

With few exceptions, PCBs were manufactured as a mixture of individual PCB congeners. These mixtures were created by adding progressively more chlorine to batches of biphenyl until a certain target percentage of chlorine by weight was achieved. Commercial mixtures with higher percentages of chlorine contained higher proportions of the more heavily chlorinated congeners, but all congeners could be expected to be present at some level in all mixtures. While PCBs were manufactured and sold under many names, the most common was the Aroclor series.

Aroclor

Aroclor is a PCB mixture produced from approximately 1930 to 1979. It is one of the most commonly known trade names for PCB mixtures. There are many types of Aroclors and each has a distinguishing suffix number that indicates the degree of chlorination. The numbering standard for the different Aroclors is as follows:

- The first two digits usually refer to the number of carbon atoms in the phenyl rings (for PCBs this is 12)

- The second two numbers indicate the percentage of chlorine by mass in the mixture. For example, the name Aroclor 1254 means that the mixture contains approximately 54 percent chlorine by weight.

PCB Trade Names

PCBs were manufactured and sold under many different names. The names in the following table have been used to refer to PCBs or to products containing PCBs. Please note:

- Some of these names may be used for substances or mixtures not containing PCBs

- Many of these names were used with distinguishing suffixes, indicating the degree of chlorination, type of formulation, or other properties (e.g., Aroclor 1254; Clophen A60)

- Some of these names may be misspellings of the correct names but are included here for completeness

Table 32.2. PCB Trade Names

Aceclor	Diaclor	PCB
Adkarel	Dicolor	PCB's
ALC	Diconal	PCBs
Apirolio	Diphenyl, chlorinated	Pheaoclor
Apirorlio	DK	Phenochlor
Arochlor	Duconal	Phenoclor
Arochlors	Dykanol	Plastivar
Aroclor	Educarel	Polychlorinated biphenyl
Aroclors	EEC-18	Polychlorinated biphenyls
Arubren	Elaol	Polychlorinated diphenyl
Asbestol	Electrophenyl	Polychlorinated diphenyls
ASK	Elemex	Polychlorobiphenyl
Askael	Elinol	Polychlorodiphenyl
Askarel	Eucarel	Prodelec
Auxol	Fenchlor	Pydrau
Bakola	Fenclor	Pyraclor
Biphenyl, chlorinated	Fenocloro	Pyralene
Chlophen	Gilotherm	Pyranol
Chloretol	Hydol	Pyroclor
Chlorextol	Hyrol	Pyronol
Chlorinated biphenyl	Hyvol	Saf-T-Kuhl
Chlorinated diphenyl	Inclor	Saf-T-Kohl
Chlorinol	Inerteen	Santosol

Table 32.2. Continued

Chlorobiphenyl	Inertenn	Santotherm
Chlorodiphenyl	Kanechlor	Santothern
Chlorphen	Kaneclor	Santovac
Chorextol	Kennechlor	Solvol
Chorinol	Kenneclor	Sorol
Clophen	Leromoll	Soval
Clophenharz	Magvar	Sovol
Cloresil	MCS 1489	Sovtol
Clorinal	Montar	Terphenychlore
Clorphen	Nepolin	Therminal
Decachlorodiphenyl	No-Flamol	Therminol
Delor	NoFlamol	Turbinol
Delorene	Non-Flamol	-
-	Olex-sf-d	-
-	Orophene	-

Health Effects of PCBs

PCBs have been demonstrated to cause a variety of adverse health effects. They have been shown to cause cancer in animals as well as a number of serious noncancer health effects in animals, including: effects on the immune system, reproductive system, nervous system, endocrine system and other health effects. Studies in humans support evidence for potential carcinogenic and noncarcinogenic effects of PCBs. The different health effects of PCBs may be interrelated. Alterations in one system may have significant implications for the other systems of the body. The potential health effects of PCB exposure are discussed in greater detail below.

Cancer

PCBs are one of the most widely studied environmental contaminants. Many studies in animals and human populations have been performed to assess the potential carcinogenicity of PCBs. The EPA's first assessment of PCB carcinogenicity was completed in 1987. At that time, data was limited to Aroclor 1260. In 1996, at the direction of Congress, the EPA completed a reassessment of PCB carcinogenicity titled PCBs: Cancer Dose-Response Assessment and Application to Environmental Mixtures. The EPA's cancer reassessment reflected the Agency's commitment to the use of the best science in evaluating health effects of PCBs. The reassessment was peer reviewed by 15 experts on PCBs, including scientists from government, academia, and industry. The peer reviewers agreed with the EPA's conclusion that PCBs are probable human carcinogens.

The EPA uses an approach that permits evaluation of the complete carcinogenicity database and allows the results of individual studies to be viewed in the context of all of the other available studies. Studies in animals provide conclusive evidence that PCBs cause cancer. Studies in humans raise further concerns regarding the potential carcinogenicity of PCBs. Taken together, the data strongly suggest that PCBs are probable human carcinogens.

The cancer reassessment determined that PCBs are probable human carcinogens, based on the following information:

- The EPA reviewed all of the available literature on the carcinogenicity of PCBs in animals as an important first step in the cancer reassessment, which presented clear evidence that PCBs causes cancer in animals. An industry scientist commented that "all significant studies have been reviewed and are fairly represented in the document." An industry-sponsored peer-reviewed rat study, characterized as the "gold standard study" by one peer reviewer, demonstrated that every commercial PCB mixture tested caused cancer. The new studies reviewed in the PCB reassessment allowed the EPA to develop more accurate potency estimates than previously available for PCBs. The reassessment provided the EPA with sufficient information to develop a range of potency estimates for different PCB mixtures, based on the incidence of liver cancer and in consideration of the mobility of PCBs in the environment.

The reassessment resulted in a slightly decreased cancer potency estimate for Aroclor 1260 relative to the 1987 estimate due to the use of additional dose-response information for PCB mixtures and refinements in risk assessment techniques (e.g., use of a different animal-to-human scaling factor for dose). The reassessment concluded that the types of PCBs likely to be bioaccumulated in fish and bound to sediments are the most carcinogenic PCB mixtures.

In addition to the animal studies, a number of epidemiological studies of workers exposed to PCBs have been performed. Results of human studies raise concerns for the potential carcinogenicity of PCBs. Studies of PCB workers found increases in rare liver cancers and malignant melanoma. The presence of cancer in the same target organ (liver) following exposures to PCBs both in animals and in humans and the finding of liver cancers and malignant melanomas across multiple human studies adds weight to the conclusion that PCBs are probable human carcinogens.

Some of the studies in humans have not demonstrated an association between exposures to PCBs and disease. However, epidemiological studies share common methodological limitations that can affect their ability to discern important health effects (or define them as statistically significant) even when they are present. Often, the number of individuals in a study is too small for an effect to be revealed, or there are difficulties in determining actual exposure levels, or there are multiple confounding factors (factors that tend to co-occur with PCB exposure, including smoking, drinking alcohol, and exposure to other chemicals in the workplace).

Epidemiological studies may not be able to detect small increases in cancer over background unless the cancer rate following contaminant exposure is very high or the exposure produces a very unusual type of cancer. However, studies that do not demonstrate an association between exposure to PCBs and disease should not be characterized as negative studies. These studies are most appropriately viewed as inconclusive. Limited studies that produce inconclusive findings for cancer in humans do not mean that PCBs are safe.

It is very important to note that the composition of PCB mixtures changes following their release into the environment. The types of PCBs that tend to bioaccumulate in fish and other animals and bind to sediments happen to be the most carcinogenic components of PCB mixtures. As a result, people who ingest PCB-contaminated fish or other animal products and contact PCB-contaminated sediment may be exposed to PCB mixtures that are even more toxic than the PCB mixtures contacted by workers and released into the environment.

EPA's peer-reviewed cancer reassessment concluded that PCBs are probable human carcinogens. the EPA is not alone in its conclusions regarding PCBs. The International Agency for Research on Cancer has declared PCBs to be probably carcinogenic to humans. The National Toxicology Program (NTP) has stated that it is reasonable to conclude that PCBs are carcinogenic in humans. The National Institute for Occupational Safety and Health (NIOSH) has determined that PCBs are a potential occupational carcinogen.

Noncancer Effects

The EPA evaluates all of the available data in determining the potential noncarcinogenic toxicity of environmental contaminants, including PCBs. Based on extensive studies conducted using environmentally relevant doses, the EPA found clear evidence that PCBs have significant toxic effects in animals, including nonhuman primates. PCBs can affect an animal's immune system, reproductive system, nervous system and endocrine system. The body's regulation of all of these systems is complex and interrelated. As a result, it is not surprising that PCBs can exert a multitude of serious adverse health effects.

Immune Effects

The immune system is critical for fighting infections, and diseases of the immune system have very serious potential implications for the health of humans and animals. The immune effects of PCB exposure have been studied in Rhesus monkeys and other animals. It is important to note that the immune systems of Rhesus monkeys and humans are very similar. Studies in monkeys and other animals have revealed a number of serious effects on the immune system following exposures to PCBs:

- Significant decrease in the size of the thymus gland, which is critical to the immune system in infant monkeys

- Reductions in the response of the immune system following a challenge with sheep red blood cells. This is a standard laboratory test that determines the ability of an animal to mount a primary antibody response and develop protective immunity.

- Decreased resistance to Epstein-Barr virus (EBV) and other infections in PCB-exposed animals

Individuals with diseases of the immune system may be more susceptible to pneumonia and viral infections. The animal studies were not able to identify a level of PCB exposure that did not cause effects on the immune system.

In humans, a recent study found that individuals infected with EBV had a greater association of increased exposures to PCBs. It also increased the risk of non-Hodgkins lymphoma more than for those who had no EBV infection. This finding is consistent with increases in infection with EBV in animals exposed to PCBs.

Since PCBs suppress the immune system and immune system suppression has been demonstrated as a risk factor for non-Hodgkin's lymphoma, suppression of the immune system is a possible mechanism for PCB-induced cancer. Immune effects were also noted in humans who experienced exposure to rice oil contaminated with PCBs, dibenzofurans, and dioxins.

Taken together, the studies in animals and humans suggest that PCBs may have serious potential effects on the immune systems of exposed individuals.

Reproductive Effects

Reproductive effects of PCBs have been studied in a variety of animal species, including Rhesus monkeys, rats, mice, and mink. Rhesus monkeys are generally regarded as the best laboratory species for predicting adverse reproductive effects in humans. Potentially serious effects on the reproductive system were seen in monkeys and a number of other animal species following exposures to PCB mixtures. Most significantly, PCB exposures were found to reduce the birth weight, conception rates and live birth rates of monkeys and other species; and PCB exposure reduced sperm counts in rats. Effects in monkeys were long lasting and were observed long after the dosing with PCBs occurred.

Studies of reproductive effects have also been carried out in human populations exposed to PCBs. Children born to women who worked with PCBs in factories showed decreased birth weight and a significant decrease in gestational age with increasing exposures to PCBs. Studies in fishing populations believed to have high exposures to PCBs also suggest similar decreases. This same effect was seen in multiple species of animals exposed to PCBs and suggests that reproductive effects may be important in humans following exposures to PCBs.

Neurological Effects

Proper development of the nervous system is critical for early learning and can have potentially significant implications for the health of individuals throughout their lives. Effects of PCBs on nervous system development have been studied in monkeys and a variety of other animal species. Newborn monkeys exposed to PCBs showed persistent and significant deficits in neurological development, including visual recognition, short-term memory, and learning. Some of these studies were conducted using the types of PCBs most commonly found in human breast milk.

Studies in humans have suggested effects similar to those observed in monkeys exposed to PCBs, including learning deficits and changes in activity associated with exposures to PCBs. The similarity in effects observed in humans and animals provide additional support for the potential neurobehavioral effects of PCBs.

Endocrine Effects

There has been significant discussion and research on the effects of environmental contaminants on the endocrine system ("endocrine disruption"). While the significance of endocrine disruption as a widespread issue in humans and animals is a subject of ongoing study, PCBs have been demonstrated to exert effects on thyroid hormone levels in animals and humans. Thyroid hormone levels are critical for normal growth and development, and alterations in thyroid hormone levels may have significant implications.

It has been shown that PCBs decrease thyroid hormone levels in rodents. Research has also shown that these decreases result in developmental deficits in rodents, including deficits in hearing. PCB exposures have been associated with changes in thyroid hormone levels in infants in studies conducted in the Netherlands and Japan. Additional research will be required to determine the significance of these effects in the human population.

Other Noncancer Effects

A variety of other noncancer effects of PCBs have been reported, including the following:

- Dermal and ocular effects in monkeys and humans

- Liver toxicity in rodents

- Elevated blood pressure, serum triglyceride and serum cholesterol in humans

Section 32.3

Dioxins and Furan

This section contains text excerpted from the following sources: Text
in this section begins with excerpts from "Dioxins," National Institute
of Environmental Health Sciences (NIEHS), August 28, 2017; Text
beginning with the heading "What Is Furan?" is excerpted from
"Questions and Answers on the Occurrence of Furan in Food," U.S.
Food and Drug Administration (FDA), January 25, 2018.

Dioxins are mainly by-products of industrial practices. They are produced through a variety of incineration processes, including improper municipal waste incineration and burning of trash, and can be released into the air during natural processes, such as forest fires and volcanoes. Almost every living creature has been exposed to dioxins or dioxin-like compounds (DLCs).

Strict regulatory controls on major industrial sources of dioxin have reduced emissions into the air by 90 percent, compared to levels in 1987. As of date, people are exposed to dioxins primarily by eating food, in particular, animal products, contaminated by these chemicals. Dioxins are absorbed and stored in fat tissue and, therefore, accumulate in the food chain. More than 90 percent of human exposure is through food.

Before safeguards and regulations were introduced, dioxin releases were a major problem in the United States. The Polychlorinated Biphenyls (PCBs) worked with industry to ban products containing dioxin and to curb dioxin emissions. In 1979, the EPA banned the manufacture of products containing Polychlorinated Biphenyls (PCBs) some of which are included under the term dioxin.

Consumers should eat a balanced diet and follow the *2015 Dietary Guidelines for Americans* (DGA). Each food group provides important nutrients needed for health. The following steps can reduce the potential for exposure to dioxin:

- Remove skin from fish and chicken.

- Select cuts of meat that are naturally lean, or trim visible fat.

- When catching your own fish, check local fishing advisories, as there may be consumption limits for particular kinds of fish, in particular bodies of water where local contamination has occurred.

• Use fat-free or low-fat milk and use butter in moderation.

However, dioxins break down very slowly and emissions released long ago remain in the environment. Some dioxins endure a long time, are extremely resistant to environmental degradation, and, therefore, are classified as persistent organic pollutants (POPs). Dioxin contamination is an increasing problem in some developing countries, particularly with uncontrolled burning, and dismantling, and recycling of electronic products, such as computers.

Health Effects

The dioxin tetrachlorodibenzo-p-dioxin (TCDD), or mutagen, is a known cancer-causing agent, and other DLCs are known to cause cancer in laboratory animals. Additionally, dioxin exposure has been linked to a number of other diseases, including type 2 diabetes, ischemic heart disease, and an acne-like skin disease called chloracne, a hallmark of dioxin exposure.

Dioxins can cause developmental problems in children, lead to reproductive and infertility problems in adults, resulting in miscarriages, damage the immune system, and interfere with hormones.

Exposure to dioxins has widespread effects in nearly every vertebrate species, at nearly every stage of development, including in the womb.

The Science of Dioxins

Dioxins are a family of compounds that share distinct chemical structures and characteristics. Numerous dioxin-like compounds have been identified that are considered to have significant toxicity and can cause disease. The singular term dioxin refers to the most toxic compound, TCDD.

NIEHS researchers continue to explore the detailed chemical pathway through which dioxin damages the body, but scientists are now confident that the first step takes place when dioxin binds to an intracellular protein known as the aryl hydrocarbon receptor (AhR). When that happens, the AhR can alter the expression, or function, of certain genes. The resulting cellular imbalance leads to a disruption in normal cell function and ultimately adverse health effects.

In addition to TCDD, many other chemicals bind to AhR. About 400 compounds in the environment act on the body through the AhR

413

receptor. Public health officials around the world are concerned about the combined effects of multiple chemicals that activate the AhR and are developing health standards that take into account the fact that people are exposed to mixtures of DLCs, not just one at a time.

Dioxins' Impact

The public health threats posed by dioxins were highlighted dramatically in the public consciousness in the late 1970s and early 1980s. Newspapers and television broadcasts were full of stories about ailing veterans who had been exposed to dioxins through Agent Orange, an herbicide and defoliant used in the Vietnam War.

Concerns about Agent Orange and other DLCs continue today. Research supported by the National Institute of Environmental Health Sciences (NIEHS) and many others, examining the link between dioxin and serious illnesses, has helped lead the U.S. Department of Veterans Affairs (VA) to recognize certain cancers and other health problems as presumptive diseases associated with exposure to Agent Orange or other herbicides during military service. Presumptive diseases are certain diseases that the VA assumes can be related to a Veteran's qualifying military service.

Dioxins were also brought to light in 1982, when the town of Times Beach, Mo., was declared off-limits, because of dioxin contamination. This incident in Missouri, as well as others, helped spark passage of legislation that created Superfund, the environmental program established to address abandoned hazardous waste sites. In addition to funding work in labs across the nation, the NIEHS administers the Superfund Research Program (SRP). SRP involves a network of university grants that are designed to seek solutions to the complex health and environmental issues associated with the nation's hazardous waste sites.

The research conducted by the SRP is a coordinated effort with the U.S. Environmental Protection Agency (EPA), the federal entity charged with cleaning up the worst hazardous waste sites in the country, including those contaminated with dioxins. As of date, the hazards posed by dioxins have faded from public view. And, in fact, the extent of the hazard has diminished in the United States, as environmental controls significantly reduced the introduction of new industrial sources of dioxin. However, the problem has not vanished, and the scientific community has continued its work to reduce exposures and treat diseases that arise from them.

Dioxins, Furans, and PCBs Contain Phenyl Rings of Carbon Atoms

Dioxins, furans, and polychlorinated biphenyls (PCBs) are a class of similar chlorinated aromatic organic compounds. Dioxins have two phenyl rings connected by two oxygen atoms. Furans have one or two phenyl rings connected to a furan ring. PCBs have two phenyl rings attached at one point. One or more chlorine atoms can attach to any available carbon atom, allowing for 100–200 forms of each. Dioxins and dioxin-like furans have no known commercial or natural use. They are produced primarily during the incineration or burning of waste; the bleaching processes used in pulp and paper mills; and the chemical syntheses of trichlorophenoxyacetic acid, hexachlorophene, vinyl chloride, trichlorophenol, and pentachlorophenol. PCBs were once synthesized for use as heat-exchanger, transformer, and hydraulic fluids, and also used as additives to paints, oils, window caulking, and floor tiles. Production of PCBs peaked in the early 1970s and was banned in the United States after 1979.

What Is Furan?

Furan is a colorless, volatile liquid used in some chemical manufacturing industries. Furan has occasionally been reported to be found in foods. Now scientists at U.S. Food and Drug Administration (FDA) have discovered that furan forms in some foods more commonly than previously thought. This discovery is likely a result of the ability to detect compounds at exceedingly low levels with the latest analytical instruments rather than a change in the presence of furan. The scientists think the furan forms in the food during traditional heat treatment techniques, such as cooking, jarring, and canning.

Furan: Not a Dioxin-Like Compound

No, furan is not a dioxin-like compound. The term "furans" is sometimes used as shorthand for a group of environmental contaminants called the dibenzofurans, which have dioxin-like activity. In addition "furans" refers to a large class of compounds of widely varying structures including, for example, nitrofurans. These chemicals have different effects than the furan that is now being studied.

Furan in Food

So far, FDA has focused on testing canned or jarred foods, because these foods are heated in sealed containers. Furan has been found in such canned or jarred foods as soups, sauces, beans, pasta meals, and baby foods.

Can Cause Cancer

Furan causes cancer in animals in studies where animals are exposed to furan at high doses. Because furan levels have been measured in only a few foods to date, it is difficult for FDA scientists to accurately calculate levels of furan exposure in food and to estimate a risk to consumers. However, FDA's preliminary estimate of consumer exposure is well below what FDA expects would cause harmful effects. FDA will continue to thoroughly evaluate these preliminary data and conduct additional studies to better determine the potential risk to human health.

Furan in Baby Food

The new data show furan in baby foods. It is not a matter of concern. These data are exploratory and provide only a very limited and incomplete picture of the levels of furan in foods. These data alone do not indicate exposure or risk. FDA's preliminary estimate of consumer exposure is well below what FDA expects would cause harmful effects. FDA has no evidence that consumers should alter their infants' and children's diets and eating habits to avoid exposure to furan.

In the course of investigations to confirm the accuracy of a report that furan may be formed in food under certain circumstances, FDA scientists discovered that a wider variety of foods that were heat treated than previously thought contained varying levels of furan.

Why Is Furan a Concern?

Furan is listed in the U.S. Department of Health and Human Services (HHS) list of carcinogens, and considered as possibly carcinogenic by the International Agency for Research on Cancer (IARC), based on studies in laboratory animals at high exposures. The concern is whether furan may also cause cancer in humans through long-term exposure to very low levels of furan in foods.

Did Furan Suddenly Appear in Food?

No, furan did not suddenly appear in food and has likely been present in food for many years. Furan appears to result from heat treatment techniques, such as canning and jarring, which have long been essential methods of safe food preparation and preservation. Scientists have previously reported finding furan in a small number of foods. What's new now is that FDA scientists have developed a new method that can measure exceedingly low levels of furan and applied that method to a wide variety of foods.

FDA on Furan in Foods

Since first investigating furan in foods with a semi-quantitative method, FDA has refined its method to give quantitative furan measurements, applied that method to a limited number of foods, and begun planning for a larger survey of foods. FDA has also published in the Federal Register a call for data on furan from the scientific community. FDA will evaluate the available data and will develop an action plan that will outline the agency's goals and planned activities on the issue of furan in food. The action plan will consider such items as an expanded food survey, studies to identify mechanisms of formation in foods and potential strategies to reduce furan levels, and toxicology studies to address mechanisms of furan toxicity and dose-response.

How Does Furan Form in Foods?

Exactly how furan forms in food are unknown. Early indications are that there are probably multiple mechanisms of furan formation. Heating is probably an important contributing factor to furan formation in foods, but heat may not be the only pathway to furan formation.

How Do the Levels of Furan in Canned Foods Relate to Foods as Eaten?

It is possible that canned or jarred foods that have measurable furan levels right after opening may contain lower levels of furan after they are heated in open containers, as they typically would be prior to consumption. Furan is volatile, and a portion may evaporate when foods are heated in an open container, such as a pot. To test this hypothesis, FDA will compare furan levels in foods directly from a can or jar and after heating them as a consumer ordinarily would before consumption.

Will More Foods Be Tested?

Yes, FDA will test more foods and different types of foods, such as noncanned foods and home prepared foods, in the future. FDA will also look at the effect on furan levels of opening and heating canned and jarred foods.

Should Consumers Change Their Eating Habits?

No. FDA's preliminary exposure data suggest that the levels of furan being found in food are well below levels that would cause harmful effects. Until more is known, FDA recommends that consumers eat a balanced diet, choosing a variety of foods that are low in trans fat and saturated fat, and rich in high-fiber grains, fruits, and vegetables.

Chapter 33

Contaminants in Fish and Shellfish

Chapter Contents

Section 33.1

Mercury in Seafood

This section contains text excerpted from the following sources:
Text beginning with the heading "Mercury in Fish and Shellfish" is
excerpted from "What You Need to Know about Mercury in Fish and
Shellfish," U.S. Food and Drug Administration (FDA), January 25,
2018; Text under the heading "Eating Fish That Contain Mercury" is
excerpted from "Guidelines for Eating Fish That Contain Mercury,"
U.S. Environmental Protection Agency (EPA), January 11, 2018.

Mercury in Fish and Shellfish

Fish and shellfish are an important part of a healthy diet. Fish and
shellfish contain high-quality protein and other essential nutrients, are
low in saturated fat and contain omega-3 fatty acids. A well-balanced
diet that includes a variety of fish and shellfish can contribute to heart
health and children's proper growth and development. So, women and
young children, in particular, should include fish or shellfish in their
diets due to the many nutritional benefits.

However, nearly all fish and shellfish contain traces of mercury. For
most people, the risk from mercury by eating fish and shellfish is not
a health concern. Yet, some fish and shellfish contain higher levels of
mercury that may harm an unborn baby or young child's developing
nervous system. The risks from mercury in fish and shellfish depend
on the amount of fish and shellfish eaten and the levels of mercury
in the fish and shellfish. Therefore, the U.S. Food and Drug Administration (FDA) and U.S. Environmental Protection Agency (EPA) are
advising women who may become pregnant, pregnant women, nursing
mothers, and young children to avoid some types of fish and eat fish
and shellfish that are lower in mercury.

By following these 3 recommendations for selecting and eating
fish or shellfish, women, and young children will receive the benefits
of eating fish and shellfish and be confident that they have reduced
their exposure to the harmful effects of mercury.

1. Do not eat shark, swordfish, king mackerel, or tilefish because
    they contain high levels of mercury.

2. Eat up to 12 ounces (2 average meals) a week of a variety of fish and shellfish that are lower in mercury.

   - Five of the most commonly eaten fish that are low in mercury are shrimp, canned light tuna, salmon, pollock, and catfish

   - Another commonly eaten fish, albacore ("white") tuna has more mercury than canned light tuna. So, when choosing your two meals of fish and shellfish, you may eat up to 6 ounces (one average meal) of albacore tuna per week.

3. Check local advisories about the safety of fish caught by family and friends in your local lakes, rivers, and coastal areas. If no advice is available, eat up to 6 ounces (one average meal) per week of fish you catch from local waters, but don't consume any other fish during that week.

Follow these same recommendations when feeding fish and shellfish to your young child, but serve smaller portions.

Frequently Asked Questions about Mercury in Fish and Shellfish

What Is Mercury and Methylmercury?

Mercury occurs naturally in the environment and can also be released into the air through industrial pollution. Mercury falls from the air and can accumulate in streams and oceans and is turned into methylmercury in the water. It is this type of mercury that can be harmful to your unborn baby and young child. Fish absorb the methylmercury as they feed in these waters and so it builds up in them. It builds up more in some types of fish and shellfish than others, depending on what the fish eat, which is why the levels vary.

I'm a Woman Who Could Have Children but I'm Not Pregnant—So Why Should I Be Concerned about Methylmercury?

If you regularly eat types of fish that are high in methylmercury, it can accumulate in your blood stream over time. Methylmercury is removed from the body naturally, but it may take over a year for the levels to drop significantly. Thus, it may be present in a woman even before she becomes pregnant. This is the reason why women who are trying to become pregnant should also avoid eating certain types of fish.

Is There Methylmercury in All Fish and Shellfish?

Nearly all fish and shellfish contain traces of methylmercury. However, larger fish that have lived longer have the highest levels of methylmercury because they've had more time to accumulate it. These large fish (swordfish, shark, king mackerel and tilefish) pose the greatest risk. Other types of fish and shellfish may be eaten in the amounts recommended by FDA and EPA.

What about Fish Sticks and Fast Food Sandwiches?

Fish sticks and "fast-food" sandwiches are commonly made from fish that are low in mercury.

The Advice about Canned Tuna Is in the Advisory, but What's the Advice about Tuna Steaks?

Because tuna steak generally contains higher levels of mercury than canned light tuna, when choosing your two meals of fish and shellfish, you may eat up to 6 ounces (one average meal) of tuna steak per week.

What If I Eat More than the Recommended Amount of Fish and Shellfish in a Week?

One week's consumption of fish does not change the level of methylmercury in the body much at all. If you eat a lot of fish one week, you can cut back for the next week or two. Just make sure you average the recommended amount per week.

Where Do I Get Information about the Safety of Fish Caught Recreationally by Family or Friends?

Before you go fishing, check your Fishing Regulations Booklet for information about recreationally caught fish. You can also contact your local health department for information about local advisories. You need to check local advisories because some kinds of fish and shellfish caught in your local waters may have higher or much lower than average levels of mercury. This depends on the levels of mercury in the water in which the fish are caught. Those fish with much lower levels may be eaten more frequently and in larger amounts.

Eating Fish That Contain Mercury

To enjoy the benefits of eating fish while minimizing exposure to mercury, you should:

- Eat mainly types of fish low in mercury.

- Limit your consumption of types of fish with typically higher levels of mercury.

Fish are important for a healthy diet. They are a lean, low-calorie source of protein. However, some fish may contain mercury or other harmful chemicals at sufficiently high levels to be a concern.

Federal, state and local governments issue fish consumption advisories when fish are unsafe to eat. The advisories may suggest that people avoid eating certain kinds or certain amounts of fish.

- Some advisories apply to specific water types (like specific lakes)

- Some may focus on groups of particularly sensitive people (e.g., women of childbearing age)

- Some advisories include notices of "no restriction" to tell us that certain fish are safe to eat

The degree of exposure to mercury depends on both the amount and the type of fish eaten. If you are concerned about your health or your family's as a result of a potential exposure to mercury, get in touch with your healthcare provider. She will be able to tell you if the degree of mercury exposure is a concern, and what to do about it.

Section 33.2

Food Poisoning from Marine Toxins

This section includes text excerpted from "Food Poisoning from Marine Toxins," Centers for Disease Control and Prevention (CDC), May 31, 2017.

Seafood poisoning from marine toxins is an underrecognized hazard for travelers, particularly in the tropics and subtropics. Furthermore, the risk is increasing as a result of factors such as climate change, coral reef damage, and spread of toxic algal blooms.

Ciguatera Fish Poisoning (CFP)

Ciguatera fish poisoning occurs after eating reef fish contaminated with toxins such as ciguatoxin or maitotoxin. These potent toxins originate from Gambierdiscus toxicus (G. toxicus), a small marine organism (dinoflagellate) that grows on and around coral reefs. Dinoflagellates are ingested by herbivorous fish. The toxins produced by G. toxicus are then modified and concentrated as they pass up the marine food chain to carnivorous fish and finally to humans. Ciguatoxins are concentrated in the fish liver, intestines, roe, and heads.

G. toxicus may proliferate on dead coral reefs more effectively than other dinoflagellates. The risk of ciguatera is likely to increase as more coral reefs deteriorate because of climate change, ocean acidification, construction, and nutrient runoff.

Risk for Travelers

Ciguatera poisoning is underrecognized and underreported; up to 50,000 cases occur globally every year. The incidence in travelers to highly endemic areas has been estimated as high as 3 per 100. Ciguatera is widespread in tropical and subtropical waters, usually between the latitudes of 35°N and 35°S; it is particularly common in the Pacific and Indian Oceans and the Caribbean Sea.

The incidence and geographic distribution of ciguatera poisoning are increasing. Newly recognized areas of risk include the Canary Islands, the eastern Mediterranean, and the western Gulf of Mexico. Medical practitioners must be aware that cases of ciguatera fish poisoning acquired by travelers in endemic areas may present in nonendemic (temperate) areas. In addition, cases of ciguatera fish poisoning are seen with increasing frequency in nonendemic areas as a result of the increasing global trade in seafood products.

Fish that are most likely to cause ciguatera poisoning are large carnivorous reef fish, such as barracuda, grouper, moray eel, amberjack, sea bass, or sturgeon. Omnivorous and herbivorous fish such as parrot-fish, surgeonfish, and red snapper can also be a risk.

Clinical Presentation

Ciguatera poisoning may cause gastrointestinal, cardiovascular, neurologic, and neuropsychiatric illness. The first symptoms usually develop within 3–6 hours after eating contaminated fish, but may be delayed for up to 30 hours. Symptoms include:

- Gastrointestinal: diarrhea, nausea, vomiting, and abdominal pain

- Cardiovascular: bradycardia, heart block, hypotension

- Neurologic: paresthesias, weakness, pain in the teeth or a sensation that the teeth are loose, burning or metallic taste in the mouth, generalized itching, sweating, and blurred vision

- Cold allodynia (abnormal sensation when touching cold water or objects) has been reported as characteristic, but there can be acute sensitivity to both hot and cold. Neurologic symptoms usually last a few days to several weeks but may persist for months or even years.

- Neuropsychiatric: fatigue, general malaise, and insomnia

The overall death rate from ciguatera poisoning is <0.1 percent but varies according to the toxin dose and availability of medical care to deal with complications. The diagnosis of ciguatera poisoning is based on the characteristic signs and symptoms and a history of eating species of fish that are known to carry ciguatera toxin. Fish testing can be done by the U.S. Food and Drug Administration (FDA) in their laboratory at Dauphin Island. There is no readily available test for ciguatera toxins in human clinical specimens.

Prevention

Travelers can take the following precautions to prevent ciguatera fish poisoning:

- Avoid or limit consumption of reef fish.

- Never eat high-risk fish such as barracuda or moray eel.

- Avoid the parts of the fish that concentrate ciguatera toxin: liver, intestines, roe, and head.

Remember that ciguatera toxins do not affect the texture, taste, or smell of fish, and they are not destroyed by gastric acid, cooking, smoking, freezing, canning, salting, or pickling.

Treatment

There is no specific antidote for ciguatoxin or maitotoxin poisonings. Symptomatic treatment may include gabapentin or pregabalin (neuropathic symptoms), amitriptyline (chronic paresthesias, depression, and pruritus), fluoxetine (chronic fatigue), and nifedipine or acetaminophen (headaches). Intravenous mannitol has been reported in uncontrolled studies to reduce the severity and duration of neurologic symptoms, particularly if given within 48 hours of the appearance of symptoms. It should only be given to hemodynamically stable, well-hydrated patients.

After recovering from ciguatera poisoning, patients may want to avoid any fish, nuts, alcohol, or caffeine for at least 6 months as they may cause a relapse in symptoms.

Scombroid

Scombroid, one of the most common fish poisonings, occurs worldwide in both temperate and tropical waters. The illness occurs after eating improperly refrigerated or preserved fish containing high levels of histamine and often resembles a moderate to a severe allergic reaction.

Fish typically associated with scombroid have naturally high levels of histidine in the flesh and include tuna, mackerel, mahi-mahi (dolphin fish), sardine, anchovy, herring, bluefish, amberjack, and marlin. Histidine is converted to histamine by bacterial overgrowth in fish that has been improperly stored after capture. Histamine and other scombrotoxins are resistant to cooking, smoking, canning, or freezing.

Clinical Presentation

Symptoms of scombroid poisoning resemble an acute allergic reaction and usually appear 10–60 minutes after eating contaminated fish. They include flushing of the face and upper body (resembling sunburn), severe headache, palpitations, itching, blurred vision, abdominal cramps, and diarrhea. Untreated, symptoms usually resolve within 12 hours but may last up to 48 hours. Rarely, there may be a respiratory compromise, malignant arrhythmias, and hypotension requiring hospitalization. There are no long-term sequelae. Diagnosis is usually clinical. A clustering of cases helps exclude the possibility of true fish allergy.

Prevention

Fish contaminated with histamine may have a peppery, sharp, salty, taste or "bubbly" feel but will usually look, smell, and taste normal. The key to prevention is to make sure that the fish is properly iced or refrigerated at temperatures <38°F (<3.3°C), or immediately frozen after it is caught. Cooking, smoking, canning, or freezing will not destroy histamine in contaminated fish.

Treatment

Scombroid poisoning usually responds well to antihistamines (H1-receptor blockers, although H2-receptor blockers may also be of benefit).

Shellfish Poisoning

Several forms of poisoning may occur after ingesting toxin-containing shellfish, such as filter-feeding bivalve mollusks (such as mussels, oysters, clams, scallops, and cockles), gastropod mollusks (such as abalone, whelks, and moon snails), or crustaceans (such as Dungeness crabs, shrimp, and lobsters). The toxins originate in small marine organisms (dinoflagellates or diatoms) that are ingested and are concentrated by shellfish.

Risk for Travelers

Contaminated (toxic) shellfish may be found in temperate and tropical waters, typically during or after phytoplankton blooms, also called harmful algal blooms (HABs). One example of a HAB is the Florida red tide caused by Karenia brevis.

Clinical Presentation

Poisoning results in gastrointestinal and neurologic illness of varying severity. Symptoms typically appear 30–60 minutes after ingesting toxic shellfish but can be delayed for several hours. Diagnosis is usually one of exclusion and is typically made clinically in patients who have recently eaten shellfish.

Paralytic Shellfish Poisoning (PSP)

Paralytic shellfish poisoning (PSP) is the most common and most severe form of shellfish poisoning. PSP is caused by eating shellfish contaminated with saxitoxins. These potent neurotoxins are produced by various dinoflagellates. A wide range of shellfish may cause PSP, but most cases occur after eating mussels or clams.

PSP occurs worldwide but is most common in temperate waters, especially off the Pacific and Atlantic Coasts of North America, including

Alaska. Cases have also been reported from countries such as the Philippines, China, Chile, Scotland, Ireland, New Zealand, and Australia.

Symptoms usually appear 30–60 minutes after eating toxic shellfish and include numbness and tingling of the face, lips, tongue, arms, and legs. There may be headache, nausea, vomiting, and diarrhea. Severe cases are associated with ingestion of large doses of toxin and clinical features such as ataxia, dysphagia, mental status changes, flaccid paralysis, and respiratory failure. The case-fatality ratio is dependent on the availability of modern medical care, including mechanical ventilation. The death rate may be particularly high in children.

Neurotoxic Shellfish Poisoning (NSP)

Neurotoxic shellfish poisoning (NSP) is caused by eating shellfish contaminated with brevetoxins produced by the dinoflagellate K. brevis. NSP has been reported from the southeastern coast of the United States, the Gulf of Mexico, the Caribbean, and New Zealand.

NSP usually presents 30 minutes to 3 hours after eating toxic shellfish. Most cases present with gastroenteritis accompanied by minor neurologic symptoms resembling mild ciguatera poisoning or mild paralytic shellfish poisoning. A syndrome known as aerosolized red tide respiratory irritation (ARTRI) occurs when aerosolized brevetoxins are inhaled in sea spray. This has been reported in association with a red tide (K. brevis bloom) in Florida. It can induce bronchoconstriction and may cause acute, temporary respiratory discomfort in healthy people. People with asthma may experience more severe and prolonged respiratory effects.

Diarrheic Shellfish Poisoning

Diarrheic shellfish poisoning (DSP) is caused by eating shellfish contaminated with toxins such as okadaic acid. It occurs worldwide, and outbreaks have been reported from China, Japan, Scandinavia, France, Belgium, Spain, Chile, Uruguay, Ireland, the United States, and Canada.

Most cases result from eating toxic bivalve mollusks such as mussels and scallops. Symptoms usually occur within 2 hours of eating contaminated shellfish and include chills, diarrhea, nausea, vomiting, and abdominal pain. Symptoms usually resolve within 2–3 days. No deaths have been reported.

Amnesic Shellfish Poisoning

Amnesic shellfish poisoning (ASP) is a rare form of shellfish poisoning caused by eating shellfish contaminated with domoic acid, produced by the diatom Pseudonitzchia spp. ASP has been reported from Canada, Scotland, Ireland, France, Belgium, Spain, Portugal, New Zealand, Australia, and Chile. Toxic mussels, scallops, razor clams, and crustaceans were responsible in those outbreaks.

In most cases, gastrointestinal symptoms such as diarrhea, vomiting, and abdominal pain develop within 24 hours of eating toxic shellfish, followed by headache, memory loss, and cognitive impairment. In severe cases there may be hypotension, arrhythmias, ophthalmoplegia, coma, and death. Survivors may have severe anterograde, short-term memory deficits.

Prevention

Shellfish poisoning can be prevented by avoiding potentially contaminated shellfish. This is particularly important in areas during or shortly after algal blooms, which may be locally referred to as "red tides" or "brown tides." Travelers to developing countries should avoid eating all shellfish because they also carry a high risk of viral and bacterial infections. Marine shellfish toxins cannot be destroyed by cooking or freezing.

Treatment

Treatment is symptomatic and supportive. Severe cases of PSP may require mechanical ventilation.

Section 33.3

Fresh and Frozen Seafood: Selecting and Serving It Safely

This section includes text excerpted from "Imported
Seafood Safety Program," U.S. Food and Drug
Administration (FDA), November 24, 2017.

The U.S. Food and Drug Administration (FDA) is responsible for the safety of all fish and fishery products entering the United States.

The agency uses every available tool to identify immediate or potential threats as well as the best course of action to protect public health and safety. As part of the FDA's import safety effort, the agency provides as much available information and guidance as possible to consumers, industry, and government about seafood safety.

Hazard Analysis and Critical Control Points

The FDA's multifaceted and risk-informed seafood safety program relies on various measures of compliance with its seafood Hazard Analysis and Critical Control Points (HACCP) regulations, which describe a management system in which food safety is addressed through the analysis and control of biological, chemical, and physical hazards from raw material production, procurement and handling, to manufacturing, distribution and consumption of the finished product.

For imported seafood, these measures include:

- inspections of foreign processing facilities
- sampling of seafood offered for import into the United States
- domestic surveillance sampling of imported products
- inspections of seafood importers
- evaluations of filers of seafood products
- foreign country program assessments
- relevant information from our foreign partners and the FDA overseas offices

Foreign Inspections and Global Presence

The FDA has increased the number of foreign site inspections in recent years, and is working globally to better accomplish its domestic mission to promote and protect the public health of the United States. The FDA has strengthened and better coordinated its international engagements by establishing permanent the FDA posts abroad in strategic locations. The posting of the FDA staff in certain overseas regions is a key part of the agency's strategy for expanding oversight of imported food.

Predictive Risk-based Evaluation for Dynamic Import Compliance Targeting (PREDICT)

The FDA is also implementing a new screening system for imports, the Predictive Risk-based Evaluation for Dynamic Import

Compliance Targeting (PREDICT), which will improve the current electronic screening system by targeting higher-risk products for exam and sampling and minimizing the delays of shipments of lower risk products. PREDICT will improve the agency's ability to detect trends and investigate patterns. This, in turn, will help to make more efficient use of the FDA's import resources and allow the FDA to adjust import sampling levels for seafood products over time and as appropriate.

Foreign Country Assessments

Foreign country assessments are systems reviews that offer the FDA a broad view of the ability of the country's industry and regulatory infrastructure to control aquaculture drugs. These assessments allow the FDA to become familiar with the controls that a country's competent authority is implementing for the distribution, availability, and use of animal drugs. The FDA uses country assessments to evaluate the country's laws for, and implementation of, control of animal drug residues in the aquaculture products it ships to the United States.

The country assessment program helps the FDA direct its foreign inspection and border surveillance resources more effectively and efficiently and allows the FDA to work directly with countries to resolve drug residue problems.

The FDA uses information from country assessments to:

- better target (i.e., increase or decrease) surveillance sampling of imported aquaculture products inform its decisions on what new analytical methods it needs to develop and what drugs or chemicals it should target for surveillance sampling

- inform its planning of foreign seafood HACCP inspections

- provide additional evidence for potential regulatory actions, such as an import alert

- improve collaboration with foreign government and industry contacts to achieve better compliance with FDA's regulatory requirements

- better understand the causes for significant changes in a country's drug residue problems, such as a sudden spike in noncompliant samples

Results of Country Assessments

- The assessment trip to China in 2006 was a key consideration in issuance of the China country-wide import alert for specific aquaculture products from China in 2007.

- The country assessments for China in 2006, Chile in 2008, and India in 2010 were considered and resulted in increased sampling and testing under the compliance program and special assignments for aquaculture products from these countries (e.g., eel from China, salmon from Chile, and shrimp from India).

Food Safety Modernization Act of 2011

The FDA conducts its seafood safety oversight activities in conformance with its statutory authorities, which have recently been expanded by the Food Safety Modernization Act (FSMA). FSMA represents the first major overhaul of the FDA's food safety law in more than 70 years and will transform the FDA's food safety program. FSMA closes significant and longstanding gaps in the FDA's food safety authority, with new safeguards to prevent, rather than react, to food safety problems, and gives the FDA important new tools to ensure that imported seafood is as safe as domestic seafood.

Integrated Food Safety System

The FDA collaborates with the President's Food Safety Working Group (FSWG) to modernize food safety by building collaborative partnerships with consumers, industry and regulatory partners.

For example, the FDA and National Marine Fisheries Service's (NMFS) Seafood Inspection Program have certain common and related objectives in carrying out their respective regulatory and service activities that lend themselves to cooperation under a Memorandum of Understanding (MoU) that sets forth the working arrangements between the agencies that facilitate each agency's efforts to discharge its responsibilities related to the inspection of fish and fishery products.

National Residue Monitoring Program

In addition to implementing the new FSMA authorities, the FDA will continue the national residue monitoring program and recognizes the benefit of such a program to ensure that foods are not contaminated with illegal animal drug residues. FSMA directs the FDA to establish a program for testing of food by accredited laboratories and will require that food be tested by accredited laboratories in some circumstances, such as in support of admission of imported food. The FDA is developing the laboratory accreditation program as part of its FSMA implementation efforts.

Consumer Information

The government website FoodSafety.gov provides a widget that displays the latest recalls and food safety alerts from both the FDA and USDA. If you have a mobile device, such as an android phone, you may be able to download an application to get recalls direct to your phone by going to Recalls.gov.

Chapter 34

Antibiotics and Hormones in Dairy and Meat

Chapter Contents

Section 34.1

Antibiotics Resistance and Food Safety

This section contains text excerpted from the following
sources: Text under the heading "What Are Antibiotics?" is
excerpted from "Antibiotics," MedlinePlus, National Institutes of
Health (NIH), May 19, 2015; Text under the heading "Antibiotic
Resistance" is excerpted from "Be Antibiotics Aware: Smart Use, Best
Care," Centers for Disease Control and Prevention (CDC),
December 15, 2017.

What Are Antibiotics?

Antibiotics are powerful medicines that fight bacterial infections.
Used properly, antibiotics can save lives. They either kill bacteria or
keep them from reproducing. Your body's natural defenses can usually
take it from there.

Antibiotics do not fight infections caused by viruses, such as

- Colds

- Flu

- Most coughs and bronchitis

- Sore throats, unless caused by strep

If a virus is making you sick, taking antibiotics may do more harm
than good. Using antibiotics when you don't need them, or not using
them properly, can add to antibiotic resistance. This happens when
bacteria change and become able to resist the effects of an antibiotic.

When you take antibiotics, follow the directions carefully. It is
important to finish your medicine even if you feel better. If you stop
treatment too soon, some bacteria may survive and re-infect you. Do
not save antibiotics for later or use someone else's prescription.

Antibiotic Resistance

Antibiotic resistance is one of the most urgent threats to the public's
health. Antibiotic resistance occurs when bacteria develop the ability

to defeat the drugs designed to kill them. Each year in the United States, at least 2 million people get infected with antibiotic-resistant bacteria, and at least 23,000 people die as a result.

Antibiotics save lives but any time antibiotics are used, they can cause side effects and lead to antibiotic resistance. About 30 percent of antibiotics, or 47 million prescriptions, are prescribed unnecessarily in doctors' offices and emergency departments in the United States, which makes improving antibiotic prescribing and use a national priority.

Helping healthcare professionals improve the way they prescribe antibiotics, and improving the way we take antibiotics, helps keep us healthy now, helps fight antibiotic resistance, and ensures that these life-saving drugs will be available for future generations.

When Antibiotics Are Needed

Antibiotics are only needed for treating certain infections caused by bacteria. We rely on antibiotics to treat serious infections, such as pneumonia, and life-threatening conditions including sepsis, the body's extreme response to an infection. Effective antibiotics are also needed for people who are at high risk for developing infections. Some of those at high risk for infections include patients undergoing surgery, patients with end-stage kidney disease, or patients receiving cancer therapy (chemotherapy).

When Antibiotics Aren't Needed

Antibiotics won't help for some common bacterial infections including most cases of bronchitis, many sinus infections, and some ear infections. An antibiotic will not make you feel better if you have a virus. Antibiotics do not work on viral infections, such as colds, flu, or runny noses, even if the mucus is thick, yellow or green.

Antibiotics save lives, and when a patient needs antibiotics, the benefits outweigh the risk of side effects. When antibiotics aren't needed, they won't help you, and the side effects could still hurt you. Common side effects of antibiotics can include:

- rash

- dizziness

- nausea

- diarrhea

- yeast infections

More serious side effects include *Clostridium* difficile infection (also called *C. difficile* or *C. diff*), which causes diarrhea that can lead to severe colon damage and death. People can also have severe and life-threatening allergic reactions.

What You Can Do to Feel Better

Talk with your healthcare professional about the best treatment for your or your loved one's illness. If you need antibiotics, take them exactly as prescribed. Talk with your healthcare professional if you have any questions about your antibiotics, or if you develop any side effects especially diarrhea since that could be a C. difficile infection, which needs to be treated immediately.

Respiratory viruses usually go away in a week or two without treatment. Ask your healthcare professional about the best way to feel better while your body fights off the virus. To stay healthy and keep others healthy:

- Clean your hands

- Cover coughs

- Stay home when sick

- Get recommended vaccines

Section 34.2

Recombinant Bovine Growth Hormone (rBGH)

This section includes text excerpted from "Report on
the U.S. Food and Drug Administration's (FDA) Review of the
Safety of Recombinant Bovine Somatotropin," U.S. Food and Drug
Administration (FDA), October 27, 2017.

Report on the U.S. Food and Drug Administration's (FDA) Review of the Safety of Recombinant Bovine Somatotropin

Following an extensive review of the data to support the safety and
effectiveness of the product, the U.S. Food and Drug Administration
(FDA) approved the Monsanto Company's New Animal Drug Application for Posilac containing a recombinant bovine growth hormone
(rBGH) (also known as recombinant bovine somatotropin, rBST, or
Sometribove).

Growth hormone (GH) is a protein hormone produced in the pituitary gland of animals including humans and is essential for normal
growth, development, and health maintenance. Approximately 60
years ago, it was discovered that injecting cows with GH extracted
from cattle pituitary glands increased milk production. In the 1980s, it
became technically possible and economically feasible to produce large
quantities of bovine GH (bGH) using recombinant deoxyribonucleic
acid (DNA) processes. The Posilac product contains a recombinant
bGH (rBGH) which is essentially the same as (pituitary-derived) bGH.

In order to grant approval of Posilac, the FDA determined, among
other things, that food products from cows treated with rBGH are
safe for consumption by humans. Vermont Public Interest Research
Group (VPIRG) and Rural Vermont have questioned the validity of
this finding based on an analysis by reviewers at Health Canada (the
Canadian counterpart of the FDA). This analysis, based in large part
on a 90-day rat study, challenges the FDA's human health findings
and argues that possible adverse health effects of Posilac were not

addressed because long-term toxicology studies to ascertain human health safety were not required by the FDA or conducted by Monsanto.

The FDA has completed a comprehensive, page by page audit of the human food safety sections of the investigational new animal drug file and master file supporting the rBGH approval. This audit examined all the studies used in determining the human food safety of rBGH, including the 90-day rat oral toxicity study and the report of the antibody response to oral rBGH upon which the Canadian reviewers relied. Upon determining that a review had not been performed on the antibody data during the course of the original review of the Monsanto application, these data were reviewed in their entirety. As set forth in detail below, the FDA believes that the Canadian reviewers did not interpret the study results correctly and that there are no new scientific concerns regarding the safety of milk from cows treated with rBGH. The determination that long-term studies were not necessary for assessing the safety of rBGH was based on studies which show that: bGH is biologically inactive in humans even if injected, rBGH is orally inactive, and bGH and rBGH are biologically indistinguishable.

Absorption

When taken orally, proteins typically are broken down in the digestive process and are not absorbed into the body. To determine whether a rBGH product had biologically significant oral activity, the FDA's required the drugs sponsor to perform short-term toxicology studies to assess whether biologically active rBGH was being absorbed into the body. Absorption of biologically active rBGH into the body could indicate a need for long-term studies to assess the possible impact on various body organs, particularly the liver. The study was conducted by orally administering rBGH to rats for 28 days at 100 times the daily dose administered to dairy cattle. The FDA determined that there was no evidence for the absorption of biologically active rBGH following oral administration because there were no dose-related trends associated with oral administration of rBGH to rats for 28 days.

The Canadian analysis takes issue with the FDA's findings regarding a 90-day rat oral toxicity study performed by Monsanto to fulfill a requirement of the European Union (EU) for rBGH approval. The study was conducted by a Searle laboratory of Monsanto and submitted to the FDA pursuant to the FDA's requirement that all relevant safety information for an investigational new animal drug is included in the sponsor's application. The FDA reviewed the study in 1989, except as noted below, and it was determined that there were no observed effects from oral administration at any dose. In this study, there was evidence that oral administration of rBGH produced an antibody response; however, such response was consistent with that produced by a number of food proteins and is not necessarily an indication of absorption of intact rBGH.

As rBGH produces significant biological effects when injected into rats, this study supported the inability of rBGH to cause significant biological effects following oral administration even at doses 50 times greater than the injected dose.

The report of the 90-day rat oral toxicity study included discussion of a satellite study group of rats. This satellite study was conducted to investigate the antibody response to rBGH as an indirect measure of the possible absorption of rBGH from the rat gastrointestinal tract. This satellite study was not reviewed when originally submitted. Once this oversight was detected, the FDA immediately undertook the review of the data.

FDA's review of the antibody response study "Determination of Sometribove immunoglobulin in rat serum" was completed on November 30, 1998. The study showed:

- Six out of 30 rats receiving 5 mg (10^{-3} grams)/kg/day oral rBGH, and 9 out of 30 rats receiving 50 mg/kg/day produced antibodies, while there was no measurable response at 0.5 mg/kg/day (500 μg (10^{-6} grams)/kg/day). Thus, at high doses, these data appear to show some systemic anti-rBGH response to the oral administration of rBGH to rats.

- The methodology used in this study, however, was inadequate to determine the systemic bioavailability of oral rBGH. Immune cells throughout the body, including cells in the gastrointestinal tract and in the systemic circulation, produce antibodies. Antibodies produced in the gastrointestinal tract, however, can travel from the gastrointestinal tract to the systemic circulation. Thus the presence of antibodies in the systemic circulation is not proof of systemic absorption of rBGH from the gastrointestinal tract.

- The level of antibodies present in rat plasma is relatively low and would not be expected to have any adverse effect on the host

- It may be calculated, based upon consumption of 1.5 liters of milk per day, by a 10 kg child, with a concentration of approximately 5 micrograms (μg: 10^{-6}) rBST per liter of milk, that children are exposed to 7.5 μg/kg/day. This concentration is several hundred-fold below the lowest dose that elicited antibody production in the submitted study (0.5 mg/kg/day). Thus, the daily amount of rBGH needed to result in systemic antibody levels are orders of magnitude above that which could reasonably be expected to be consumed on a daily basis.

It is noted that there were no dose-related effects on body weight or organ weight found in either the 90-day oral exposure study or the pivotal 28-day oral exposure study in rats, demonstrating a lack of biological activity.

In addition, a study published by Seaman demonstrated that orally administered doses of up to 40 mg/kg/day of bovine somatotropin had no effect on weight gain (while such effects were observed following injection of the drug). This study demonstrated a dose-dependent increased weight gain in hypophysectomized rats administered bovine somatotropin at doses of 0.15, 0.30, and 0.60 mg/kg/day for up to 9 days by subcutaneous injection. Oral administration of bovine somatotropin at doses up to 40 mg/kg/day had no effect on body weight gain in this sensitive bioassay. Subcutaneous administration of bovine somatotropin to hypophysectomized rats resulted in a modest increase in serum antibodies to rBGH by the end of the study (day 9) coupled with measurable plasma levels of bovine somatotropin by radioimmunoassay. Oral administration resulted in no detectable levels of bovine somatotropin in the blood while there was a detectable production of antibodies. Seaman concluded that this study does not provide evidence for the absorption of intact somatotropin following oral administration as there was no effect on weight gain nor could somatotropin be measured by the analytical method. The authors conclude that the antibody response was most likely directed toward recognizable fragments of the parent protein molecule rather than intact bovine somatotropin. As to the question of whether the antibody response itself might be considered an adverse effect, the authors cite several reports showing that the vast majority of healthy infants and 15–30 percent of adults have antibodies to various dietary proteins, especially milk-derived proteins. The FDA reviewed the study published by Seaman. and generally agreed with the reported conclusions.

FDA believes that the available data confirm that biologically significant amounts of rBGH are not absorbed in humans following the consumption of milk from cows treated with rBGH. Oral toxicity studies of longer duration are not necessary because rBGH at dietary levels found in the milk of rBGH-treated cows is not significantly biologically available.

Thyroid Cysts and Prostate Infiltration

In addition to the antibody results, concern has been raised that the 90-day rat study suggested that rBGH caused the rats to develop thyroid cysts and an infiltration of cells into the prostate. It is argued that such results, if true, would be evidence of absorption of rBGH and possible harmful effects.

An examination of the individual animal reports for gross and histopathological findings revealed thyroid cysts in all treatment groups, including the positive and negative controls. Neither frequency nor severity of these cysts appeared to be related to rBGH administration by either the oral or subcutaneous routes, at any dose, in either gender. Thyroid cysts are enlarged thyroid follicles and are not related to cancer formation.

A similar examination also was made of the prostate observations. The mononuclear cell infiltration observed is an indication of mild inflammation, and again, is not related to cancer formation. The prostate and accessory sex glands are frequent sites of inflammatory changes in male rats. These changes are common in older rats, but they also occur in young adult rats. Although there appears to be a dose-related increase in the number of rats showing mononuclear cell infiltration following oral administration, there was no difference between the negative and positive control groups. If the prostatic changes were induced by rBGH, it would be expected that the frequency and severity of changes would be significantly greater in the positive versus the negative control group. Therefore, as with the thyroid cysts, these observations do not appear to be related to the treatment of the rats with rBGH. Neither the thyroid nor prostate changes provide any evidence of an observable effect of rBGH in the rat and do not provide evidence of absorption.

IGF-I

The Canadian report indicates that milk from rBGH-treated cows contains significantly elevated levels of insulin-like growth factor I (IGF-I) in milk, and presents human health safety concerns. IGF-I is a protein normally found in all humans and is not intrinsically harmful. IGF-I is necessary for normal growth, development, and health maintenance. Circulating plasma levels of the hormone increase from birth to late puberty and subsequently decline in adults to approximately 100 ng (10-9 grams)/ml (range = 42 – 308 ng/ml for men and women >23 yrs). IGF-1 is structurally similar to insulin and, like insulin is not biologically effective following oral administration.

The safety of IGF-I in milk was thoroughly considered by the FDA in its review of the Posilac application. Some early studies suggested that treatment of dairy cows with rBGH produced a slight, but statistically significant, increase in the average milk IGF-I concentration. The FDA determined that this modest increase in milk IGF-I concentration was not a human food safety concern because it was less than the natural variation in milk IGF-I levels observed during lactation and was less than the fluctuation observed in milk from treated and control cows prior to rBGH administration.

Since making that analysis, however, the FDA has received and reviewed several more comprehensive studies designed to ascertain the effect of rBGH treatment on milk IGF-I levels. These studies have demonstrated that the levels of IGF-I found in milk from treated cows are within the range of those normally found in milk from untreated cows. In 1993, the Joint FAO/WHO Expert Committee on Food Additives (JECFA) concluded, "the most definitive and comprehensive studies demonstrate that IGF-I concentrations (in milk) are not altered after rBGH treatment." The 1998 JECFA Committee report summarized a study showing no significant difference in commercially available milk labeled as coming from non-rBGH treated cows and milk from cows presumed to be treated with rBGH but not labeled as to treatment.

A recent study has been published on the association between prostate cancer and IGF-I. This study showed a positive correlation between the level of IGF-I in plasma and the increased risk of prostate cancer. Although the mechanism responsible for induction of cancer has not been characterized fully, it is clear that IGF-I is not the causative agent.

FDA has examined the literature and finds no definitive evidence of any direct link between IGF-I and breast cancer. Some authors have hypothesized a link, whereas others have expressed that while IGF-I is one of several growth factors and hormones that can contribute to an increase in cell numbers of many cell types invitro, no one factor is responsible for changing normal cells into cancerous cells. Furthermore, the FDA has been advised that there is no substantive evidence that IGF-I causes normal breast cells to become cancerous.

In evaluating the potential for human health risk from a natural component of the body, one can examine the effect of an increased exposure to IGF-I by employing several assumptions (i.e., IGF-I levels in milk from rBGH-treated cows are increased from 4 ng/ml to 6 ng/ml, all of the IGF-I in milk is absorbed into the body, and absorbed

IGF-I is confined to the vascular compartment). Assuming 5000 ml blood plasma volume in a 60 kg person and assuming this person consumes 1.5 liters of milk containing 9000 ng IGF-I from rBGH-treated cows (as opposed to 6000 ng IGF-I in milk from untreated cows), the maximum increase in blood IGF-I would be less than 2 ng/ml of which only one-third could be attributed to the use of rBGH. This minute increase would dilute into the endogenous pool of circulating IGF-I. IGF-I entering the circulation is rapidly bound to serum binding proteins which attenuate the biological activity.

It bears repeating that the assumptions that milk levels of IGF-I are increased following treatment with rBGH and that biologically active IGF-I is absorbed into the body are not supported by the main body of science. Careful analysis of the published literature fails to provide compelling evidence that milk from rBGH-treated cows contains increased levels of IGF-1 compared to milk from untreated cows. Despite recent studies that demonstrate that milk proteins protect IGF-I from digestion, the vast majority of the published work indicates that very little IGF-I is absorbed following ingestion. The most recent 1998 review by the JECFA concluded, "the concentration of IGF-I in milk from rBGH-treated cows is orders of magnitude lower than the physiological amounts produced in the gastrointestinal tract and other parts of the body. Thus, the concentration of IGF-I would not increase either locally in the gastrointestinal tract or systemically, and the potential for IGF-I to promote tumor growth would not increase when milk from rBGH-treated cows was consumed; there is thus no appreciable risk for consumers."

Effect of rbGH on Infants and Children

Strong concerns over the potential risk to infants and children of milk containing rBGH were expressed by Vermont Public Interest Group and Rural Vermont but no specific issues were raised to substantiate this concern. The FDA considers the impact on high-risk populations in assessing the safety of new animal drugs. For rBGH in particular, issues related to levels of IGF-I in infant formula were carefully examined by the FDA. Other concerns, including the hypothetical development of insulin-dependent diabetes mellitus following the consumption of milk from rBGH-treated cows, have been reviewed by the FDA as well as other national and international scientists. To date, all of these reviews have concluded that consumption by infants and children of milk and edible products from rBGH-treated cows is safe.

Mastitis

A General Accounting Office (GAO) report found that the FDA's review of rBGH had met all established guidelines and that bovine growth hormone did not appear to represent a direct human health risk. However, because rBGH-treated cows tended to have a small but significantly greater incidence of mastitis, GAO recommended that the degree to which antibiotics must be used to treat mastitis should be evaluated in rBGH-treated cows with respect to human food safety. In response to GAO's recommendation, the FDA's Center for Veterinary Medicine convened its Veterinary Medicine Advisory Committee and other expert consultants for an open public hearing on March 31, 1993. The Committee concluded that, while rBGH treatment might cause a statistically significant increase in mastitis, the human health risk posed by the possible increased use of antibiotics to treat the mastitis was insignificant. Again, the recent Joint FAO/WHO Expert Committee on Food Additives (JECFA) report addressed the issue of antibiotic use associated with rBGH use. The Committee concluded, "The use of rBGH would not result in a higher risk to human health due to the use of antibiotics to treat mastitis and that the increased potential for drug residues in milk could be managed by practices currently in use within the dairy industry and by following directions for use."

External Reviews Have Confirmed Validity of the FDA Review

The FDA's review of rBGH has been scrutinized by both the Department of Health and Human Services' Office of Inspector General (OIG) and by GAO, as well as by JECFA. OIG announced that an audit of issues related to the FDA's review of rBGH found no evidence to question the FDA's process for determining the human food safety of rBGH. The OIG found that sufficient research had been conducted to substantiate the safety of the milk and meat of rBGH-treated cows for human consumption. In addition, the OIG found no evidence that indicated that the FDA or Monsanto engaged in manipulation or suppression of animal health test data. As noted above, GAO report found that the FDA's review of rBGH had met all established guidelines and concluded that bovine growth hormone did not pose a risk for human consumption. In its reviews, JECFA also came to the conclusion that rBGH can be used without any appreciable risk to the health of consumers.

Chapter 35

Food Additives

For centuries, ingredients have served useful functions in a variety of foods. Our ancestors used salt to preserve meats and fish, added herbs and spices to improve the flavor of foods, preserved fruit with sugar, and pickled cucumbers in a vinegar solution. Today, consumers demand and enjoy a food supply that is flavorful, nutritious, safe, convenient, colorful, and affordable. Food additives and advances in technology help make that possible.

There are thousands of ingredients used to make foods. The U.S. Food and Drug Administration (FDA) maintains a list of over 3000 ingredients in its database "Everything added to food in the United States," many of which we use at home every day (e.g., sugar, baking soda, salt, vanilla, yeast, spices, and colors).

Still, some consumers have concerns about additives because they may see the long, unfamiliar names and think of them as complex chemical compounds. In fact, every food we eat whether a just picked strawberry or a homemade cookie is made up of chemical compounds that determine flavor, color, texture and nutrient value. All food additives are carefully regulated by federal authorities and various international organizations to ensure that foods are safe to eat and are accurately labeled.

This chapter includes text excerpted from "Food—Overview of Food Ingredients, Additives and Colors," U.S. Food and Drug Administration (FDA), February 7, 2018.

This chapter provides helpful background information about food and color additives: what they are, why they are used in foods, and how they are regulated for safe use.

Why Are Food and Color Ingredients Added to Food?

Additives perform a variety of useful functions in foods that consumers often take for granted. Some additives could be eliminated if we were willing to grow our own food, harvest and grind it, spend many hours cooking and canning, or accept increased risks of food spoilage. But most consumers rely on the many technological, aesthetic, and convenient benefits that additives provide.

Following are some reasons why ingredients are added to foods:

- **To maintain or improve safety and freshness.** Preservatives slow product spoilage caused by mold, air, bacteria, fungi, or yeast. In addition to maintaining the quality of the food, they help control contamination that can cause foodborne illness, including life-threatening botulism. One group of preservatives—antioxidants—prevents fats and oils and the foods containing them from becoming rancid or developing an off-flavor. They also prevent cut fresh fruits such as apples from turning brown when exposed to air.

- **To Improve or maintain nutritional value.** Vitamins and minerals (and fiber) are added to many foods to make up for those lacking in a person's diet or lost in processing, or to enhance the nutritional quality of a food. Such fortification and enrichment has helped reduce malnutrition in the United States and worldwide. All products containing added nutrients must be appropriately labeled.

- **Improve taste, texture, and appearance.** Spices, natural and artificial flavors, and sweeteners are added to enhance the taste of food. Food colors maintain or improve appearance. Emulsifiers, stabilizers, and thickeners give foods the texture and consistency consumers expect. Leavening agents allow baked goods to rise during baking. Some additives help control the acidity and alkalinity of foods, while other ingredients help maintain the taste and appeal of foods with reduced fat content.

What Is a Food Additive?

In its broadest sense, a food additive is any substance added to food. Legally, the term refers to "any substance the intended use of which results or may reasonably be expected to result—directly or indirectly—in its becoming a component or otherwise affecting the characteristics of any food." This definition includes any substance used in the production, processing, treatment, packaging, transportation or storage of food. The purpose of the legal definition, however, is to impose a premarket approval requirement. Therefore, this definition excludes ingredients whose use is generally recognized as safe (where government approval is not needed), those ingredients approved for use by the FDA or the U.S. Department of Agriculture (USDA) prior to the food additives provisions of law, and color additives and pesticides where other legal premarket approval requirements apply.

Direct food additives are those that are added to a food for a specific purpose in that food. For example, xanthan gum—used in salad dressings, chocolate milk, bakery fillings, puddings, and other foods to add texture—is a direct additive. Most direct additives are identified on the ingredient label of foods.

Indirect food additives are those that become part of the food in trace amounts due to its packaging, storage or another handling. For instance, minute amounts of packaging substances may find their way into foods during storage. Food packaging manufacturers must prove to the FDA that all materials coming in contact with food are safe before they are permitted for use in such a manner.

What Is a Color Additive?

A color additive is any dye, pigment or substance which when added or applied to a food, drug or cosmetic, or to the human body, is capable (alone or through reactions with other substances) of imparting color. The FDA is responsible for regulating all color additives to ensure that foods containing color additives are safe to eat, contain only approved ingredients and are accurately labeled.

Color additives are used in foods for many reasons:

- to offset color loss due to exposure to light, air, temperature extremes, moisture, and storage conditions

- to correct natural variations in color

- to enhance colors that occur naturally

- to provide color to colorless and "fun" foods

Without color additives, colas wouldn't be brown, margarine wouldn't be yellow and mint ice cream wouldn't be green. Color additives are now recognized as an important part of practically all processed foods we eat.

The FDA's permitted colors are classified as subject to certification or exempt from certification, both of which are subject to rigorous safety standards prior to their approval and listing for use in foods.

- Certified colors are synthetically produced (or human-made) and used widely because they impart an intense, uniform color, are less expensive and blend more easily to create a variety of hues. There are nine certified color additives approved for use in the United States. Certified food colors generally do not add undesirable flavors to foods.

- Colors that are exempt from certification include pigments derived from natural sources such as vegetables, minerals or animals. Nature-derived color additives are typically more expensive than certified colors and may add unintended flavors to foods. Examples of exempt colors include annatto extract (yellow), dehydrated beets (bluish-red to brown), caramel (yellow to tan), beta-carotene (yellow to orange) and grape skin extract (red, green).

How Are Additives Approved for Use in Foods?

Food and color additives are more strictly studied, regulated and monitored than at any other time in history. The FDA has the primary legal responsibility for determining their safe use. To market, a new food or color additive (or before using an additive already approved for one use in another manner not yet approved), a manufacturer or other sponsor must first petition the FDA for its approval. These petitions must provide evidence that the substance is safe for the ways in which it will be used.

When evaluating the safety of a substance and whether it should be approved, the FDA considers:

- the composition and properties of the substance

- the amount that would typically be consumed

- immediate and long-term health effects

- various safety factors

The evaluation determines an appropriate level of use that includes a built-in safety margin a factor that allows for uncertainty about the levels of consumption that are expected to be harmless. In other words, the levels of use that gain approval are much lower than what would be expected to have any adverse effect.

Because of inherent limitations of science, the FDA can never be absolutely certain of the absence of any risk from the use of any substance. Therefore, the FDA must determine based on the best science available if there is a reasonable certainty of no harm to consumers when an additive is used as proposed.

If an additive is approved, the FDA issues regulations that may include the types of foods in which it can be used, the maximum amounts to be used, and how it should be identified on food labels. In 1999, procedures changed so that the FDA now consults with USDA during the review process for ingredients that are proposed for use in meat and poultry products. Federal officials then monitor the extent of Americans' consumption of the new additive and results of any new research on its safety to ensure its use continues to be within safe limits.

If new evidence suggests that a product already in use may be unsafe, or if consumption levels have changed enough to require another look, federal authorities may prohibit its use or conduct further studies to determine if the use can still be considered safe.

Regulations known as Good Manufacturing Practices (GMP) limit the amount of food ingredients used in foods to the amount necessary to achieve the desired effect.

Summing Up

Food ingredients have been used for many years to preserve, flavor, blend, thicken and color foods, and have played an important role in reducing serious nutritional deficiencies among consumers. These ingredients also help ensure the availability of flavorful, nutritious, safe, convenient, colorful, and affordable foods that meet consumer expectations year round.

Food and color additives are strictly studied, regulated, and monitored. Federal regulations require evidence that each substance is safe at its intended level of use before it may be added to foods. Furthermore, all additives are subject to ongoing safety review as scientific understanding and methods of testing continue to improve. Consumers should feel safe about the foods they eat.

Frequently Asked Questions on Food and Color Additives

How Are Ingredients Listed on a Product Label?

Food manufacturers are required to list all ingredients in the food on the label. On a product label, the ingredients are listed in order of predominance, with the ingredients used in the greatest amount first, followed in descending order by those in smaller amounts. The label must list the names of any the FDA-certified color additives (e.g., FD and C Blue No. 1 or the abbreviated name, Blue 1). But some ingredients can be listed collectively as "flavors," "spices," "artificial flavoring," or in the case of color additives exempt from certification, "artificial colors," without naming each one. Declaration of an allergenic ingredient in a collective or single color, flavor, or spice could be accomplished by simply naming the allergenic ingredient in the ingredient list.

What Are Dyes and Lakes in Color Additives?

Certified color additives are categorized as either dyes or lakes. Dyes dissolve in water and are manufactured as powders, granules, liquids or other special purpose forms. They can be used in beverages, dry mixes, baked goods, confections, dairy products, pet foods, and a variety of other products.

Lakes are the water-insoluble form of the dye. Lakes are more stable than dyes and are ideal for coloring products containing fats and oils or items lacking sufficient moisture to dissolve dyes. Typical uses include coated tablets, cake, and donut mixes, hard candies, and chewing gums.

Do Additives Cause Childhood Hyperactivity?

Although this hypothesis was popularized in the 1970's, results from studies on this issue either have been inconclusive, inconsistent, or difficult to interpret due to inadequacies in study design. A consensus development panel of the National Institutes of Health (NIH) concluded that for some children with attention deficit hyperactivity disorder (ADHD) and confirmed food allergy, a dietary modification has produced some improvement in behavior. Although the panel said that elimination diets should not be used universally to treat childhood hyperactivity, since there is no scientific evidence to predict which children may benefit, the panel recognized that initiation of a trial of dietary treatment or continuation of a diet in patients whose families and physicians perceive benefits may be warranted. However, a 1997 review published in the Journal of the American Academy of Child and Adolescent Psychiatry noted there is minimal evidence of efficacy and extreme difficulty inducing children and adolescents to comply with restricted diets. Thus, dietary treatment should not be recommended, except possibly with a small number of preschool children who may be sensitive to tartrazine, known commonly as FD&C Yellow No.5. In 2007, synthetic certified color additives again came under scrutiny following the publication of a study commissioned by the U.K. Food Standards Agency (FSA) to investigate whether certain color additives cause hyperactivity in children. Both the FDA and European Food Safety Authority (EFSA) independently reviewed the results from this study and each has concluded that the study does not substantiate a link between the color additives that were tested and behavioral effects.

What Is the Difference between Natural and Artificial Ingredients? Is a Naturally Produced Ingredient Safer than an Artificially Manufactured Ingredient?

Natural ingredients are derived from natural sources (e.g., soybeans and corn provide lecithin to maintain product consistency; beets provide beet powder used as food coloring). Other ingredients are not found in nature and, therefore, must be synthetically produced as artificial ingredients. Also, some ingredients found in nature can be manufactured artificially and produced more economically, with greater purity and more consistent quality, than their natural counterparts. For example, vitamin C or ascorbic acid may be derived from an orange or produced in a laboratory. Food ingredients are subject to the same strict safety standards regardless of whether they are naturally or artificially derived.

Are Certain People Sensitive to FD&C Yellow No. 5 in Foods?

FD&C Yellow No. 5, is used to color beverages, dessert powders, candy, ice cream, custards, and other foods. The FDA's Committee on Hypersensitivity to Food Constituents concluded in 1986 that FD&C Yellow No. 5 might cause hives in fewer than one out of 10,000 people. It also concluded that there was no evidence the color additive in food provokes asthma attacks. The law now requires Yellow No. 5 to be identified on the ingredient line. This allows the few who may be sensitive to the color to avoid it.

Do Low-Calorie Sweeteners Cause Adverse Reactions?

No. Food safety experts generally agree there is no convincing evidence of a cause and effect relationship between these sweeteners and negative health effects in humans. The FDA has monitored consumer complaints of possible adverse reactions for more than 15 years.

For example, in carefully controlled clinical studies, aspartame has not been shown to cause adverse or allergic reactions. However, persons with a rare hereditary disease known as phenylketonuria (PKU) must control their intake of phenylalanine from all sources, including aspartame. Although aspartame contains only a small amount of phenylalanine, labels of aspartame-containing foods and beverages must include a statement advising phenylketonurics of the presence of phenylalanine.

Individuals who have concerns about possible adverse effects from food additives or other substances should contact their physicians.

How Do They Add Vitamins and Minerals to Fortified Cereals?

Adding nutrients to a cereal can cause taste and color changes in the product. This is especially true with added minerals. Since no one wants cereal that tastes like a vitamin supplement, a variety of techniques are employed in the fortification process. In general, those nutrients that are heat stable (such as vitamins A and E and various minerals) are incorporated into the cereal itself (they're baked right in). Nutrients that are not stable to heat (such as B-vitamins) are applied directly to the cereal after all heating steps are completed. Each cereal is unique—some can handle more nutrients than others can. This is one reason why fortification levels are different across all cereals.

What Is the Role of Modern Technology in Producing Food Additives?

Many new techniques are being researched that will allow the production of additives in ways not previously possible. One approach is the use of biotechnology, which can use simple organisms to produce food additives. These additives are the same as food components found in nature.

Table 35.1. Types of Food Ingredients

Types of Ingredients	What They Do	Examples of Uses	Names Found on Product Labels
Preservatives	Prevent food spoilage from bacteria, molds, fungi, or yeast (antimicrobials); slow or prevent changes in color, flavor, or texture and delay rancidity (antioxidants); maintain freshness	Fruit sauces and jellies, beverages, baked goods, cured meats, oils and margarines, cereals, dressings, snack foods, fruits and vegetables	Ascorbic acid, citric acid, sodium benzoate, calcium propionate, sodium erythorbate, sodium nitrite, calcium sorbate, potassium sorbate, BHA, BHT, EDTA, tocopherols (Vitamin E)
Sweeteners	Add sweetness with or without the extra calories	Beverages, baked goods, confections, table-top sugar, substitutes, many processed foods	Sucrose (sugar), glucose, fructose, sorbitol, mannitol, corn syrup, high fructose corn syrup, saccharin, aspartame, sucralose, acesulfame potassium (acesulfame-K), neotame
Color Additives	Offset color loss due to exposure to light, air, temperature extremes, moisture and storage conditions; correct natural variations in color; enhance colors that occur naturally; provide color to colorless and "fun" foods	Many processed foods, (candies, snack foods margarine, cheese, soft drinks, jams/jellies, gelatins, pudding and pie fillings)	FD&C Blue Nos. 1 and 2, FD&C Green No. 3, FD&C Red Nos. 3 and 40, FD&C Yellow Nos. 5 and 6, Orange B, Citrus Red No. 2, annatto extract, beta-carotene, grape skin extract, cochineal extract or carmine, paprika oleoresin, caramel color, fruit and vegetable juices, saffron (Note: Exempt color additives are not required to be declared by name on labels but may be declared simply as colorings or color added)
Flavors and Spices	Add specific flavors (natural and synthetic)	Pudding and pie fillings, gelatin dessert mixes, cake mixes, salad dressings, candies, soft drinks, ice cream, BBQ sauce	Natural flavoring, artificial flavor, and spices

Table 35.1. Continued

Types of Ingredients	What They Do	Examples of Uses	Names Found on Product Labels
Flavor Enhancers	Enhance flavors already present in foods (without providing their own separate flavor)	Many processed foods, (candies, snack foods margarine, cheese, soft drinks, jams/jellies, gelatins, pudding and pie fillings)	Monosodium glutamate (MSG), hydrolyzed soy protein, autolyzed yeast extract, disodium guanylate or inosinate
Fat Replacers (and components of formulations used to replace fats)	Provide expected texture and a creamy "mouth-feel" in reduced-fat foods	Baked goods, dressings, frozen desserts, confections, cake and dessert mixes, dairy products	Olestra, cellulose gel, carrageenan, polydextrose, modified food starch, microparticulated egg white protein, guar gum, xanthan gum, whey protein concentrate
Nutrients	Replace vitamins and minerals lost in processing (enrichment), add nutrients that may be lacking in the diet (fortification)	Flour, breads, cereals, rice, macaroni, margarine, salt, milk, fruit beverages, energy bars, instant breakfast drinks	Thiamine hydrochloride, riboflavin (Vitamin B2), niacin, niacinamide, folate or folic acid, beta-carotene, potassium iodide, iron or ferrous sulfate, alpha-tocopherols, ascorbic acid, Vitamin D, amino acids (L-tryptophan, L-lysine, L-leucine, L-methionine)
Emulsifiers	Allow smooth mixing of ingredients, prevent separation Keep emulsified products stable, reduce stickiness, control crystallization, keep ingredients dispersed, and to help products dissolve more easily	Salad dressings, peanut butter, chocolate, margarine, frozen desserts	Soy lecithin, mono- and diglycerides, egg yolks, polysorbates, sorbitan monostearate

Table 35.1. Continued

Types of Ingredients	What They Do	Examples of Uses	Names Found on Product Labels
Stabilizers and Thickeners, Binders, Texturizers	Produce uniform texture, improve "mouth-feel"	Frozen desserts, dairy products, cakes, pudding and gelatin mixes, dressings, jams and jellies, sauces	Gelatin, pectin, guar gum, carrageenan, xanthan gum, whey
pH Control Agents and acidulants	Control acidity and alkalinity, prevent spoilage	Beverages, frozen desserts, chocolate, low acid canned foods, baking powder	Lactic acid, citric acid, ammonium hydroxide, sodium carbonate
Leavening Agents	Promote rising of baked goods	Bread and other baked goods	Baking soda, monocalcium phosphate, calcium carbonate
Anticaking agents	Keep powdered foods free-flowing, prevent moisture absorption	Salt, baking powder, confectioner's sugar	Calcium silicate, iron ammonium citrate, silicon dioxide
Humectants	Retain moisture	Shredded coconut, marshmallows, soft candies, confections	Glycerin, sorbitol
Yeast Nutrients	Promote growth of yeast	Bread and other baked goods	Calcium sulfate, ammonium phosphate
Dough Strengtheners and Conditioners	Produce more stable dough	Bread and other baked goods	Ammonium sulfate, azodicarbonamide, L-cysteine
Firming Agents	Maintain crispness and firmness	Processed fruits and vegetable	Calcium chloride, calcium lactate
Enzyme Preparations	Modify proteins, polysaccharides and fats	Cheese, dairy products, meat	Enzymes, lactase, papain, rennet, chymosin
Gases	Serve as propellant, aerate, or create carbonation	Oil cooking spray, whipped cream, carbonated beverages	Carbon dioxide, nitrous oxide

457

Chapter 36

Foodborne Illnesses

Chapter Contents

Section 36.1

Introduction to Foodborne Illnesses

This section includes text excerpted from "Foodborne
Illnesses," National Institute of Diabetes and Digestive and
Kidney Diseases (NIDDK), June 2014. Reviewed April 2018.

Foodborne illnesses are infections or irritations of the gastrointestinal (GI) tract caused by food or beverages that contain harmful
bacteria, parasites, viruses, or chemicals. The GI tract is a series of
hollow organs joined in a long, twisting tube from the mouth to the
anus. Common symptoms of foodborne illnesses include vomiting,
diarrhea, abdominal pain, fever, and chills.

Most foodborne illnesses are acute, meaning they happen suddenly
and last a short time, and most people recover on their own without
treatment. Rarely, foodborne illnesses may lead to more serious complications. Each year, an estimated 48 million people in the United
States experience a foodborne illness. Foodborne illnesses cause about
3,000 deaths in the United States annually.

What Causes Foodborne Illnesses?

The majority of foodborne illnesses are caused by harmful bacteria and viruses. Some parasites and chemicals also cause foodborne
illnesses.

Bacteria

Bacteria are tiny organisms that can cause infections of the GI
tract. Not all bacteria are harmful to humans.

Some harmful bacteria may already be present in foods when
they are purchased. Raw foods including meat, poultry, fish and
shellfish, eggs, unpasteurized milk and dairy products, and fresh
produce often contain bacteria that cause foodborne illnesses. Bacteria can contaminate food—making it harmful to eat—at any time
during growth, harvesting or slaughter, processing, storage, and
shipping.

Foods may also be contaminated with bacteria during food preparation in a restaurant or home kitchen. If food preparers do not thoroughly wash their hands, kitchen utensils, cutting boards, and other kitchen surfaces that come into contact with raw foods, cross-contamination—the spread of bacteria from contaminated food to uncontaminated food—may occur.

If hot food is not kept hot enough or cold food is not kept cold enough, bacteria may multiply. Bacteria multiply quickly when the temperature of food is between 40–140 degrees. Cold food should be kept below 40 degrees and hot food should be kept above 140 degrees. Bacteria multiply more slowly when food is refrigerated, and freezing food can further slow or even stop the spread of bacteria. However, bacteria in refrigerated or frozen foods become active again when food is brought to room temperature. Thoroughly cooking food kills bacteria.

Many types of bacteria cause foodborne illnesses. Examples include:

- *Salmonella*, a bacterium found in many foods, including raw and undercooked meat, poultry, dairy products, and seafood. Salmonella may also be present on egg shells and inside eggs

- *Campylobacter jejuni (C. jejuni)*, found in raw or undercooked chicken and unpasteurized milk

- *Shigella*, a bacterium spread from person to person. These bacteria are present in the stools of people who are infected. If people who are infected do not wash their hands thoroughly after using the bathroom, they can contaminate food that they handle or prepare. Water contaminated with infected stools can also contaminate produce in the field.

- *Escherichia coli (E. coli)*, which includes several different strains, only a few of which cause illness in humans. *E. coli O157:H7* is the strain that causes the most severe illness. Common sources of *E. coli* include raw or undercooked hamburger, unpasteurized fruit juices and milk, and fresh produce.

- *Listeria monocytogenes (L. monocytogenes)*, which has been found in raw and undercooked meats, unpasteurized milk, soft cheeses, and ready-to-eat deli meats and hot dogs

- *Vibrio*, a bacterium that may contaminate fish or shellfish

- *Clostridium botulinum (C. botulinum)*, a bacterium that may contaminate improperly canned foods and smoked and salted fish

Viruses

Viruses are tiny capsules, much smaller than bacteria, that contain genetic material. Viruses cause infections that can lead to sickness. People can pass viruses to each other. Viruses are present in the stool or vomit of people who are infected. People who are infected with a virus may contaminate food and drinks, especially if they do not wash their hands thoroughly after using the bathroom.

Common sources of foodborne viruses include:

- food prepared by a person infected with a virus
- shellfish from contaminated water
- produce irrigated with contaminated water

Common foodborne viruses include:

- norovirus, which causes inflammation of the stomach and intestines
- hepatitis A, which causes inflammation of the liver

Parasites

Parasites are tiny organisms that live inside another organism. In developed countries such as the United States, parasitic infections are relatively rare.

Cryptosporidium parvum and *Giardia intestinalis* are parasites that are spread through water contaminated with the stools of people or animals who are infected. Foods that come into contact with contaminated water during growth or preparation can become contaminated with these parasites. Food preparers who are infected with these parasites can also contaminate foods if they do not thoroughly wash their hands after using the bathroom and before handling food.

Trichinella spiralis is a type of roundworm parasite. People may be infected with this parasite by consuming raw or undercooked pork or wild game.

Chemicals

Harmful chemicals that cause illness may contaminate foods such as:

- fish or shellfish, which may feed on algae that produce toxins, leading to high concentrations of toxins in their bodies. Some types of fish, including tuna and mahi-mahi, may be contaminated with bacteria that produce toxins if the fish are not properly refrigerated before they are cooked or served.

- certain types of wild mushrooms
- unwashed fruits and vegetables that contain high concentrations of pesticides

Who Gets Foodborne Illnesses?

Anyone can get a foodborne illness. However, some people are more likely to develop foodborne illnesses than others, including:

- infants and children
- pregnant women and their fetuses
- older adults
- people with weak immune systems

These groups also have a greater risk of developing severe symptoms or complications of foodborne illnesses.

What Are the Symptoms of Foodborne Illnesses?

Symptoms of foodborne illnesses depend on the cause. Common symptoms of many foodborne illnesses include:

- vomiting
- diarrhea or bloody diarrhea
- abdominal pain
- fever
- chills

Symptoms can range from mild to serious and can last from a few hours to several days. *C. botulinum* and some chemicals affect the nervous system, causing symptoms such as:

- headache
- tingling or numbness of the skin
- blurred vision
- weakness
- dizziness
- paralysis

463

What Are the Complications of Foodborne Illnesses?

Foodborne illnesses may lead to dehydration, hemolytic uremic syndrome (HUS), and other complications. Acute foodborne illnesses may also lead to chronic—or long-lasting—health problems.

Dehydration

When someone does not drink enough fluids to replace those that are lost through vomiting and diarrhea, dehydration can result. When dehydrated, the body lacks enough fluid and electrolytes—minerals in salts, including sodium, potassium, and chloride—to function properly. Infants, children, older adults, and people with weak immune systems have the greatest risk of becoming dehydrated.

Signs of dehydration are:

- excessive thirst
- infrequent urination
- dark-colored urine
- lethargy, dizziness, or faintness

Signs of dehydration in infants and young children are:

- dry mouth and tongue
- lack of tears when crying
- no wet diapers for 3 hours or more
- high fever
- unusually cranky or drowsy behavior
- sunken eyes, cheeks, or soft spot in the skull

Also, when people are dehydrated, their skin does not flatten back to normal right away after being gently pinched and released.

Severe dehydration may require intravenous (IV) fluids and hospitalization. Untreated severe dehydration can cause serious health problems such as organ damage, shock, or coma—a sleeplike state in which a person is not conscious.

Hemolytic Uremic Syndrome (HUS)

HUS is a rare disease that mostly affects children younger than 10 years of age. HUS develops when *E. coli* bacteria lodged in the digestive tract make toxins that enter the bloodstream. The toxins start to destroy red blood cells, which help the blood to clot, and the lining of the blood vessels.

In the United States, *E. coli O157:H7* infection is the most common cause of HUS, but infection with other strains of *E. coli*, other bacteria, and viruses may also cause HUS. A study found that about 6 percent of people with *E. coli O157:H7* infections developed HUS. Children younger than age 5 have the highest risk, but females and people age 60 and older also have increased risk.

Symptoms of *E. coli O157:H7* infection include diarrhea, which may be bloody, and abdominal pain, often accompanied by nausea, vomiting, and fever. Up to a week after *E. coli* symptoms appear, symptoms of HUS may develop, including irritability, paleness, and decreased urination. HUS may lead to acute renal failure, which is a sudden and temporary loss of kidney function. HUS may also affect other organs and the central nervous system. Most people who develop HUS recover with treatment. Research shows that in the United States between 2000–2006, fewer than 5 percent of people who developed HUS died of the disorder. Older adults had the highest mortality rate—about one-third of people age 60 and older who developed HUS died.

Studies have shown that some children who recover from HUS develop chronic complications, including kidney problems, high blood pressure, and diabetes.

Other Complications

Some foodborne illnesses lead to other serious complications. For example, *C. botulinum* and certain chemicals in fish and seafood can paralyze the muscles that control breathing. L. monocytogenes can cause spontaneous abortion or stillbirth in pregnant women.

Research suggests that acute foodborne illnesses may lead to chronic disorders, including:

- **Reactive arthritis** is a type of joint inflammation that usually affects the knees, ankles, or feet. Some people develop this disorder following foodborne illnesses caused by certain bacteria, including *C. jejuni* and *Salmonella*. Reactive arthritis usually lasts fewer than 6 months, but this condition may recur or become chronic arthritis.

- **Irritable bowel syndrome (IBS)** is a disorder of unknown cause that is associated with abdominal pain, bloating, and diarrhea or constipation or both. Foodborne illnesses caused by bacteria increase the risk of developing IBS.

- **Guillain-Barré syndrome (GBS)** is a disorder characterized by muscle weakness or paralysis that begins in the lower body and progresses to the upper body. This syndrome may occur after foodborne illnesses caused by bacteria, most commonly *C. jejuni*. Most people recover in 12 months.

A study found that adults who had recovered from *E. coli O157:H7* infections had increased risks of high blood pressure, kidney problems, and cardiovascular disease.

When Should People with Foodborne Illnesses See a Healthcare Provider?

People with any of the following symptoms should see a healthcare provider immediately:

- signs of dehydration
- prolonged vomiting that prevents keeping liquids down
- diarrhea for more than 2 days in adults or for more than 24 hours in children
- severe pain in the abdomen or rectum
- a fever higher than 101 degrees
- stools containing blood or pus
- stools that are black and tarry
- nervous system symptoms
- signs of HUS

If a child has a foodborne illness, parents or guardians should not hesitate to call a healthcare provider for advice.

How Are Foodborne Illnesses Diagnosed?

To diagnose foodborne illnesses, healthcare providers ask about symptoms, foods and beverages recently consumed, and medical history. Healthcare providers will also perform a physical examination to look for signs of illness.

Diagnostic tests for foodborne illnesses may include a stool culture, in which a sample of stool is analyzed in a laboratory to check for signs of infections or diseases. A sample of vomit or a sample of the suspected food, if available, may also be tested. A healthcare provider may perform additional medical tests to rule out diseases and disorders that cause symptoms similar to the symptoms of foodborne illnesses.

If symptoms of foodborne illnesses are mild and last only a short time, diagnostic tests are usually not necessary.

How Are Foodborne Illnesses Treated?

The only treatment needed for most foodborne illnesses is replacing lost fluids and electrolytes to prevent dehydration.

Over-the-counter (OTC) medications such as loperamide (Imodium) and bismuth subsalicylate (Pepto-Bismol and Kaopectate) may help stop diarrhea in adults. However, people with bloody diarrhea—a sign of bacterial or parasitic infection—should not use these medications. If diarrhea is caused by bacteria or parasites, OTC medications may prolong the problem. Medications to treat diarrhea in adults can be dangerous for infants and children and should only be given with a healthcare provider's guidance.

If the specific cause of the foodborne illness is diagnosed, a health-care provider may prescribe medications, such as antibiotics, to treat the illness. Hospitalization may be required to treat life threatening symptoms and complications, such as paralysis, severe dehydration, and HUS.

Eating, Diet, and Nutrition

The following steps may help relieve the symptoms of foodborne illnesses and prevent dehydration in adults:

- drinking plenty of liquids such as fruit juices, sports drinks, caffeine-free soft drinks, and broths to replace fluids and electrolytes

- sipping small amounts of clear liquids or sucking on ice chips if vomiting is still a problem

- gradually reintroducing food, starting with bland, easy-to-digest foods such as rice, potatoes, toast or bread, cereal, lean meat, applesauce, and bananas

- avoiding fatty foods, sugary foods, dairy products, caffeine, and alcohol until recovery is complete

Infants and children present special concerns. Infants and children are likely to become dehydrated more quickly from diarrhea and vomiting because of their smaller body size. The following steps may help relieve symptoms and prevent dehydration in infants and children:

- giving oral rehydration solutions such as Pedialyte, Naturalyte, Infalyte, and CeraLyte to prevent dehydration

- giving food as soon as the child is hungry

- giving infants breast milk or full strength formula, as usual, along with oral rehydration solutions

Older adults and adults with weak immune systems should also drink oral rehydration solutions to prevent dehydration.

How Are Foodborne Illnesses Prevented?

Foodborne illnesses can be prevented by properly storing, cooking, cleaning, and handling foods.

- Raw and cooked perishable foods—foods that can spoil—should be refrigerated or frozen promptly. If perishable foods stand at room temperature for more than 2 hours, they may not be safe to eat. Refrigerators should be set at 40 degrees or lower and freezers should be set at 0 degrees.

- Foods should be cooked long enough and at a high enough temperature to kill the harmful bacteria that cause illnesses. A meat thermometer should be used to ensure foods are cooked to the appropriate internal temperature:

  - 145 degrees for roasts, steaks, and chops of beef, veal, pork, and lamb, followed by 3 minutes of rest time after the meat is removed from the heat source

  - 160 degrees for ground beef, veal, pork, and lamb

  - 165 degrees for poultry

- Cold foods should be kept cold and hot foods should be kept hot

- Fruits and vegetables should be washed under running water just before eating, cutting, or cooking. A produce brush can be used under running water to clean fruits and vegetables with firm skin.

- Raw meat, poultry, seafood, and their juices should be kept away from other foods

- People should wash their hands for at least 20 seconds with warm, soapy water before and after handling raw meat, poultry, fish, shellfish, produce, or eggs. People should also wash their hands after using the bathroom, changing diapers, or touching animals.

- Utensils and surfaces should be washed with hot, soapy water before and after they are used to prepare food. Diluted bleach—1 teaspoon of bleach to 1 quart of hot water—can also be used to sanitize utensils and surfaces.

Traveler's Diarrhea

People who visit certain foreign countries are at risk for traveler's diarrhea, which is caused by eating food or drinking water contaminated with bacteria, viruses, or parasites. Traveler's diarrhea can be a problem for people traveling to developing countries in Africa, Asia, Latin America, and the Caribbean. Visitors to Canada, most European countries, Japan, Australia, and New Zealand do not face much risk for traveler's diarrhea.

To prevent traveler's diarrhea, people traveling from the United States to developing countries should avoid:

- drinking tap water, using tap water to brush their teeth, or using ice made from tap water

- drinking unpasteurized milk or milk products

- eating raw fruits and vegetables, including lettuce and fruit salads, unless they peel the fruits or vegetables themselves

- eating raw or rare meat and fish

- eating meat or shellfish that is not hot when served

- eating food from street vendors

Travelers can drink bottled water, bottled soft drinks, and hot drinks such as coffee or tea.

People concerned about traveler's diarrhea should talk with a healthcare provider before traveling. The healthcare provider may recommend that travelers bring medication with them in case they develop diarrhea during their trip. Healthcare providers may advise some people—especially people with weakened immune systems—to take antibiotics before and during a trip to help prevent traveler's diarrhea. Early treatment with antibiotics can shorten a bout of traveler's diarrhea.

Section 36.2

Bovine Spongiform Encephalopathy (Mad Cow Disease)

This section includes text excerpted from "Animal and Veterinary—
All about BSE (Mad Cow Disease)," U.S. Food and Drug
Administration (FDA), December 22, 2017.

The word bovine spongiform encephalopathy (BSE) is short but it stands for a disease with a long name, bovine spongiform encephalopathy. "Bovine" means that the disease affects cows, "spongiform" refers to the way the brain from a sick cow looks spongy under a microscope, and "encephalopathy" indicates that it is a disease of the brain. BSE is commonly called "mad cow disease." it is a progressive neurologic disease of cows. Progressive means that it gets worse over time. Neurologic means that it damages a cow's central nervous system (brain and spinal cord).

Causes of Bovine Spongiform Encephalopathy (BSE)

Most scientists think that BSE is caused by a protein called a prion. For reasons that are not completely understood, the normal prion protein changes into an abnormal prion protein that is harmful. The body of a sick cow does not even know the abnormal prion is there. Without knowing it is there, the cow's body cannot fight off the disease.

Signs of BSE in Cows

A common sign of BSE in cows is incoordination. A sick cow has trouble walking and getting up. A sick cow may also act very nervous or violent, which is why BSE is often called "mad cow disease."

It usually takes 4–6 years from the time a cow is infected with the abnormal prion to when it first shows symptoms of BSE. This is called the incubation period. During the incubation period, there is no way to tell that a cow has BSE by looking at it. Once a cow starts to show symptoms, it gets sicker and sicker until it dies, usually within two weeks to six months. There is no treatment for BSE and no vaccine to prevent it.

Currently, there is no reliable way to test for BSE in a live cow. After a cow has died, scientists can tell if it had BSE by looking at its brain under a microscope and seeing the spongy appearance. Scientists can also tell if a cow had BSE by using test kits that can detect the abnormal prion in the brain.

How a Cow Gets BSE

The parts of a cow that are not eaten by people are cooked, dried, and ground into a powder. The powder is then used for a variety of purposes, including as an ingredient in animal feed. A cow gets BSE by eating feed contaminated with parts that came from another cow that was sick with BSE. The contaminated feed contains the abnormal prion, and a cow becomes infected with the abnormal prion when it eats the feed. If a cow gets BSE, it most likely ate the contaminated feed during its first year of life. Remember, if a cow becomes infected with the abnormal prion when it is one-year-old, it usually will not show signs of BSE until it is five-years-old or older.

Can People Get BSE?

People can get a version of BSE called variant Creutzfeldt-Jakob disease (vCJD). As of December 4, 2017, 231 people worldwide are known to have become sick with vCJD according to the University of Edinburgh's National CJD Research and Surveillance Unit. It is thought that they got the disease from eating food made from cows sick with BSE. Most of the people who have become sick with vCJD lived in the United Kingdom at some point in their lives. Only four lived in the United States, and most likely, these four people became infected when they were living or traveling overseas.

Neither vCJD nor BSE is contagious. This means that it is not like catching a cold. A person (or a cow) cannot catch it from being near a sick person or cow. Also, research studies have shown that people cannot get BSE from drinking milk or eating dairy products, even if the milk came from a sick cow.

How the U.S. Food and Drug Administration (FDA) Contributes to Your Food Safety

The U.S. Food and Drug Administration (FDA) is doing many things to keep the food in the United States safe for both people and cows. Since August 1997, the FDA has not allowed most parts from cows and certain other animals to be used to make food that is fed to cows. This protects healthy cows from getting BSE by making sure that the food they eat is not contaminated with the abnormal prion.

In April 2009, the FDA took additional steps to make sure the food in the United States stays safe. Certain high-risk cow parts are not allowed to be used to make any animal feed, including pet food. This prevents all animal feed from being accidentally contaminated with the abnormal prion. High-risk cow parts are those parts of the cow that have the highest chance of being infected with the abnormal prion, such as the brains and spinal cords from cows that are 30 months of age or older.

By keeping the food that is fed to cows safe, the FDA is protecting people by making sure that the food they eat comes from healthy cows.

The FDA also works with the U.S. Department of Agriculture (USDA) to keep cows in the United States healthy and free of BSE. The USDA prevents high-risk cows and cow products from entering the U.S. from other countries. The USDA also makes sure that high-risk cow parts, such as the brains and spinal cords, and cows that are unable to walk or that show other signs of disease are not used to make food for people.

The steps the FDA and USDA have taken to prevent cows in the United States from getting BSE are working very well. Only five cows with BSE have been found in the United States. Four of these cows were born in the United States, and one was born in Canada. The USDA reports that the last cow with BSE in the United States was found in July 2017.

It is worth noting that there are two types of BSE, classical and atypical. Classical is caused by contaminated feed fed to cows. Atypical is rarer and happens spontaneously, usually in cows 8-years-old or older. Of the five U.S. cows found with BSE, four were atypical.

Can Other Animals Get BSE?

Sheep, goats, mink, deer, and elk can get sick with their own versions of BSE. Cats are the only common household pet known to have a version of BSE. It is called feline spongiform encephalopathy, and the same things that are being done to protect people and cows are also protecting cats. No cat in the United States has ever been found to have this disease.

Section 36.3

Campylobacter

This section includes text excerpted from "*Campylobacter* (Campylobacteriosis)—Questions and Answers," Centers for Disease Control and Prevention (CDC), October 2, 2017.

Campylobacter infection, or campylobacteriosis, is an infectious disease caused by *Campylobacter* bacteria. It is one of the most common causes of diarrheal illness in the United States. The Foodborne Diseases Active Surveillance Network (FoodNet) indicates that about 14 cases are diagnosed each year for every 100,000 people. Many more cases go undiagnosed or unreported. The Centers for Disease Control and Prevention (CDC) estimates *Campylobacter* infection affects more than 1.3 million people every year. Most cases are not part of recognized outbreaks, and more cases occur in summer than in winter.

Campylobacter are bacteria that can make people and animals sick. Most human illness is caused by one species, called *Campylobacter* jejuni, but other species also can cause human illness.

Symptoms of Campylobacter *Infection*

People with *Campylobacter* infection usually have diarrhea (often bloody), fever, and abdominal cramps. The diarrhea may be accompanied by nausea and vomiting. These symptoms usually start within two to five days after exposure and last about a week. Some infected people do not have any symptoms. In people with weakened immune systems, such as people with the blood disorders thalassemia and hypogammaglobulinemia, acquired immunodeficiency syndrome (AIDS), or people receiving some kinds of chemotherapy, *Campylobacter* occasionally spreads to the bloodstream and causes a life-threatening infection.

Contamination of Food and Water Campylobacter

Many chickens, cows, and other birds and animals that show no signs of illness carry *Campylobacter*. *Campylobacter* can be carried in the intestines, liver, and giblets of animals and can be transferred to other edible parts of an animal when it's slaughtered. In 2014, National Antimicrobial Resistance Monitoring System (NARMS) testing found *Campylobacter* on 33 percent of raw chicken bought from retailers.

Milk can become contaminated when a cow has a *Campylobacter* infection in her udder or when milk is contaminated with manure. Other foods, such as fruits and vegetables, can be can become contaminated through contact with soil containing feces from cows, birds, or other animals. Animal feces can also contaminate lakes and streams. Pasteurization of milk, washing or scrubbing of fruits and vegetables, and disinfection of drinking water helps prevent illness.

How People Get Infected with Campylobacter *Bacteria*

Most *Campylobacter* infections are associated with eating raw or undercooked poultry or from contamination of other foods by these items. People can get infected when a cutting board that has been used to cut and prepare raw chicken isn't washed before it is used to prepare foods that are served raw or lightly cooked, such as salad or fruit. People also can get infected through contact with the feces of a dog or cat. *Campylobacter* does not usually spread from one person to another.

Outbreaks of *Campylobacter* infections have been associated most often with poultry, raw (unpasteurized) dairy products, untreated water, and produce. *Campylobacter* infection is common in the developing world, and people who travel abroad have a greater chance of becoming infected. About 1 in 5 *Campylobacter* infections reported to the Foodborne Diseases Active Surveillance Network (FoodNet) are associated with international travel.

Even more rarely, people may become infected through contaminated blood during a transfusion.

Diagnosis and Treatment of Campylobacter *Infection*

Campylobacter infection is diagnosed when a laboratory test detects *Campylobacter* bacteria in stool, body tissue, or fluids. The test could be a culture that isolates the bacteria or a rapid diagnostic test that detects genetic material of the bacteria.

Most people with *Campylobacter* infection recover without specific treatment. Patients should drink extra fluids as long as the diarrhea lasts. Antibiotics are needed only for patients who are very ill or at high risk for severe disease, such as people with severely weakened immune systems, such as people with the blood disorders thalassemia and hypogammaglobulinemia, acquired immune deficiency syndrome (AIDS), or people receiving chemotherapy.

Is Campylobacter *Infection Serious?*

Most people with a *Campylobacter* infection recover completely within a week, although they may shed (get rid of) *Campylobacter* bacteria in their stool for several weeks after recovery, which might result in person-to-person transmission. *Campylobacter* infection rarely results in long-term consequences. Some studies have esti-mated that 5–20 percent of people with *Campylobacter* infection develop irritable bowel syndrome for a limited time and 1–5 percent develop arthritis.

About 1 in every 1,000 reported *Campylobacter* illnesses leads to Guillain-Barré syndrome (GBS). GBS happens when a person's immune system is triggered by an earlier infection, such as *Campy-lobacter* infection. GBS can lead to muscle weakness and sometimes paralysis that can last for a few weeks to several years, and often requires intensive medical care. Most people recover fully, but some have permanent nerve damage, and some have died of GBS. As many as 40 percent of GBS cases in the United States may be triggered by *Campylobacter* infection.

Public Health Agencies and Their Role in Controlling Campylobacter *and Preventing Infections*

CDC tracks all reported human *Campylobacter* infections and works to identify the source of infections transmitted by food and other routes. Through the surveillance systems listed below, CDC monitors cases, estimates the total number of people infected each year, targets prevention measures to meet food safety goals, and provides data and analyses that inform food safety action and policy.

- PulseNet, a national laboratory network that detects foodborne disease outbreaks, compares the deoxyribonucleic acid (DNA) fingerprints of *Campylobacter* from patients to find clusters of illnesses that may represent an outbreak.

- FoodNet, a collaboration among CDC, 10 state health departments, the U.S. Department of Agriculture's Food Safety and Inspection Service (USDA-FSIS), and U.S. Food and Drug Administration (FDA), collects data on human infections caused by *Campylobacter*.

- National Antimicrobial Resistance Monitoring System (NARMS), a collaboration among the state and local public health departments, CDC, FDA, and U.S. Department of Agriculture (USDA), tracks changes in antibiotic resistance among *Campylobacter* bacteria isolated from humans, retail meats, and food animals.

- National Outbreak Reporting System (NORS) collects data from state health departments for *Campylobacter* outbreaks.

- Laboratory Enteric Disease Surveillance (LEDS) collects data for laboratory-confirmed *Campylobacter* infections from state public health laboratories.

The USDA-FSIS regulates meat, poultry, and processed eggs. In 2011, USDA-FSIS established performance standards to limit *Campylobacter* contamination of whole broiler chickens, requiring contamination rates to be no more than 10.4 percent of samples in processing plants. In 2016, USDA-FSIS implemented further measures, requiring *Campylobacter* contamination rates to be no more than 1.9 percent in ground chicken and turkey products and 7.7 percent in raw chicken parts in processing plants. USDA-FSIS also is posting contamination testing results online.

The FDA regulates all foods other than those regulated by USDA-FSIS. The FDA publishes the Food Code, a model for regulating retail and food service establishments, including restaurants, grocery stores, and institutions, such as nursing homes. The FDA Food Safety Modernization Act (FSMA), passed in 2011, aims to ensure the U.S. food supply is safe by shifting the focus to preventing contamination.

Section 36.4

Escherichia coli

This section includes text excerpted from "*E.coli (Escherichia coli),*" Centers for Disease Control and Prevention (CDC), January 25, 2018.

Escherichia coli (abbreviated as *E. coli*) are bacteria found in the environment, foods, and intestines of people and animals. *E. coli* are a large and diverse group of bacteria. Although most strains of *E. coli* are harmless, others can make you sick. Some kinds of *E. coli* can cause diarrhea, while others cause urinary tract infections, respiratory illness, and pneumonia, and other illnesses.

E. coli consists of a diverse group of bacteria. Pathogenic *E. coli* strains are categorized into pathotypes. Six pathotypes are associated with diarrhea and collectively are referred to as diarrheagenic *E. coli*.

1. Shiga toxin-producing *E. coli* (STEC)—STEC may also be referred to as Verocytotoxin-producing *E. coli* (VTEC) or enterohemorrhagic *E. coli* (EHEC). This pathotype is the one most commonly heard about in the news in association with foodborne outbreaks.

2. Enterotoxigenic *E. coli* (ETEC)

3. Enteropathogenic *E. coli* (EPEC)

4. Enteroaggregative *E. coli* (EAEC)

5. Enteroinvasive *E. coli* (EIEC)

6. Diffusely adherent *E. coli* (DAEC)

What Are Shiga Toxin-Producing Eschericia coli (STEC)?

Some kinds of *E. coli* cause disease by making a toxin called Shiga toxin. The bacteria that make these toxins are called "Shiga toxin-producing" *E. coli*, or STEC for short. You might hear these bacteria called verocytotoxic *E. coli* (VTEC) or enterohemorrhagic *E. coli* (EHEC);

these all refer generally to the same group of bacteria. The strain of Shiga toxin-producing *E. coli O104:H4* that caused a large outbreak in Europe in 2011 was frequently referred to as EHEC. The most commonly identified STEC in North America is *E. coli O157:H7* (often shortened to *E. coli O157* or even just "O157"). When you hear news reports about outbreaks of *"E. coli"* infections, they are usually talking about *E. coli O157*.

In addition to *E. coli O157*, many other kinds (called serogroups) of STEC cause disease. Other *E. coli* serogroups in the STEC group, including *E. coli O145*, are sometimes called "non-O157 STECs." Currently, there are limited public health surveillance data on the occurrence of non-O157 STECs, including STEC O145; many STEC O145 infections may go undiagnosed or unreported.

Compared with STEC O157 infections, identification of non-O157 STEC infections is more complex. First, clinical laboratories must test stool samples for the presence of Shiga toxins. Then, the positive samples must be sent to public health laboratories to look for non-O157 STEC. Clinical laboratories typically cannot identify non-O157 STEC. Other non-O157 STEC serogroups that often cause illness in people in the United States include O26, O111, and O103. Some types of STEC frequently cause severe disease, including bloody diarrhea and hemolytic uremic syndrome (HUS), which is a type of kidney failure.

Are There Important Differences E. coli *O157 and Other STEC?*

Most of what we know about STEC comes from studies of *E. coli O157* infection, which was first identified as a pathogen in 1982. Less is known about the non-O157 STEC, partly because older laboratory practices did not identify non-O157 infections. As a whole, the non-O157 serogroups are less likely to cause severe illness than *E. coli O157*, though sometimes they can. For example, *E. coli O26* produces the same type of toxins that *E. coli O157* produces, and causes a similar illness, though it is typically less likely to lead to kidney problems (called HUS).

Who Gets STEC Infections?

People of any age can become infected. Very young children and the elderly are more likely to develop severe illness and HUS than others, but even healthy older children and young adults can become seriously ill.

What Are the Symptoms of STEC Infections?

The symptoms of STEC infections vary for each person but often include severe stomach cramps, diarrhea (often bloody), and vomiting. If there is fever, it usually is not very high (less than 101°F/less than 38.5°C). Most people get better within 5–7 days. Some infections are very mild, but others are severe or even life-threatening.

What Is Hemolytic Uretic Syndrome (HUS), a Complication of STEC Infections?

Around 5–10 percent of those who are diagnosed with STEC infection develop a potentially life-threatening complication known as HUS. Clues that a person is developing HUS include decreased frequency of urination, feeling very tired, and losing pink color in cheeks and inside the lower eyelids. Persons with HUS should be hospitalized because their kidneys may stop working and they may develop other serious problems. Most persons with HUS recover within a few weeks, but some suffer permanent damage or die.

How Soon Do Symptoms Appear after Exposure?

The time between ingesting the STEC bacteria and feeling sick is called the "incubation period." The incubation period is usually 3–4 days after the exposure, but may be as short as 1 day or as long as 10 days. The symptoms often begin slowly with mild belly pain or nonbloody diarrhea that worsens over several days. HUS, if it occurs, develops an average 7 days after the first symptoms, when the diarrhea is improving.

Where Do STEC Come From?

STEC live in the guts of ruminant animals, including cattle, goats, sheep, deer, and elk. The major source for human illnesses is cattle. STEC that cause human illness generally do not make animals sick. Other kinds of animals, including pigs and birds, sometimes pick up STEC from the environment and may spread it.

How Are These Infections Spread?

Infections start when you swallow STEC—in other words, when you get tiny (usually invisible) amounts of human or animal feces in your mouth. Unfortunately, this happens more often than we would like to think about. Exposures that result in illness include consumption of contaminated food, consumption of unpasteurized (raw) milk, consumption of water that has not been disinfected, contact with cattle, or contact with the feces of infected people. Some foods are considered to carry such a high risk of infection with *E. coli O157* or another germ that health officials recommend that people avoid them completely. These foods include unpasteurized (raw) milk, unpasteurized apple cider, and soft cheeses made from raw milk. Sometimes the contact is pretty obvious (working with cows at a dairy or changing diapers, for example), but sometimes it is not (like eating an undercooked hamburger or a contaminated piece of lettuce). People have gotten infected by swallowing lake water while swimming, touching the environment in petting zoos and other animal exhibits, and by eating food prepared by people who did not wash their hands well after using the toilet. Almost everyone has some risk of infection.

Where Did My Infection Come from?

Because there are so many possible sources, for most people we can only guess. If your infection happens to be part of the about 20 percent of cases that are part of a recognized outbreak, the health department might identify the source.

How Common Are STEC Infections?

An estimated 265,000 STEC infections occur each year in the United States. STEC O157 causes about 36 percent of these infections, and non-O157 STEC cause the rest. Public health experts rely on estimates rather than actual numbers of infections because not all STEC infections are diagnosed, for several reasons. Many infected people do not seek medical care; many of those who do seek care do not provide a stool specimen for testing, and many labs do not test for non-O157 STEC. However, this situation is changing as more labs have begun using newer, simpler tests that can help detect non-O157 STEC.

How Are STEC Infections Diagnosed and When Should I Contact My Healthcare Provider?

STEC infections are usually diagnosed through laboratory testing of stool specimens (feces). Identifying the specific strain of STEC is essential for public health purposes, such as finding outbreaks. Many labs can determine if STEC are present, and most can identify *E. coli O157*. Labs that test for the presence of Shiga toxins in stool can detect non-O157 STEC infections. However, for the O group (serogroup) and other characteristics of non-O157 STEC to be identified, Shiga toxin-positive specimens must be sent to a state public health laboratory.

Contact your healthcare provider if you have diarrhea that lasts for more than 3 days, or it is accompanied by high fever, blood in the stool, or so much vomiting that you cannot keep liquids down and you pass very little urine.

What Is the Best Treatment for STEC Infection?

Nonspecific supportive therapy, including hydration, is important. Antibiotics should not be used to treat this infection. There is no evidence that treatment with antibiotics is helpful, and taking antibiotics may increase the risk of HUS. Antidiarrheal agents like Imodium® may also increase that risk.

Should an Infected Person Be Excluded from School or Work?

School and work exclusion policies differ by local jurisdiction. Check with your local or state health department to learn more about the laws where you live. In any case, good hand-washing after changing diapers, after using the toilet, and before preparing food is essential to prevent the spread of these and many other infections.

How Can STEC Infections Be Prevented?

- Wash your hands thoroughly after using the bathroom or changing diapers and before preparing or eating food. Wash your hands after contact with animals or their environments (at farms, petting zoos, fairs, even your own backyard)

- Cook meats thoroughly. Ground beef and meat that has been needle-tenderized should be cooked to a temperature of at least 160°F/70°C. It's best to use a thermometer, as color is not a very reliable indicator of "doneness"

- Avoid raw milk, unpasteurized dairy products, and unpasteurized juices (like fresh apple cider)

- Avoid swallowing water when swimming or playing in lakes, ponds, streams, swimming pools, and backyard "kiddie" pools

- Prevent cross-contaminated in food preparation areas by thoroughly washing hands, counters, cutting boards, and utensils after they touch raw meat

Section 36.5

Salmonella

This section includes text excerpted from
"*Salmonella*," Centers for Disease Control and
Prevention (CDC), March 9, 2015.

Salmonella is a bacteria that makes people sick. It was discovered by an American scientist named Dr. Salmon, and has been known to cause illness for over 125 years. The illness people get from a *Salmonella* infection is called salmonellosis.

Most people infected with *Salmonella* develop diarrhea, fever, and abdominal cramps between 12–72 hours after infection. The illness usually lasts 4–7 days, and most individuals recover without treatment. In some cases, diarrhea may be so severe that the patient needs to be hospitalized. In these patients, the *Salmonella* infection may spread from the intestines to the bloodstream, and then to other body sites. In these cases, *Salmonella* can cause death unless the person is treated promptly with antibiotics. The elderly, infants, and those with impaired immune systems are more likely to have a severe illness.

How Common Is Salmonella Infection?

The Centers for Disease Control and Prevention (CDC) estimates *Salmonella* causes about 1.2 million illnesses, 23,000 hospitalizations, and 450 deaths in the United States every year. Among these illnesses, about 1.1 million are acquired in the United States. Among the illnesses acquired in the United States, CDC estimates that food is the source for about 1 million illnesses, 19,000 hospitalizations, and 380 deaths.

There are many different kinds of *Salmonella* bacteria. *Salmonella* serotype Typhimurium and *Salmonella* serotype Enteritidis are the most common in the United States. *Salmonella* infections are more common in the summer than winter.

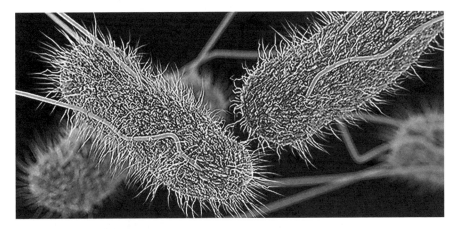

Figure 36.1. *Medical Illustration of* Salmonella

Who Is at Highest Risk for Salmonella Infection?

Children are at the highest risk for *Salmonella* infection. Children under the age of 5 have higher rates of *Salmonella* infection than any other age group. Young children, older adults, and people with weakened immune systems are the most likely to have severe infections.

Are There Long-Term Consequences to a Salmonella Infection?

People with diarrhea due to a *Salmonella* infection usually recover completely, although it may be several months before their bowel habits are entirely normal.

A small number of people with *Salmonella* develop pain in their joints. This is called reactive arthritis. Reactive arthritis can last for months or years and can lead to chronic arthritis, which can be difficult to treat. Antibiotic treatment of the initial *Salmonella* infection does not make a difference in whether or not the person develops arthritis. People with reactive arthritis can also develop irritation of the eyes and painful urination.

Prevention

Quick Tips for Preventing **Salmonella**

- Cook poultry, ground beef, and eggs thoroughly. Do not eat or drink foods containing raw eggs, or raw (unpasteurized) milk.

- If you are served undercooked meat, poultry, or eggs in a restaurant, don't hesitate to send it back to the kitchen for further cooking

- Wash hands, kitchen work surfaces, and utensils with soap and water immediately after they have been in contact with raw meat or poultry

- Be particularly careful with foods prepared for infants, the elderly, and the immunocompromised. Wash hands with soap after handling reptiles, birds, or baby chicks, and after contact with pet feces.

- Avoid direct or even indirect contact between reptiles (turtles, iguanas, other lizards, snakes) and infants or immunocompromised persons.

- Don't work with raw poultry or meat, and an infant (e.g., feed, change diaper) at the same time.

- Mother's milk is the safest food for young infants.

- Breastfeeding prevents salmonellosis and many other health problems.

More about Prevention

There is no vaccine to prevent salmonellosis. Because foods of animal origin may be contaminated with *Salmonella*, people should not eat raw or undercooked eggs, poultry, or meat. Raw eggs may be unrecognized in some foods, such as homemade Hollandaise sauce, Caesar and other homemade salad dressings, tiramisu, homemade ice cream, homemade mayonnaise, cookie dough, and frostings. Poultry and meat, including hamburgers, should be well-cooked, not pink in the middle. Persons also should not consume raw or unpasteurized milk or other dairy products. Produce should be thoroughly washed.

Cross-contamination of foods should be avoided. Uncooked meats should be kept separate from produce, cooked foods, and ready-to-eat foods. Hands, cutting boards, counters, knives, and other utensils should be washed thoroughly after touching uncooked foods. Hand should be washed before handling food, and between handling different food items.

People who have salmonellosis should not prepare food or pour water for others until their diarrhea has resolved. Many health departments require that restaurant workers with *Salmonella* infection have a stool test showing that they are no longer carrying the *Salmonella* bacterium before they return to work.

People should wash their hands after contact with animal feces. Because reptiles are particularly likely to have *Salmonella*, and it can contaminate their skin, everyone should immediately wash their hands after handling reptiles. Reptiles (including turtles) are not appropriate pets for small children and should not be in the same house as an infant. *Salmonella* carried in the intestines of chicks and ducklings contaminates their environment and the entire surface of the animal. Children can be exposed to the bacteria by simply holding, cuddling, or kissing the birds. Children should not handle baby chicks or other young birds. Everyone should immediately wash their hands after touching birds, including baby chicks and ducklings, or their environment.

Some prevention steps occur everyday without you thinking about it. Pasteurization of milk and treatment of municipal water supplies are highly effective prevention measures that have been in place for decades. In the 1970s, small pet turtles were a common source of salmonellosis in the United States, so in 1975, the sale of small turtles was banned in this country. However, in 2008, they were still being sold, and cases of *Salmonella* associated with pet turtles have been reported. Improvements in farm animal hygiene, in slaughter plant practices, and in vegetable and fruit harvesting and packing operations may help prevent salmonellosis caused by contaminated foods. Better education of food industry workers in basic food safety and restaurant inspection procedures may prevent cross-contamination and other food handling errors that can lead to outbreaks. Wider use of pasteurized egg in restaurants, hospitals, and nursing homes is an important prevention measure. In the future, irradiation or other treatments may greatly reduce contamination of raw meat.

Diagnosis and Treatment

How Can Salmonella Infections Be Diagnosed?

Diagnosing salmonellosis requires testing a clinical specimen (such as stool or blood) from an infected person to distinguish it from other illnesses that can cause diarrhea, fever, and abdominal cramps. Once *Salmonella* is identified in the specimen, additional testing can be done to further characterize the *Salmonella*.

Steps in Laboratory Testing and Reporting Salmonella

- Laboratory scientists identify *Salmonella* infection by culturing a patient's sample. If *Salmonella* bacteria grow, then the diagnosis is confirmed, or in laboratory-terms, "culture confirmed"

- Clinical diagnostic laboratories report the test results to the treating clinician and submit *Salmonella* isolates to state and territorial public health laboratories for serotyping and DNA fingerprinting

- The public health laboratories report the results to CDC's Laboratory-based Enteric Disease Surveillance and to PulseNet

- The public health laboratories forward atypical serotypes to CDC's National *Salmonella* Reference Laboratory for more characterization or confirmation

Serotyping Salmonella

Salmonella are divided into serotypes according to structures on the bacteria's surface. Serotyping is used in outbreak investigations to link cases of illness with similar bacteria and track them to the source (example: a contaminated food or an infected animal). Some serotypes are only found in one kind of animal or in a single place. Others are found in many different animals and all over the world. Some serotypes can cause especially severe illnesses when they infect people; most typically cause milder illnesses.

Serotyping has played an important role in the understanding the epidemiologic and molecular characterization of *Salmonella* for decades. Today, modern genetic subtyping methods provide scientists with additional information to understand common serotypes and identify, investigate, and trace outbreaks.

Pulsenet and Pulsed-Field Gel Electrophoresis (PFGE)

In addition to serotyping, state public health laboratories routinely subtype *Salmonella* isolates using pulsed-field gel electrophoresis (PFGE) to create a "DNA fingerprint."

The laboratories submit these fingerprint patterns to a dynamic database maintained by PulseNet, a national network of public health and food regulatory agency laboratories coordinated by CDC. The network includes state health departments, local health departments, and federal agencies (CDC, U.S. Department of Agriculture's Food Safety and Inspection Service (USDA/FSIS), and FDA).

PulseNet data are available to participating health departments for comparing PFGE patterns. Finding a group of infections with the same pattern could indicate an outbreak. Finding the same pattern in a food could help link illness to a specific food source.

Sequence-Based Subtyping with Multiple Locus Variable-Number Tandem Repeat Analysis (MLVA) Collapsed

In addition to PFGE, Multiple Locus Variable-number Tandem Repeat Analysis, or MLVA, is another technique used by PulseNet to further characterize *Salmonella* isolates.

Next Generation of Laboratory Testing Collapsed

New methods for subtyping. PulseNet is working with other federal and state agencies to evaluate the use of whole-genome sequencing (WGS) to replace PFGE as its standard method for subtyping *Salmonella* and other bacteria that cause diarrheal disease. It is hoped that WGS will make the PulseNet process faster, more accurate, and more efficient.

New methods for diagnosis. CDC is also working to adapt its processes to important changes in how *Salmonella* is diagnosed in patients. Until recently, culture (laboratory procedures to grow living *Salmonella* from patient specimens) was the diagnostic standard and the cornerstone of public health surveillance.

FDA has approved culture-independent diagnostic testing (CIDT) methods for diagnosing *Salmonella* infections, but they are not widely used yet. These new methods do not depend on culturing the specimen, so they do not yield an isolate for serotyping or PFGE. When adopted, these new tests could impact surveillance in a number of ways. PulseNet hopes to develop sequence-based tests that are themselves culture-independent using new systems developed for WGS.

Section 36.6

Listeria

This section includes text excerpted from
"*Listeria* (Listeriosis)," Centers for Disease Control
and Prevention (CDC), December 12, 2016.

Listeriosis is a serious infection caused by the germ *Listeria* monocytogenes. People usually become ill with listeriosis after eating contaminated food. The disease primarily affects pregnant women, newborns, older adults, and people with weakened immune systems. It's rare for people in other groups to get sick with *Listeria* infection.

Listeriosis is usually a mild illness for pregnant women, but it causes severe disease in the fetus or newborn baby. Some people with *Listeria* infections, most commonly adults 65 years and older and people with weakened immune systems, develop severe infections of the bloodstream (causing sepsis) or brain (causing meningitis or encephalitis). *Listeria* infections can sometimes affect other parts of the body, including bones, joints, and sites in the chest and abdomen.

Every year, about 1,600 people get listeriosis in the United States.

Symptoms of Listeriosis

Listeriosis can cause a variety of symptoms, depending on the person and the part of the body affected. *Listeria* can cause fever and diarrhea similar to other foodborne germs, but this type of *Listeria* infection is rarely diagnosed. Symptoms in people with invasive listeriosis, meaning the bacteria has spread beyond the gut, depend on whether the person is pregnant.

- **Pregnant women.** Pregnant women typically experience only fever and other flu-like symptoms, such as fatigue and muscle aches. However, infections during pregnancy can lead to miscarriage, stillbirth, premature delivery, or life-threatening infection of the newborn.

- **People other than pregnant women.** Symptoms can include headache, stiff neck, confusion, loss of balance, and convulsions in addition to fever and muscle aches.

People with invasive listeriosis usually report symptoms starting 1–4 weeks after eating food contaminated with *Listeria*; some people have reported symptoms starting as late as 70 days after exposure or as early as the same day of exposure.

Diagnosis and Treatment of Listeriosis

Listeriosis is usually diagnosed when a bacterial culture (a type of laboratory test) grows *Listeria* monocytogenes from a body tissue or fluid, such as blood, spinal fluid, or the placenta.

Listeriosis is treated with antibiotics.

How People Get Infected with Listeria

Listeriosis is usually caused by eating food contaminated with *Listeria* monocytogenes. If infection occurs during pregnancy, *Listeria* bacteria can spread to the baby through the placenta.

What Should I Do If I Ate a Food That May Have Been Contaminated with Listeria?

You should seek medical care and tell the doctor about eating possibly contaminated food if you have a fever and other symptoms of possible listeriosis, such as fatigue and muscle aches, within two months after eating possibly contaminated food. This is especially important if you are pregnant, age 65 or older, or have a weakened immune system.

If you ate food possibly contaminated with *Listeria* and do not feel sick, most experts believe you do not need tests or treatment. Talk with your medical provider if you have questions about what to do after eating possibly contaminated food.

Is Listeriosis a Serious Disease?

Most people with invasive listeriosis require hospital care, and about one in five people with the infection die. When listeriosis occurs during pregnancy, it can cause miscarriage, stillbirth, or newborn death. Listeriosis during pregnancy results in fetal loss in about 20 percent and newborn death in about 3 percent of cases.

Outbreaks of Listeriosis

A few outbreaks of listeriosis are identified most years. Even though most cases of listeriosis are not part of recognized outbreaks, outbreak investigations help show which foods are sources of listeriosis.

Public Health Agencies and Their Role in Preventing or Control Listeriosis

Federal, state, and local governments are doing the following:

- Providing guidance to industry and developing and enforcing regulations, like the Food Safety Modernization Act (FSMA), to focus food safety efforts on safer production and handling of foods

- Tracking *Listeria* infections to identify opportunities to improve policies and practices, particularly to protect groups of people who are more likely to get sick with listeriosis

- Investigating and stopping outbreaks by recalling contaminated foods and warning the public

- Applying Centers for Disease Control and Prevention's (CDC) enhanced approach to investigating *Listeria* infections in all states so disease detectives can rapidly solve outbreaks by:

  - Deoxyribonucleic acid (DNA) fingerprinting the germ to identify outbreaks and contaminated foods, and interviewing people who are sick—quickly and with the same questions—about what they ate

  - Helping health departments get the technology and training for whole-genome sequencing and analysis, which will make it possible to find *Listeria* infections and outbreaks more quickly, and track them to their sources

Protecting Myself and My Family from Infection

People who are more likely to get a *Listeria* infection (pregnant women, people 65 years or older, and people with a weakened immune system and those who prepare food for them can:

- Know which foods are risky and avoid these foods

- Avoid drinking raw (unpasteurized) milk or eating soft cheeses made from it

- Be aware that Mexican-style cheeses made from pasteurized milk, such as queso fresco, have caused *Listeria* infections, likely because they were contaminated during cheese-making

- Heat deli meats and hot dogs until steaming hot before eating

- Refrigerate leftovers within 2 hours in shallow, covered containers and use within 3–4 days

- Avoid cross-contamination in the refrigerator or other places in the kitchen

- Use a thermometer to make sure your refrigerator is 40°F or lower and your freezer is 0°F or lower

Section 36.7

Shigella

This section includes text excerpted from "*Shigella*—Shigellosis," Centers for Disease Control and Prevention (CDC), October 12, 2017.

Shigellosis is a diarrheal disease caused by a group of bacteria called *Shigella*. *Shigella* causes about 500,000 cases of diarrhea in the United States annually. There are four different species of *Shigella*:

1. *Shigella sonnei* (the most common species in the United States)

2. *Shigella flexneri*

3. *Shigella boydii*

4. *Shigella dysenteriae*

S. dysenteriae and S. boydii are rare in the United States, though they continue to be important causes of disease in the developing world. *Shigella* dysenteriae type 1 can be deadly.

How Shigellosis Spreads

Shigella germs are in the stool (poop) of sick people while they have diarrhea and for up to a week or two after the diarrhea has gone away. *Shigella* germs are very contagious; it takes just a small number of *Shigella* germs to make someone sick. People can get shigellosis when they put something in their mouths or swallow something that

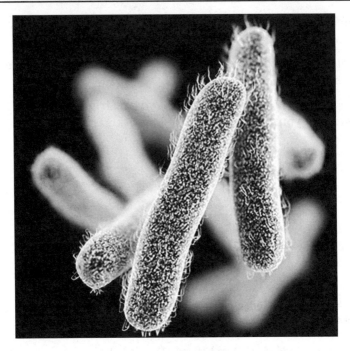

Figure 36.2. *Medical Illustration of Shigellosis*

has come into contact with the stool of someone else who is sick with shigellosis. People could get sick by:

- Getting *Shigella* germs on their hands and then touching your food or mouth. You can get *Shigella* germs on your hands after:

  - Touching surfaces contaminated with germs from stool from a sick person, such as toys, bathroom fixtures, changing tables, or diaper pails

  - Changing the diaper of a sick child or caring for a sick person

- Eating food that was prepared by someone who is sick with shigellosis

- Swallowing recreational water (for example, lake or river water) while swimming or drinking water that is contaminated with stool (poop) containing the germ

- Having exposure to stool during sexual contact with someone who is sick or recently (several weeks) recovered from shigellosis

Symptoms of Shigellosis

Symptoms of shigellosis typically start 1–2 days after exposure to the germ and include:

- Diarrhea (sometimes bloody)

- Fever

- Stomach pain

- Feeling the need to pass stool [poop] even when the bowels are empty

For most people, symptoms usually last about 5–7 days. In some cases, it may take several months before bowel habits (for example, how often someone passes stool and the consistency of their stool) are entirely normal.

Population That Is Likely to Get Shigellosis

- **Young children** are the most likely to get shigellosis, but people of all ages are affected. Many outbreaks are related to child care settings and schools, and illness commonly spreads from young children to their family members and others in their communities because it is so contagious.

- **Travelers** to developing countries may be more likely to get shigellosis, and to become infected with strains of *Shigella* bacteria that are resistant to important antibiotics. Travelers may be exposed through contaminated food, water (both drinking and recreational water), or surfaces. Travelers can protect themselves by strictly following food and water precautions, and washing hands with soap frequently.

- **Gay and bisexual men and other men who have sex with men** (MSM)* are more likely to acquire shigellosis than the general adult population. *Shigella* passes from feces or soiled fingers of one person to the mouth of another person, which can happen during sexual activity. Many shigellosis outbreaks among MSM have been reported in the United States, Canada, Japan, and Europe since 1999.

- **People who have weakened immune systems due to illness (such as human immunodeficiency virus (HIV)) or medical treatment (such as chemotherapy for cancer)** can get a more serious illness. A severe shigellosis may involve the infection spreading into the blood, which can be life-threatening.

- **Large outbreaks** of shigellosis often start in child care settings and spread among small social groups such as in traditionally observant Jewish communities. Similar outbreaks could occur among any race, ethnicity or community social circle because *Shigella* germs can spread easily from one person to another.

*The term "men who have sex with men" is used in CDC surveillance systems because it indicates men who engage in behaviors that may transmit Shigella *infection, rather than how someone identifies their sexuality.*

Diagnosis of Shigellosis

Many kinds of germs can cause diarrhea. Knowing which germ is causing an illness is important to help guide appropriate treatment. Healthcare providers can order laboratory tests to identify *Shigella* germs in the stool of an infected person.

Treatment of Shigellosis

People who have shigellosis usually get better without antibiotic treatment in 5–7 days. People with mild shigellosis may need only fluids and rest. Bismuth subsalicylate (for example, Pepto-Bismol) may be helpful but people sick with shigellosis should not use medications that cause the gut to slow down and interfere with the way the body digests food, such as loperamide (for example, Imodium) or diphenoxylate with atropine (for example, Lomotil).

Healthcare providers may prescribe antibiotics for people with severe cases of shigellosis to help them get better faster. However, some antibiotics are not effective against certain types of *Shigella*. Healthcare providers can order laboratory tests to determine which antibiotics are likely to work. Tell your healthcare provider if you do not get better within a couple of days after starting antibiotics. They can do more tests to learn whether your type of *Shigella* bacteria can be treated effectively with the antibiotic you are taking. If not, your doctor may prescribe another type of antibiotic.

How I Can Reduce My Chance of Getting Shigellosis

You can reduce your chance of getting sick from *Shigella* by taking these steps:

- Carefully washing your hands with soap and water during key times:

  - Before preparing food and eating

  - After changing a diaper or helping to clean another person who has defecated (pooped)

- If you care for a child in diapers who has shigellosis, promptly throw away the soiled diapers in a covered, lined garbage can. Wash your hands and the child's hands carefully with soap and water right after changing the diapers. Clean up any leaks or spills of diaper contents immediately.

- Avoid swallowing water from ponds, lakes, or untreated swimming pools.

- When traveling internationally, stick to safe eating and drinking habits, and wash hands often with soap and water.

- Avoid having sex (vaginal, anal, and oral) for one week after your partner recovers from diarrhea. Because *Shigella* germs may be in stool for several weeks, follow safe sexual practices, or ideally avoid having sex, for several weeks after your partner has recovered.

I Was Diagnosed with Shigellosis. What Can I Do to Avoid Giving It to Other People?

- Wash your hands carefully and frequently with soap and water, especially after using the bathroom.

- Do not prepare food for others while you are sick. After you get better, wash your hands carefully with soap and water before preparing food for others.

- Stay home from child care, school and food service facilities while sick. Your local health department may have a policy on when to return to child care or school. Avoid swimming until you have fully recovered.

495

- Wait to have sex (vaginal, anal, and oral) for one week after you no longer have diarrhea. Because *Shigella* germs may be in stool for several weeks, follow safe sexual practices, or ideally avoid having sex, for several weeks after you have recovered.

My Child Was Diagnosed with Shigellosis. How Can I Keep Others from Catching It?

- Supervise handwashing of toddlers and small children after they use the bathroom. Wash your hands and your infant's hands with soap and water after diaper changes.

- Throw away soiled diapers in a covered, lined garbage can. Clean diaper changing areas after using them.

- Keep your child out of child care and group play settings while sick with diarrhea, and follow the guidance of your local health department about returning your child to their child care facility.

- Avoid taking your child swimming or to group water play venues until after they no longer have diarrhea.

  - Have children and staff shower with soap before swimming.

    - If a child is too young to shower independently, have staff wash the child, particularly the rear end, with soap and water.

    - Take frequent bathroom breaks or check their diapers often.

    - Change diapers in a diaper-changing area or bathroom and not by the water.

    - Discourage children from getting the water in their mouths and swallowing it.

Section 36.8

Botulism

This section includes text excerpted from "Botulism,"
Centers for Disease Control and Prevention (CDC), May 8, 2017.

Botulism is a rare but serious illness caused by a toxin that attacks the body's nerves and causes difficulty breathing, muscle paralysis, and even death. This toxin is made by *Clostridium botulinum* and sometimes *Clostridium butyricum* and *Clostridium baratii* bacteria. These bacteria can be spread by food and sometimes by other means.

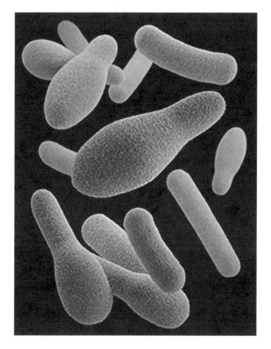

Figure 36.3. *Medical Illustration of Botulism*

The bacteria that make botulinum toxin are found naturally in many places, but it's rare for them to make people sick. These bacteria make spores, which act like protective coatings. Spores help the bacteria survive in the environment, even in extreme conditions. The spores usually do not cause people to become sick, even when they're eaten. But under certain conditions, these spores can grow and make one of the most lethal toxins known. The conditions in which the spores can grow and make toxin are:

- Low-oxygen or no oxygen (anaerobic) environment

- Low acid

- Low sugar

- Low salt

- A certain temperature range

- A certain amount of water

For example, improperly home-canned, preserved, or fermented foods can provide the right conditions for spores to grow and make botulinum toxin. When people eat these foods, they can become seriously ill, or even die, if they don't get proper medical treatment quickly.

Kinds of Botulism

There are five main kinds of botulism:

1. **Foodborne botulism** can happen by eating foods that have been contaminated with botulinum toxin. Common sources of foodborne botulism are homemade foods that have been improperly canned, preserved, or fermented. Though uncommon, store-bought foods also can be contaminated with botulinum toxin.

2. **Wound botulism** can happen if the spores of the bacteria get into a wound and make a toxin. People who inject drugs have a greater chance of getting wound botulism. Wound botulism has also occurred in people after a traumatic injury, such as a motorcycle accident, or surgery.

3. **Infant botulism** can happen if the spores of the bacteria get into an infant's intestines. The spores grow and produce the toxin which causes illness.

4. **Adult intestinal toxemia** (also known as adult intestinal toxemia) botulism is a very rare kind of botulism that can happen if the spores of the bacteria get into an adult's intestines, grow, and produce the toxin (similar to infant botulism).

Although it's not known why people get this kind of botulism, people who have serious health conditions that affect the gut may be more likely to get sick.

5. **Iatrogenic botulism** can happen if too much botulinum toxin is injected for cosmetic reasons, such as for wrinkles, or medical reasons, such as for migraine headaches.

All kinds of botulism can be fatal and are medical emergencies. If you or someone you know has symptoms of botulism, see your doctor or go to the emergency room immediately.

Symptoms

The symptoms of botulism are:

- double vision
- blurred vision
- drooping eyelids
- slurred speech
- difficulty swallowing
- a thick-feeling tongue
- dry mouth
- muscle weakness

Infants with botulism:

- appear lethargic
- feed poorly
- are constipated
- have a weak cry
- have poor muscle tone (appear "floppy")

These symptoms all result from muscle paralysis caused by the toxin. If untreated, the disease may progress and symptoms may worsen to cause paralysis of certain muscles, including those used in breathing and those in the arms, legs, and trunk (part of the body from the neck to the pelvis area, also called the torso). People with botulism may not show all of these symptoms at once.

In foodborne botulism, symptoms generally begin 18–36 hours after eating a contaminated food. However, symptoms can begin as soon as 6 hours after or up to 10 days later.

If you or someone you know has symptoms of botulism, see your doctor or go to the emergency room immediately.

Diagnosis

If you or someone you know has symptoms of botulism, see your doctor or go to the emergency room immediately.

To make a diagnosis, your doctor will ask questions and examine you to find out the cause of your symptoms. However, these clues are usually not enough for your doctor to diagnose you because some diseases have symptoms similar to those of botulism, such as Guillain-Barré syndrome (GBS), stroke, myasthenia gravis, and opioid overdose. Your doctor may perform special tests to make a diagnosis. Some of these tests are:

- Brain scan

- Spinal fluid examination

- Nerve and muscle function tests (nerve conduction study (NCS) and electromyography (EMG))

- Tensilon test for myasthenia gravis

If these tests don't determine what is making you sick, your doctor may order laboratory tests to look for the toxin and the bacteria that cause botulism. These laboratory tests are the only way to know for certain whether you have botulism. It may take several days to get the results of your tests from the laboratory. If your doctor suspects you have botulism, you may start treatment right away.

Treatment

Doctors treat botulism with a drug called an antitoxin. The toxin attacks the body's nerves, and the antitoxin prevents it from causing any more harm. It does not heal the damage the toxin has already done. Depending on how severe your symptoms are, you may need to stay in the hospital for weeks or even months before you are well enough to go home.

If your disease is severe, you may have breathing problems and even respiratory (breathing) failure if the toxin paralyzes the muscles involved in breathing. If that happens, your doctor may put you on a breathing machine (ventilator) until you are able to breathe on your own. The paralysis caused by the toxin will improve slowly. The medical and nursing care you receive in the hospital will help you recover.

If you have wound botulism, your doctor may need to surgically remove the source of the toxin-producing bacteria and give you antibiotics.

Survival and Complications

Botulism can result in death due to respiratory failure. However, because of the development of antitoxin and modern medical care, people with botulism today have a much lower chance of dying than people did in the past. Fifty years ago, for every 100 people with botulism, 50 would die. Now, with antitoxin and proper medical treatment, fewer than 5 of every 100 people with botulism die.

Even with antitoxin and intensive medical and nursing care, some patients die from infections or other problems that are caused by being paralyzed for weeks or months. Patients who survive botulism may have fatigue and shortness of breath for years afterward, and may need long-term therapy to help them recover.

Prevention

Many cases of botulism are preventable.

Foodborne Botulism

Many cases of foodborne botulism have happened after people eating home-canned, preserved, or fermented foods that were contaminated with toxin. The foods might have become contaminated if they were not canned (processed) correctly.

Foods with low acid content are the most common sources of home canning-related botulism cases. Examples of low-acid foods are:

- Asparagus
- Green beans
- Beets
- Corn
- Potatoes

New sources of foodborne botulism continue to be identified. Contamination can happen when food is handled improperly when it is made, when it is stored, or when it is used by consumers. Some examples of foods that have been contaminated are:

- Chopped garlic in oil
- Canned cheese sauce
- Canned tomatoes
- Carrot juice
- Baked potatoes wrapped in foil

In Alaska, most cases of foodborne botulism are caused by fermented fish and other aquatic animals.

If you preserve, can, or ferment your own foods, you can reduce the chance of these foods giving you, your family, or friends botulism by:

- Following safe home canning instructions as recommended by the U.S. Department of Agriculture (USDA)
- Following all instructions for washing, cleaning, and sterilizing items used in canning
- Using pressure canners for low-acid foods like potatoes, most other vegetables, and meats

Everyone can reduce their chances of getting botulism by:

- Refrigerating homemade oils infused with garlic or herbs and throwing away any unused oils after 4 days
- Keeping potatoes that have been baked while wrapped in aluminum foil hot (at temperatures above 140°F) until they are served, or refrigerating them with the foil loosened

Wound Botulism

Prevent wound botulism by keeping wounds clean. If wounds appear infected, seek medical care quickly. A wound might be infected if it is:

- Red
- Swollen
- Painful
- Warm to the touch

- Full of pus or other drainage

- Accompanied by fever

Not all wounds with botulism show these general symptoms of a wound infection. If you have a wound and begin to have symptoms of botulism, seek medical care immediately.

People who inject illicit drugs, such as black tar heroin, are more likely to get wound botulism than people who do not inject drugs. People who get botulism from injecting illicit drugs might not have an obviously infected injection site. Learn more about preventing wound botulism caused by injecting drugs.

Wound botulism may happen after traumatic injuries, such as motorcycle crashes, and surgeries. Be alert to signs of infection.

Infant Botulism

Most infant botulism cases cannot be prevented because the bacteria that causes the disease is in soil and dust. The bacteria can be found inside homes on floors, carpet, and countertops—even after cleaning. For almost all children and adults who are healthy, ingesting botulism spores is not dangerous and will not cause botulism (it's the toxin that is dangerous). For reasons unknown, some infants get botulism when the spores get into their digestive tracts, grow, and produce the toxin.

Honey can contain the bacteria that causes infant botulism, so do not feed honey to children younger than 12 months. Honey is safe for people 1 year of age and older.

Adult Intestinal Colonization

Adult intestinal colonization (also called adult intestinal toxemia) is a very rare type of botulism. People who have health conditions that change the structure or proper workings of their intestines (gut) may be at higher risk. Only a handful of people have been diagnosed with adult intestinal toxemia, and scientists do not fully understand how a person gets this type of botulism. It may be similar to infant botulism, which cannot be prevented.

Iatrogenic Botulism

You can prevent iatrogenic (an illness caused by medical examination or treatment) botulism by getting injections of botulinum toxin only by licensed practitioners:

- If you need an injection of botulinum toxin for a medical condition, your doctor will choose the safest dose

- If you get an injection of botulinum toxin for cosmetic reasons, be sure to go to a licensed professional

Section 36.9

Staphylococcus

This section includes text excerpted from "Food Safety—Staphylococcal Food Poisoning," Centers for Disease Control and Prevention (CDC), September 19, 2016.

Staphylococcal food poisoning is a gastrointestinal illness caused by eating foods contaminated with toxins produced by the bacterium *Staphylococcus aureus* (Staph). Staph is found on the skin and in the nose of about 25 percent of healthy people and animals. It usually does not cause illness in healthy people, but Staph has the ability to make toxins that can cause food poisoning.

How People Get Staphylococcal Food Poisoning

People who carry Staph can contaminate food if they don't wash their hands before touching it. Staph can also be found in unpasteurized milk and cheese products. Because Staph is salt tolerant, it can grow in salty foods like ham. As it multiplies in food, Staph produces toxins. Although Staph bacteria are easily killed by cooking, the toxins are resistant to heat and so cannot be destroyed by cooking.

Foods at highest risk of transmitting Staph toxins are those that people handle and then do not cook. Examples are sliced meat, puddings, pastries, and sandwiches. Food contaminated with Staph toxin may not smell bad or look spoiled.

Symptoms of Staphylococcal Food Poisoning

Staphylococcal toxins are fast-acting, symptoms usually develop within 30 minutes to 6 hours. Patients typically experience vomiting, nausea, stomach cramps, and diarrhea. The illness cannot be passed to other people and typically lasts for only 1 day. Severe illness is rare.

How I Can Know If I Have Staphylococcal Food Poisoning

Toxin-producing Staph can be identified in stool or vomit using specialized techniques. The toxins can also be detected in foods. Suspicion of staphylococcal food poisoning is generally based only on the signs and symptoms of the patient. Testing for the toxin-producing bacteria or the toxin is not usually done in individual patients, but can be done for outbreaks. If you think you may have food poisoning, contact your doctor.

Treatment for Staphylococcal Food Poisoning

For most patients, staphylococcal food poisoning is a brief illness. The most important treatment is plenty of fluids. Medicines may be given to decrease vomiting and nausea. Patients with severe illness may require intravenous fluids in a hospital.

Antibiotics are not useful in treating this illness because the toxin is not affected by antibiotics.

Are Patients Sick with Staphyococcal Food Poisoning Contagious?

Patients with this illness are not contagious because the toxins are not transmitted from one person to another.

How Staphylococcal Food Poisoning Can Be Prevented

Staphylococcal food poisoning can be prevented by preventing the contamination of food with Staph. The following food safety tips can help protect you and your family:

- Wash hands and under fingernails thoroughly with soap and water before handling and preparing food.

- Do not prepare food if you are ill.

- If you have wounds or infections on your hands or wrists, wear gloves while preparing food.

- Keep kitchens and food serving areas clean.

- If food is to be stored longer than two hours, keep hot foods hot (warmer than 140°F) and cold foods cold (40°F or colder).

- Store cooked food in a wide, shallow container and refrigerate as soon as possible.

Staphylococcal Toxins and Bioterrorist Attack

Staph toxins could be used as a biological agent either by contamination of food or water or by aerosolization (using pressure to produce a fine mist) and inhalation. Breathing in low doses of staphylococcal enterotoxin B may cause fever, cough, difficulty breathing, headache, and some vomiting and nausea. High doses of the toxin have a much more serious effect.

Chapter 37

Foodborne Viruses

Chapter Contents

Section 37.1

Hepatitis A

This section includes text excerpted from "Hepatitis A Questions and Answers for the Public," Centers for Disease Control and Prevention (CDC), November 2, 2017.

About Hepatitis A

What Is Hepatitis?

Hepatitis means inflammation of the liver. When the liver is inflamed or damaged, its function can be affected. Heavy alcohol use, toxins, some medications, and certain medical conditions can cause hepatitis but a virus often causes hepatitis. In the United States, the most common hepatitis viruses are hepatitis A virus, hepatitis B virus, and hepatitis C virus.

What Is Hepatitis A?

Hepatitis A is a highly contagious liver infection caused by the hepatitis A virus. It can range from a mild illness lasting a few weeks to a severe illness lasting several months. Although rare, hepatitis A can cause death in some people. Hepatitis A usually spreads when a person unknowingly ingests the virus from objects, food, or drinks contaminated by small, undetected amounts of stool from an infected person.

What Is the Difference between Hepatitis A, Hepatitis B, and Hepatitis C?

Hepatitis A, hepatitis B, and hepatitis C are liver infections caused by three different viruses. Although each can cause similar symptoms, they have different modes of transmission and can affect the liver differently. Hepatitis A is usually a short-term infection and does not become chronic. Hepatitis B and hepatitis C can also begin as short-term, acute infections, but in some people, the virus remains in the body, resulting in chronic disease and long-term liver problems. There are vaccines to prevent hepatitis A and hepatitis B; however, there is no vaccine for hepatitis C.

How Serious Is Hepatitis A?

Most people who get hepatitis A feel sick for several weeks, but they usually recover completely and do not have lasting liver damage. In rare cases, hepatitis A can cause liver failure and death; this is more common in people older than 50 and in people with other liver diseases.

How Common Is Hepatitis a in the United States?

In 2015, there were an estimated 2,800 hepatitis A cases in the United States. Hepatitis A rates have declined by more than 95 percent since the hepatitis A vaccine first became available in 1995.

Transmission/Exposure

How Is Hepatitis A Spread?

Hepatitis A usually spreads when a person unknowingly ingests the virus from objects, food, or drinks contaminated by small, undetected amounts of stool from an infected person. Hepatitis A can also spread from close personal contact with an infected person such as through sex or caring for someone who is ill.

Contamination of food (this can include frozen and undercooked food) by hepatitis A can happen at any point: growing, harvesting, processing, handling, and even after cooking. Contamination of food or water is more likely to occur in countries where hepatitis A is common and in areas where there are poor sanitary conditions or poor personal hygiene. In the United States, chlorination of water kills hepatitis A virus that enters the water supply. The U.S. Food and Drug Administration (FDA) routinely monitors natural bodies of water used for recreation for fecal contamination so there is no need for monitoring for hepatitis A virus specifically.

Who Is at Risk for Hepatitis A?

Although anyone can get hepatitis A, in the United States, certain groups of people are at higher risk, such as:

- People with direct contact with someone who has hepatitis A

- Travelers to countries where hepatitis A is common

- Men who have sexual contact with men
- People who use drugs, both injection and noninjection drugs
- Household members or caregivers of adoptees from countries where hepatitis A is common
- People with clotting factor disorders, such as hemophilia
- People working with nonhuman primates

I Think I Have Been Exposed to Hepatitis A. What Should I Do?

If you have any questions about potential exposure to hepatitis A, call your health professional or your local or state health department. If you were recently exposed to hepatitis A virus and have not been vaccinated against hepatitis A, you might benefit from an injection of either immune globulin or hepatitis A vaccine. However, the vaccine or immune globulin is only effective if given within the first 2 weeks after exposure. A health professional can decide what is best based on your age and overall health.

What Is Postexposure Prophylaxis (PEP)?

Postexposure prophylaxis (PEP) refers to trying to prevent or treat a disease after an exposure. For hepatitis A, postexposure prophylaxis is an injection of either immune globulin or hepatitis A vaccine. However, the vaccine or immune globulin is only effective in preventing hepatitis A if given within the first 2 weeks after exposure.

If I Have Had Hepatitis A in the Past, Can I Get It Again?

No. Once you recover from hepatitis A, you develop antibodies that protect you from the virus for life. An antibody is a substance found in the blood that the body produces in response to a virus. Antibodies protect the body from the disease by attaching to the virus and destroying it.

How Long Does Hepatitis A Virus Survive Outside the Body?

The hepatitis A virus is able to survive outside the body for months. High temperatures, such as boiling or cooking food or liquids for at least 1 minute at 185°F (85°C), kill the virus, although freezing temperatures do not.

Symptoms

What Are the Symptoms of Hepatitis A?

Older children and adults typically have symptoms. If symptoms develop, they can appear abruptly and can include:

- Fever
- Fatigue
- Loss of appetite
- Nausea
- Vomiting
- Abdominal pain
- Dark urine
- Clay-colored stools
- Joint pain
- Jaundice (yellowing of the skin and eyes)

Most children younger than age 6 do not have symptoms when they have hepatitis A. When symptoms are present, young children typically do not have jaundice but most older children and adults with hepatitis A have jaundice.

How Soon after Exposure to Hepatitis A Will Symptoms Appear?

If symptoms occur, they usually start appearing 4 weeks after exposure, but can occur as early as 2 and as late as 7 weeks after exposure. Symptoms usually develop over a period of several days.

How Long Do Hepatitis A Symptoms Last?

Symptoms usually last less than 2 months, although some people (10–15%) with hepatitis A can have symptoms for as long as 6 months.

Can a Person Spread Hepatitis A Without Having Symptoms?

Yes. Many people, especially children, have no symptoms. In addition, a person can transmit the virus to others up to 2 weeks before symptoms appear.

Diagnosis/Treatment

How Will I Know If I Have Hepatitis A? How Is Hepatitis A Diagnosed?

A doctor can determine if you have hepatitis A by discussing your symptoms and taking a blood sample.

How Is Hepatitis A Treated?

Unvaccinated people who have been exposed (within 2 weeks) to the hepatitis A virus should get the hepatitis A vaccine or a shot of immune globulin to prevent severe illness. To treat the symptoms of hepatitis A, doctors usually recommend rest, adequate nutrition, and fluids. Some people will need medical care in a hospital. It can take a few months before people with hepatitis A begin to feel better.

Prevention/Vaccination

Can Hepatitis A Be Prevented?

Yes. The best way to prevent hepatitis A is through vaccination with the hepatitis A vaccine. To get the full benefit of the hepatitis A vaccine, more than one shot is needed. The number and timing of these shots depend on the type of vaccine you are given. Practicing good hand hygiene—including thoroughly washing hands after using the bathroom, changing diapers, and before preparing or eating food—plays an important role in preventing the spread of hepatitis A.

Who Should Get Vaccinated against Hepatitis A?

The Advisory Committee on Immunization Practices (ACIP) recommends hepatitis A vaccination for the following people:

- All children at age 1 year
- Travelers to countries where hepatitis A is common
- Family and caregivers of adoptees from countries where hepatitis A is common
- Men who have sexual encounters with other men
- Users of recreational drugs, whether injected or not

- People with chronic or long-term liver disease, including hepatitis B or hepatitis C
- People with clotting-factor disorders
- People with direct contact with others who have hepatitis A
- Any person wishing to obtain immunity (protection)

How Is the Hepatitis A Vaccine Given?

The hepatitis A vaccine is safe and effective and given as 2 shots, 6 months apart. Both shots are needed for long-term protection. The hepatitis A vaccine also comes in a combination form, containing both hepatitis A and B vaccine, that can be given to anyone 18 years of age and older. This combination vaccine is given as 3 shots, over 6 months. All three shots are needed for long-term protection for both hepatitis A and B.

Is the Hepatitis A Vaccine Effective?

Yes, the hepatitis A vaccine is highly effective in preventing hepatitis A virus infection. A second hepatitis A shot results in long-term protection.

Is the Hepatitis A Vaccine Safe?

Yes, the hepatitis A vaccine is safe. No serious side effects have been reported from the hepatitis A vaccine. Soreness at the injection site is the most common side effect reported. As with any medicine, there is always a small risk that a serious problem could occur after someone gets the vaccine. However, the potential risks associated with hepatitis A are much greater than the potential risks associated with the hepatitis A vaccine. Since the licensure of the first hepatitis A vaccine in 1995, millions of doses of hepatitis A vaccine have been given in the United States and worldwide.

Who Should Not Receive the Hepatitis A Vaccine?

People who have ever had a serious allergic reaction to the hepatitis A vaccine or who are known to be allergic to any part of the hepatitis A vaccine should not receive the vaccine. Tell your doctor if you have any severe allergies. Also, the vaccine is not licensed for use in infants under age 1 year.

513

What Is Immune Globulin (IG)?

Immune globulin (IG) is a substance made from human blood plasma that contains antibodies that protect against infection. Immune globulin is a shot and provides short-term protection against hepatitis A for up to 2 months depending on the dosage given. IG is sometimes used before traveling to a country where hepatitis A is common. IG is also used to prevent infection after exposure to the hepatitis A virus but must be given within 2 weeks after exposure for the best protection.

Will the Hepatitis A Vaccine Protect Me from Other Forms of Hepatitis?

No, the hepatitis A vaccine will only protect you against hepatitis A. There is a separate vaccine available for hepatitis B. There is also a combination hepatitis A and hepatitis B vaccine that offers protection for both viruses. There is no vaccine for hepatitis C at this time.

Can Hepatitis A Vaccine Be Given to People with Compromised Immune Systems, Such as Hemodialysis Patients or People with Acquired Immunodeficiency Syndrome (AIDS)?

Yes. The hepatitis A vaccine is inactivated (not "live"), so it can be given to people with compromised immune systems.

Is It Harmful to Have an Extra Dose of Hepatitis A Vaccine or to Repeat the Entire Hepatitis A Vaccine Series?

No, getting extra doses of hepatitis A vaccine is not harmful.

What Should Be Done If the Last Dose of Hepatitis A Vaccine Is Delayed?

If the second dose has been delayed (more than 6 months since the first dose was given), the second, or last dose, should be given as soon as possible. The first dose does not need to be given again.

Where Can I Get the Hepatitis A Vaccine?

Speak with your health professional or call your local public health department, where free or low-cost vaccines for adults may be offered. For children, check the Vaccines for Children Program.

Hepatitis A Vaccine and International Travel

Who Should Get the Hepatitis A Vaccine before Traveling Internationally?

Anyone who is susceptible (unvaccinated or never had hepatitis A) and planning to travel to countries where hepatitis A is common should be vaccinated with the hepatitis A vaccine or immune globulin (IG) before traveling. Even travelers to urban areas, resorts, and luxury hotels in countries where hepatitis A is common are at high risk. Even travelers reporting that they maintained good hand hygiene and were careful about what they drank and ate have been infected when traveling to countries where hepatitis A is common.

How Soon before Travel Should I Get the Hepatitis A Vaccine?

You should get the first dose of hepatitis A vaccine as soon as you plan international travel to a country where hepatitis A is common. Two weeks or more before departure is ideal, but getting the vaccine any time before travel will provide some protection.

For optimal protection, older adults, people who are immunocompromised, and people with chronic liver disease or other chronic medical conditions who are planning to depart in less than 2 weeks should receive the first dose of vaccine and can get a shot of immune globulin at the same time, at a separate injection site.

I'm Leaving for My Trip in a Few Days; Can I Still Get the Hepatitis A Vaccine?

Experts say that the first dose of hepatitis A vaccine can be given any time before departure. This will provide some protection for most healthy people.

What Should I Do If I Am Traveling Internationally but Cannot Receive Hepatitis A Vaccine?

Travelers who are allergic to a vaccine component or who are younger than 12 months should receive a single dose of IG. IG provides effective protection against hepatitis A virus infection for up to 2 months, depending on the dosage given. If you are staying longer than two months, you can get another dose of IG for continued protection.

Section 37.2

Noroviruses

This section contains text excerpted from the following sources:
Text in this section begins with excerpts from "Norovirus Infections,"
MedlinePlus, National Institutes of Health (NIH), August 25, 2016;
Text beginning with the heading "Symptoms" is excerpted from
"About Norovirus," Centers for Disease Control
and Prevention (CDC), August 30, 2016.

Noroviruses are a group of related viruses. Infection with these viruses causes an illness called gastroenteritis, an inflammation of the stomach and intestines. It can spread from person to person, or through contaminated food or water. You can also get it if you touch a contaminated surface. Norovirus can be serious, especially for young children and older adults.

Treatment includes bed rest and lots of liquids to prevent dehydration. There is no specific medicine to treat norovirus infections.

Proper hand washing and safe food preparation may help prevent infections.

Symptoms

Norovirus causes inflammation of the stomach or intestines or both. This is called acute gastroenteritis.

The most common symptoms:

- diarrhea

- throwing up

- nausea

- stomach pain

Other symptoms:
- fever

- headache

- body aches

A person usually develops symptoms 12–48 hours after being exposed to norovirus. Most people with norovirus illness get better within 1–3 days.

If you have norovirus illness, you can feel extremely ill and throw up or have diarrhea many times a day. This can lead to dehydration, especially in young children, older adults, and people with other illnesses.

Symptoms of dehydration:

- decrease in urination

- dry mouth and throat

- feeling dizzy when standing up

Children who are dehydrated may cry with few or no tears and be unusually sleepy or fussy.

Transmission

Norovirus is a highly contagious virus. Anyone can get infected with norovirus and get sick. Also, you can get norovirus illness many times in your life. One reason for this is that there are many different types of noroviruses. Being infected with one type of norovirus may not protect you against other types.

Norovirus can be found in your stool (feces) even before you start feeling sick. The virus can stay in your stool for 2 weeks or more after you feel better.

You are most contagious:

- when you are sick with norovirus illness, and

- during the first few days after you recover from norovirus illness

You can become infected with norovirus by accidentally getting stool or vomit from infected people in your mouth. This usually happens by:

- eating food or drinking liquids that are contaminated with norovirus, touching surfaces or objects contaminated with norovirus then putting your fingers in your mouth

- having contact with someone who is infected with norovirus (for example, caring for or sharing food or eating utensils with someone with norovirus illness)

Norovirus can spread quickly in closed places like daycare centers, nursing homes, schools, and cruise ships. Most norovirus outbreaks happen from November to April in the United States.

Treatment

- There is no specific medicine to treat people with norovirus illness. Norovirus infection cannot be treated with antibiotics because it is a viral (not a bacterial) infection.

- If you have norovirus illness, you should drink plenty of liquids to replace fluid lost from throwing up and diarrhea. This will help prevent dehydration.

- Sports drinks and other drinks without caffeine or alcohol can help with mild dehydration. But, these drinks may not replace important nutrients and minerals. Oral rehydration fluids that you can get over the counter are most helpful for mild dehydration.

- Dehydration can lead to serious problems. Severe dehydration may require hospitalization for treatment with fluids given through your vein (intravenous or IV fluids). If you think you or someone you are caring for is severely dehydrated, call the doctor.

Preventing Norovirus Infection

Practice Proper Hand Hygiene

Wash your hands carefully with soap and water:

- especially after using the toilet and changing diapers
- always before eating, preparing, or handling food

Noroviruses can be found in your vomit or stool even before you start feeling sick. The virus can stay in your stool for 2 weeks or more after you feel better, so it is important to continue washing your hands often during this time.

Alcohol-based hand sanitizers can be used in addition to hand washing, but they should not be used as a substitute for washing with soap and water.

Wash Fruits and Vegetables and Cook Seafood Thoroughly

Carefully wash fruits and vegetables before preparing and eating them. Cook oysters and other shellfish thoroughly before eating them.

Be aware that noroviruses are relatively resistant. They can survive temperatures as high as 140°F and quick steaming processes that are often used for cooking shellfish.

Food that might be contaminated with norovirus should be thrown out.

Keep sick infants and children out of areas where food is being handled and prepared.

When You Are Sick, Do Not Prepare Food or Care for Others Who Are Sick

You should not prepare food for others or provide healthcare while you are sick and for at least 2 days after symptoms stop. This also applies to sick workers in settings such as schools and daycares where they may expose people to norovirus.

Many local and state health departments require that food workers and preparers with norovirus illness not work until at least 48 hours after symptoms stop. If you were recently sick, you can be given different duties in the restaurant, such as working at a cash register or hosting.

Clean and Disinfect Contaminated Surfaces

After throwing up or having diarrhea, immediately clean and disinfect contaminated surfaces. Use a chlorine bleach solution with a concentration of 1000–5000 ppm (5–25 tablespoons of household bleach (5.25%) per gallon of water) or other disinfectant registered as effective against norovirus by the U.S. Environmental Protection Agency (EPA).

Wash Laundry Thoroughly

Immediately remove and wash clothes or linens that may be contaminated with vomit or stool (feces).

You should:

- handle soiled items carefully without agitating them

- wear rubber or disposable gloves while handling soiled items and wash your hands after

- wash the items with detergent at the maximum available cycle length then machine dry them

Chapter 38

Acrylamide from High-Temperature Cooking

Frequently Asked Questions about Acrylamide

What Is Acrylamide?

Acrylamide is a chemical that can form in some foods during high-temperature cooking processes, such as frying, roasting, and baking. Acrylamide in food forms from sugars and an amino acid that are naturally present in food; it does not come from food packaging or the environment.

Is Acrylamide Something New in Food? When Was Acrylamide First Detected in Food?

Acrylamide has probably always been present in cooked foods. However, acrylamide was first detected in certain foods in April 2002.

This chapter contains text excerpted from the following sources: Text under the heading "Frequently Asked Questions about Acrylamide" is excerpted from "Food—Acrylamide Questions and Answers," U.S. Food and Drug Administration (FDA), November 29, 2017; Text under the heading "Tips for Cutting Down on Acrylamide" is excerpted from "You Can Help Cut Acrylamide in Your Diet," U.S. Food and Drug Administration (FDA), December 14, 2017.

How Does Acrylamide Form in Food?

Acrylamide forms from sugars and an amino acid (asparagine) during certain types of high-temperature cooking, such as frying, roasting, and baking.

What Kinds of Cooking Lead to Acrylamide Formation? In What Foods?

High-temperature cooking, such as frying, roasting, or baking, is most likely to cause acrylamide formation. Boiling and steaming do not typically form acrylamide. Acrylamide is found mainly in foods made from plants, such as potato products, grain products, or coffee. Acrylamide does not form, or forms at lower levels, in dairy, meat, and fish products. Generally, acrylamide is more likely to accumulate when cooking is done for longer periods or at higher temperatures.

Are Acrylamide Levels in Organic Foods Different from Levels in Other Foods?

Since acrylamide is formed through cooking, acrylamide levels in cooked organic foods should be similar to levels in cooked nonorganic foods.

What Is the U.S. Food and Drug Administration (FDA) Doing about Acrylamide in Food?

The FDA has initiated a number of activities on acrylamide since the discovery of acrylamide in food, including toxicology research, analytical methodology development, food surveys, exposure assessments, formation and mitigation research, and guidance for industry.

Should I Stop Eating Foods That Are Fried, Roasted, or Baked?

No. FDA's best advice for acrylamide and eating is that consumers adopt a healthy eating plan, consistent with the *Dietary Guidelines for Americans* (DGA) (2015–2020), that emphasizes fruits, vegetables, whole grains, and fat-free or low-fat milk and milk products; includes lean meats, poultry, fish, beans, eggs, and nuts; and limits saturated fats, trans fats, cholesterol, salt (sodium), and added sugars.

Is Acrylamide Found Anywhere Else?

Acrylamide is produced industrially for use in products such as plastics, grouts, water treatment products, and cosmetics. Acrylamide is also found in cigarette smoke.

Tips for Cutting Down on Acrylamide

Given the widespread presence of acrylamide in foods, it isn't feasible to completely eliminate acrylamide from one's diet. Nor is it necessary. Removing any one or two foods from your diet would not have a significant effect on overall exposure to acrylamide.

However, here are some steps you can take to help decrease the amount of acrylamide that you and your family consume:

- Frying causes acrylamide formation. If frying frozen fries, follow manufacturers' recommendations on time and temperature and avoid overcooking, heavy crisping or burning.

- Toast bread to a light brown color rather than a dark brown color. Avoid very brown areas.

- Cook cut potato products such as frozen french fries to a golden yellow color rather than a brown color. Brown areas tend to contain more acrylamide.

- Do not store potatoes in the refrigerator, which can increase acrylamide during cooking. Keep potatoes outside the refrigerator in a dark, cool place, such as a closet or a pantry.

FDA also recommends that you adopt a healthy eating plan, consistent with the Dietary Guidelines for Americans, that:

- Emphasizes fruits, vegetables, whole grains, and fat-free or low-fat milk and milk products;

- Includes lean meats, poultry, fish, beans, eggs, and nuts; and

- Limits saturated fats, trans fats, cholesterol, salt (sodium), and added sugars.

Chapter 39

Aflatoxins

What Are Aflatoxins?

Aflatoxins are a family of toxins produced by certain fungi that are found on agricultural crops such as maize (corn), peanuts, cottonseed, and tree nuts. The main fungi that produce aflatoxins are *Aspergillus flavus* and *Aspergillus parasiticus*, which are abundant in warm and humid regions of the world. Aflatoxin-producing fungi can contaminate crops in the field, at harvest, and during storage.

How Are People Exposed to Aflatoxins?

People can be exposed to aflatoxins by eating contaminated plant products (such as peanuts) or by consuming meat or dairy products from animals that ate contaminated feed. Farmers and other agricultural workers may be exposed by inhaling dust generated during the handling and processing of contaminated crops and feeds.

This chapter contains text excerpted from the following sources: Text beginning with the heading "What Are Aflatoxins?" is excerpted from "Aflatoxins," National Cancer Institute (NCI), March 20, 2015; Text beginning with the heading "Aflatoxin Monitoring" is excerpted from "Breaking the Mold: New Strategies for Fighting Aflatoxins," Environmental Health Perspectives (EHP), National Institute of Environmental Health Sciences (NIEHS), September 1, 2013. Reviewed April 2018.

Aflatoxin Monitoring

By comparison, says Felicia Wu, Hannah Distinguished Professor of Food Science and Human Nutrition at Michigan State University (MSU), aflatoxin monitoring is rare in developing countries, with the exception of grains and nuts headed for export. "Even in countries where standards for aflatoxin exist, they may not always be enforced," she says. "Subsistence farmers just eat what they grow; lack of awareness about aflatoxin is a serious issue." In some cases, moldy foods are eaten simply because other foods might not be available, says Bowman.

Early harvest and rapid mechanical drying are big factors in U.S. farmers' ability to keep aflatoxin levels down in difficult years. The toxin forms at 25 percent moisture, down to about 17 percent. If the corn has to stand in the field warm and humid at these moistures, the risk is high. For the most part, aflatoxin monitoring requires expensive technologies, such as enzyme-linked immunosorbent assay (ELISA) test kits, high-performance liquid chromatography, and mass spectrometers.

The best way to minimize aflatoxin risk is to try to prevent the poison from getting into foods in the first place. Once it's in the food supply, aflatoxin becomes very difficult to manage. It tends to affect crops across very large agricultural areas.

Exposure to Aflatoxins and Health Risks

Liver Effects

Aflatoxins were first recognized as a health risk in the mid-twentieth century, when they were revealed as the cause of death among turkeys eating *A. flavus*–contaminated feed. Studies later showed that aflatoxin B1 causes liver cancer in nonhuman primates, rodents, and fish, as well as in humans. The International Agency for Research on Cancer (IARC) of the World Health Organization (WHO) classified aflatoxins as a Group 1 carcinogen (definitely carcinogenic to humans) in 1987, and analysis of additional data in 2002 reaffirmed this categorization.

Liver failure also occurs in highly exposed humans suffering from a condition known as aflatoxicosis. During an outbreak of aflatoxicosis that killed over 125 people in Kenya in 2004, victims experienced abdominal pain, pulmonary edema, liver necrosis, and finally death after ingesting doses of aflatoxin B1 estimated at 50 mg per day. People with hepatitis B face up to a roughly 30-fold elevated cancer risk from aflatoxin, compared with people exposed to aflatoxin only.

Confronting the Problem

Reducing those exposures can be accomplished by combining a number of good practices, such as early harvesting during weather patterns that favor *Aspergillus* infections (followed by rapid drying and storage of the crop), separating poor- and good-quality grain, drying to reduce grain moisture content, and using storage containers that minimize temperature and moisture conditions that favor fungal growth. In addition, it helps if farmers and others use good sampling practices and inexpensive tests for aflatoxins to remove bad grain at various points in the agricultural supply chain.

The Partnership for Aflatoxin Control in Africa (PACA), the United States Agency for International Development (USAID), and other organizations emphasize promoting field-based biocontrol methods that can prevent *Aspergillus* from taking hold. The leading biocontrol method was developed by Peter Cotty, a research plant pathologist at the U.S. Department of Agriculture (USDA) and an adjunct professor at the University of Arizona. Cotty's biocontrol method, now patented by the USDA Agricultural Research Service (USDA-ARS), is gaining in popularity.

Chapter 40

Perchlorates

The terms "perchlorate" or "perchlorate anion" refer to a negatively charged group of atoms consisting of a central chlorine atom
bonded to four oxygen atoms. Perchlorate has the molecular formula
ClO4. The terms "perchlorates" or "perchlorate salts" refer to the
inorganic compounds that contain the perchlorate anion bonded to a
positively charged group such as ammonium or an alkali or alkaline
earth metal.

Perchlorates can form naturally in the atmosphere, leading to trace
levels of perchlorate in precipitation. High levels of perchlorates occur
naturally in some locations, such as regions of west Texas and northern Chile.

Perchlorates are colorless and have no odor. Five perchlorates are
manufactured in large amounts: magnesium perchlorate, potassium
perchlorate, ammonium perchlorate, sodium perchlorate, and lithium
perchlorate. Perchlorates are found in the environment in two forms,
either as a solid or dissolved in water. If no water is present, as in
a drum or on top of the dry ground, then they will exist as solids. If
water is present, then they will quickly dissolve. When perchlorates
dissolve, they separate into two parts. One part has a positive charge,
and the other part has a negative charge. The part with the negative
charge is called the perchlorate anion or just perchlorate. This is the

This chapter includes text excerpted from "Public Health Statement for Perchlorates," Agency for Toxic Substances and Disease Registry (ATSDR), Centers
for Disease Control and Prevention (CDC), January 21, 2015.

part of the chemical that people look for in the environment or in your body.

Perchlorates are stable at normal temperatures, but when they are heated to a high temperature, they begin to react. Once they begin to react, they produce a large amount of heat. This causes more of the perchlorates to begin reacting, which makes even more heat. This chain reaction process repeats itself over and over until an explosion occurs. Because perchlorates react this way, they are used in rocket motors, fireworks, flares, gunpowder, and explosives.

Because perchlorates can react quickly at high temperatures, people did not expect to find them in the environment. But at normal Earth temperatures, perchlorates react much more slowly. It's learned only recently that perchlorates may last in the environment unreacted for several years.

One of the perchlorate salts, ammonium perchlorate, is produced in large amounts because it is used in rocket fuels. The solid booster rocket on the space shuttle is almost 70 percent ammonium perchlorate. Perchlorates are also used in explosives. Because perchlorates are used for some military applications, many countries consider the amounts that they make confidential. This is one reason why the exact amount of perchlorates produced or used in the United States or around the world is not known. As with most chemicals, private companies in the United States are not required to provide information on the amount of perchlorates that they make or use. The exact amount of perchlorates brought into the United States from other countries, although the largest amount probably comes from fireworks is also not known. It is important to note that production figures for a limited set of the larger profile of perchlorate applications do not readily translate into environmental release data or accurately characterize the universe of perchlorate uses and potential for release.

Other uses of perchlorates include temporary adhesives, electrolysis baths, batteries, airbags, drying agents, etching agents, cleaning agents and bleach, and oxygen generating systems. Little data is available on the nature, amount, and potential for release of these possible sources of perchlorate to the environment. Perchlorates are also used for making other chemicals. Many years ago, perchlorates were used as a medication in the United States to treat overactive thyroid glands, and they still have some medical uses in the United States and other parts of the world. Perchlorate is also used in the treatment of side effects of amiodarone, a drug used in the treatment of cardiac arrhythmias and angina.

What Happens to Perchlorates When They Enter the Environment?

Perchlorates are soluble in water and generally have high mobility in soils. This characteristic results in their ability to move from soil surfaces into groundwater (a process called leaching) when they enter the environment. Perchlorates are ionic substances and, therefore, do not volatilize from water or soil surfaces. Perchlorates are known to remain unreacted in the environment for long periods of time; however, there is evidence that microorganisms found in soil and water may eventually reduce perchlorate to other substances. If perchlorates are released to air, then they will eventually settle out of the air, primarily in rainfall. Perchlorates do not appear to accumulate in animals. The understanding of perchlorates continues to evolve, and scientific understanding related to perchlorates will continue to be reviewed and re-evaluated when new information becomes available.

Before 1997, it was very hard to measure perchlorates in the environment. In 1997, a much better method was developed, and low levels of perchlorates in water and other media can now be measured. Scientists first began looking for perchlorates near sites where they had been used or discarded and were surprised when they found them in many other places, including areas where there was no known perchlorate use. They did not think that perchlorates would last very long in the environment because of perchlorate's reactivity. Since then, scientists have been looking for perchlorates in water at more and more places. Perchlorates have recently been found in environmental media such as soil, plants, and animals located in areas where perchlorate was used and released, and in areas where there was no known use or man-made releases of perchlorates.

Perchlorates can enter the environment from several sources, both human-made (called anthropogenic) and natural sources. Since perchlorate is used in rockets and certain military applications, the manufacture, use, and disposal of products like rockets and missiles have led to perchlorate being released into the environment. When rockets undergo successful launches, the intense heat leads to nearly complete reaction of the perchlorate. Therefore, the release of perchlorate to the environment often occurs when its intended use does not occur (for example, dismantling and disposal of rockets, an accidental release from manufacturing facilities, or unsuccessful rocket launches). In the past, some of these activities resulted in high levels of perchlorate contamination of soil and groundwater at many military installations and rocket manufacturing facilities. Today, great effort is made to minimize the release of perchlorates when rockets or missiles are dismantled or when perchlorates are manufactured. Other human-made sources for perchlorate release into the environment include roadside safety flares and fireworks. Perchlorate has also been detected at low levels as an impurity in certain consumer products such as bleach, and the use and disposal of these products could also lead to releases.

Perchlorate is a natural component of a nitrate fertilizer from Chile that was imported and regularly used in the United States for many years. Although the use of this fertilizer has declined in recent years, perchlorate was released directly to soil and plants in areas where this fertilizer was applied. In addition, there appear to be natural sources of perchlorate in the environment. Perchlorates can form naturally in the atmosphere, leading to trace levels of perchlorate in rainfall. Higher than expected levels of perchlorates occur naturally in some locations such as regions of west Texas, New Mexico, and northern Chile. A combination of human activities and natural sources has led to the widespread presence of perchlorates in the environment.

How Might I Be Exposed to Perchlorates?

You may be exposed to perchlorates if you eat food or drink water that contains perchlorates. Perchlorates have been found in food and milk. Some plants, especially leafy green vegetables, have been found to have elevated levels of perchlorate. When water containing perchlorate is used to irrigate the plants, perchlorate is left behind when water evaporates from the leaves of the plants. Cows may eat fodder containing perchlorate and pass them on in their milk. The U.S. Food and Drug Administration (FDA) recently published the results of measurements of perchlorate and iodine levels in the food supply. The FDA found that 74 percent of the foods analyzed had at least one sample in which perchlorate was detected. The perchlorate dietary intake was estimated for 14 different age/gender groups in the United States. The FDA did not recommend any changes in eating habits of Americans based upon the measured levels of perchlorate.

Perchlorates have been found in lakes, rivers, and groundwater wells. Perchlorate has been identified at least once in approximately 4 percent of over 3,800 community water systems sampled throughout the United States.

Additional potential sources of perchlorate may be found if you live near a rocket manufacturing or testing facility, if you live near or work at a factory where they are made, or if you live near a factory that makes fireworks, flares, or other explosive devices. As mentioned earlier, perchlorate is being found in small amounts in areas where it has not been known to be manufactured, used, or released by humans. Exposure to perchlorates at these locations may be possible because natural levels of perchlorates occur in the environment.

Perchlorate has been detected at low levels as an impurity in certain products that are commonly used by humans. Some of these products include bleach and cleaning products that may contain bleach, bottled water, and tobacco products; even some nutritional supplements (vitamins and minerals) have been found to contain perchlorates. However, vitamin and mineral supplements are typically formulated to include iodine, a factor that would provide protection against any possible effect of perchlorate.

How Can Perchlorates Enter and Leave My Body?

Perchlorates can enter the body after you have swallowed food or water containing them. Since they easily dissolve in water, they quickly pass through the stomach and intestines and enter the bloodstream. If you breathe in air containing dust or droplets of perchlorate, it can pass through your lungs and enter the bloodstream. Perchlorates probably do not enter the body directly through the skin, but if present on your hands, hand-to-mouth-activity could contribute to oral exposure.

The bloodstream carries perchlorate to all parts of the body. Perchlorate is not changed inside the body. A few internal organs (for example, the thyroid, breast tissue, and salivary glands) can take up relatively large amounts of perchlorate from the bloodstream. Perchlorate generally leaves these organs in a few hours.

When perchlorates are swallowed, a small percentage is eliminated in the feces. More than 90 percent of perchlorate taken in by mouth enters the bloodstream. In the blood, perchlorate passes into the kidneys, which then release it into the urine. The body begins to clear itself of perchlorate through the kidneys within 10 minutes of exposure. Although most of the perchlorate that is taken into the body is quickly eliminated, the presence of perchlorate in many foods and in some drinking water sources means that exposure may continue to occur on a daily basis.

How Can Perchlorates Affect My Health?

The main target organ for perchlorate toxicity in humans is the thyroid gland. Perchlorate has been shown to partially inhibit the thyroid's uptake of iodine. Iodine is required as a building block for the synthesis of thyroid hormone. Thyroid hormones regulate certain body functions after they are released into the blood. Although not demonstrated in humans, it is anticipated that people exposed to excessive amounts of perchlorate for a long time may develop a decreased production of thyroid hormones. The medical name for this condition is hypothyroidism. Hypothyroidism is usually caused by conditions totally unrelated to perchlorates. In hypothyroidism, the lower amounts of thyroid hormones in your blood cause increases in pituitary hormones that can lead to an increase in the size of the thyroid gland. The medical name for this condition is goiter. Because thyroid hormones perform important functions throughout the body, many normal body activities also are affected by the lower hormone levels. Because perchlorates were known to lower thyroid hormone levels, at one time, perchlorates were given as a drug (more than 400 mg per day, which is many times higher than the doses that people receive from environmental exposures) to treat people with overactive thyroid glands (a condition known as hyperthyroidism). Side effects seen in a small number of treated patients were skin rashes, nausea, and vomiting. A few patients developed severe shortages of blood cells, and some of them died. Healthy volunteers who took approximately 35 mg of perchlorate every day (equivalent to drinking 2 liters of water containing 17 mg/L or 17 parts per million (ppm) perchlorate every day) for 2 weeks or 3 mg daily for 6 months (equivalent to drinking 2 liters of water containing 1.5 mg/L (1.5 ppm). perchlorate every day) showed no signs of abnormal functioning of their thyroid gland. A study of adults in Nevada found that the number of cases of thyroid disease in a group of people who drank water contaminated with perchlorate was no different than the number of cases found in a group of people who drank water without perchlorate. This means that levels of perchlorate in the water were not the cause of the thyroid disease, and a search of the literature confirms no evidence of perchlorate inducing thyroid disease. Two studies of people who worked for years in the production of perchlorate found no evidence of alterations in the workers' thyroids, livers, kidneys, or blood. One of these studies estimated that the workers may have taken up about 34 mg of perchlorate per day. A recent study showed that perchlorate levels to which the general population of the United States is exposed via food and drinking water, were associated with changes in thyroid hormone levels in women with low iodine intake, suggesting that the effect of perchlorate in people depends on gender, the length of exposure, and how much iodine the people consume. Further research is recommended to affirm these findings.

Perchlorate is a naturally occurring chemical that has been found in some foods and in some drinking water supplies. Other naturally occurring chemicals, such as thiocyanate (in food and cigarette smoke) and nitrate (in some food), are also known to inhibit iodide uptake. Further studies are needed to completely answer all questions about the potential toxicity of perchlorate.

The thyroid gland is also the main target organ for perchlorate toxicity in animals. The thyroid changes caused by perchlorate in animals may lead to tumors in the thyroid after a long period. This has occurred after administering high amounts (928–2,573 milligrams perchlorate/kg/day) of perchlorate to the animals. The National Academy of Sciences (NAS) concluded that based on the understanding of the biology of human and rodent thyroid tumors, it is unlikely that perchlorate poses a risk of thyroid cancer in humans. Perchlorates have not been classified for carcinogenic effects by the U.S. Department of Health and Human Services (DHHS) or the International Agency for Research on Cancer (IARC). The U.S. Environmental Protection Agency (EPA) has determined that perchlorate is not likely to pose a risk of thyroid cancer in humans, at least at doses below those necessary to alter thyroid hormone homeostasis, based on the hormonally-mediated mode of action in rodent studies and species differences in thyroid function.

Studies in animals also showed that perchlorate did not affect the reproductive organs or the animals' capacity to reproduce. The NAS found that the studies in animals provided important information, but their usefulness to predict whether harmful effects could occur in humans is small.

How Can Perchlorates Affect Children?

This section discusses potential health effects in humans from exposures during the period from conception to maturity at 18 years of age.

Children and developing fetuses may be more likely to be affected by perchlorate than adults because thyroid hormones are essential for normal growth and development. Two studies were conducted of newborn babies and school-age children from an area in Chile where levels of perchlorate in the drinking water were much higher than those detected in some U.S. water supplies due to natural sources of perchlorate. No evidence of abnormal thyroid function was found among the babies or the children. The mothers and the children may have taken approximately 0.2 mg of perchlorate per day in the drinking water. Some studies of newborn babies in areas from Arizona, California, and Nevada, where perchlorate has been found in the drinking water, have not provided convincing evidence of thyroid abnormalities associated with perchlorate. The Centers for Disease Control and Prevention (CDC) study of people all over the United States showed that all of the people that were tested had detectable concentrations of perchlorate in their urine, thus making it difficult to find an unexposed comparison group as a control population.

As indicated above, perchlorate has been found in breast milk, so that nursing mothers can transfer perchlorate to their babies. Nevertheless, the beneficial aspects (biological and psychological) of breastfeeding outweigh any risks from exposure to perchlorate from mother's milk, especially if they consume adequate iodine from food and supplements.

Animal studies have shown a low level of thyroid activity in developing animals exposed to perchlorates through the placenta before birth or through the mother's milk after birth. Modern studies of the effects of perchlorate on developing animals have been conducted mostly in rats. Several studies in which pregnant rats were given relatively low amounts of perchlorate have shown that perchlorate can alter the thyroid gland in the newborn animals. This has generally occurred when perchlorate also affected the thyroid of the mothers. In addition, a study suggested an alteration in an area of the brain of pups born to rats. The NAS indicated that rats are more sensitive to agents that disturb thyroid function than are humans, so the relevance of rat studies in quantitative terms to humans is limited.

How Can Families Reduce the Risk of Exposure to Perchlorates?

Although perchlorate is present in food, milk, and drinking water, it is very unlikely that it will be present in the air of the average home or apartment. Perchlorates are found in some consumer products that people use. They are present in highway and marine signal flares, small fireworks, gunpowder, and matches. Storing these items out of the reach of children and not igniting them in a closed environment, such as inside the house or the garage, will decrease the potential for exposure.

Although perchlorate has been detected in a few samples of bottled water, the levels have been very low. Therefore, if you live near a location where perchlorates have been found in drinking water at high levels, using bottled drinking water may reduce the risk to your family, particularly if you drink well water that may contain perchlorate. If you live in one of these areas, prevent your children from playing in the dirt and from eating dirt. Make sure your children wash their hands frequently, and before eating. Discourage your children from putting their hands in their mouths or doing other hand-to-mouth activities. You may also contact local public health authorities and follow their advice.

If you work in a factory that makes or uses perchlorates, it is possible to carry perchlorate dust from work on your clothing, skin, or hair. You may then get perchlorate dust in your car, home, or other locations outside of work where family members might be exposed. You should know about this possibility if you work with perchlorates. Taking a shower will remove any perchlorate dust from your skin or hair. Washing your clothes will remove any perchlorates dust from them.

Is There a Medical Test to Determine Whether I Have Been Exposed to Perchlorates?

Methods to measure perchlorate in the body are not routinely available, but perchlorate can be measured in the urine. Because perchlorate leaves the body fairly rapidly (in a matter of hours), perchlorate in the urine can only indicate very recent exposure. Levels of thyroid hormones in the blood can be monitored. Such tests will tell you if your hormone levels are altered, but will not tell you the cause (exposure to perchlorate is only one of many possibilities). Medical tests can also measure the capacity of the thyroid gland to take iodide from the blood to manufacture thyroid hormones. Exposure to perchlorate can decrease this capacity, but so can exposure to other chemicals, as well as iodine deficiency and medical conditions unrelated to any exposure to chemicals.

Chapter 41

Consumer Beverages

Chapter Contents

Section 41.1

Benzene in Commercial Beverages

This section includes text excerpted from "Food—
Questions and Answers on the Occurrence of Benzene in
Soft Drinks and Other Beverages," U.S. Food and
Drug Administration (FDA), January 24, 2018.

Benzene is a chemical that is released into the air from emissions from automobiles and burning coal and oil. It is also used in the manufacture of a wide range of industrial products, including chemicals, dyes, detergents, and some plastics.

Why Benzene Is a Concern

Benzene is a carcinogen that can cause cancer in humans. It has caused cancer in workers exposed to high levels from workplace air. Based on results from a Center for Food Safety and Applied Nutrition (CFSAN) survey of almost 200 samples of soft drinks and other beverages tested for benzene, a small number of products sampled contained more than 5 parts per billion (ppb) of benzene. The manufacturers have reformulated products, if still manufactured, which were identified in the survey as containing greater than 5 ppb benzene. CFSAN tested samples of these reformulated products and found that benzene levels were less than 1.5 ppb. The U.S. Environmental Protection Agency (EPA) has established a maximum allowable level (MCL) for benzene in drinking water of 5 ppb. The U.S. Food and Drug Administration (FDA) has adopted EPA's MCL for drinking water as an allowable level for bottled water.

Levels of Benzene in Beverages and Risk to Public Health

The results of CFSAN's survey indicate that the levels of benzene found in beverages to date do not pose a safety concern for consumers. Almost all samples analyzed in the survey contained either no benzene or levels below 5 ppb. Furthermore, benzene levels in hundreds of samples tested by national and international government agencies and the beverage industry are consistent with those found in the survey.

Benzene in Beverages

Benzene can form at very low levels (ppb level) in some beverages that contain both benzoate salts and ascorbic acid (vitamin C) or erythorbic acid (a closely related substance (isomer) also known as d-ascorbic acid). Exposure to heat and light can stimulate the formation of benzene in some beverages that contain benzoate salts and ascorbic acid (vitamin C). Sodium or potassium benzoate may be added to beverages to inhibit the growth of bacteria, yeasts, and molds. Benzoate salts also are naturally present in some fruits and their juices, such as cranberries, for example. Vitamin C may be present naturally in beverages or added to prevent spoilage or to provide additional nutrients.

Steps for Reducing or Eliminating Benzene in Beverages

The FDA is working with the beverage industry to minimize benzene formation in products. For example, it has met with industry to determine the factors contributing to benzene formation. The FDA has directly contacted those firms whose products were tested and found to contain more than 5 ppb benzene in the survey. Manufacturers have reformulated products to ensure benzene levels are minimized or eliminated. The International Council of Beverages Associations (ICBA) and the American Beverage Association (ABA) have developed guidance for all beverage manufacturers on ways to minimize benzene formation.

How the Problem Was Identified

The FDA first became aware that benzene was present in some soft drinks in 1990. At that time, the soft drink industry informed the agency that benzene could form at low levels in some beverages that contained both benzoate salts and ascorbic acid. The FDA and beverage industry initiated research at that time to identify factors contributing to benzene formation. This research found that elevated temperature and light can stimulate benzene formation in the presence of benzoate salts and ascorbic acid. As a result of these findings, many

541

manufacturers reformulated their products to reduce or eliminate benzene formation.

In November 2005, the FDA received reports that benzene had been detected at low levels in some soft drinks containing benzoate salts and ascorbic acid. CFSAN immediately initiated a survey of benzene levels in soft drinks and other beverages. The vast majority of the beverages sampled to date (including those containing both benzoate salts and ascorbic acid) contained either no detectable benzene or levels well below the 5 ppb EPA MCL for benzene in drinking water.

Products with Excessive Levels of Benzene

To date, the FDA has tested almost 200 soft drink and other beverages in the CFSAN survey. Benzene above 5 ppb was found in a total of ten products. Benzene above 5 ppb was found in nine of the beverage products that contain both added benzoate salts and ascorbic acid. The FDA also found benzene above 5 ppb in one cranberry juice beverage with added ascorbic acid but no added benzoates (cranberries contain natural benzoates). The manufacturers have reformulated products, if still manufactured, which were identified in the survey as containing greater than 5 ppb benzene. CFSAN tested samples of these reformulated products and found that benzene levels were less than 1.5 ppb.

Section 41.2

Juice Safety: What You Need to Know

This section includes text excerpted from "Food—Talking about Juice Safety: What You Need to Know," U.S. Food and Drug Administration (FDA), November 15, 2017.

When fruits and vegetables are fresh-squeezed or used raw, bacteria from the produce can end up in your juice or cider. Unless the produce or the juice has been pasteurized or otherwise treated to destroy any harmful bacteria, the juice could be contaminated. The U.S. Food and Drug Administration (FDA) has received, in the past, reports of outbreaks of foodborne illness, often called "food poisoning," that have been traced to drinking fruit and vegetable juice and cider that has not been treated to kill harmful bacteria.

While most people's immune systems can usually fight off the effects of foodborne illness, children, older adults, pregnant women, and people with weakened immune systems (such as transplant patients and individuals with human immunodeficiency virus (HIV)/acquired immunodeficiency syndrome (AIDS), cancer, or diabetes) risk serious illnesses or even death from drinking untreated juices.

Warning Labels

Most of the juice sold in the United States is pasteurized (heat-treated) to kill harmful bacteria. Juice products may also be treated by nonheat processes for the same purpose. However, some grocery stores, health food stores, cider mills, farmers' markets, and juice bars sell packaged juice that was made on site that has not been pasteurized or otherwise treated to ensure its safety. These untreated products should be kept under refrigeration and are required to carry the following warning on the label:

WARNING. This product has not been pasteurized and, therefore, may contain harmful bacteria that can cause serious illness in children, the elderly, and persons with weakened immune systems.

However, the FDA does not require warning labels for juice or cider that is sold by the glass—for example, at apple orchards, farmers' markets, roadside stands, juice bars, and some restaurants.

Steps to Prevent Illness

Follow these simple steps to prevent illness.
When purchasing juice:

- Look for the warning label to avoid the purchase of untreated juices. You can find pasteurized or otherwise treated products in your grocers' refrigerated sections, frozen food cases, or in nonrefrigerated containers, such as juice boxes, bottles, or cans. Untreated juice is most likely to be sold in the refrigerated section of a grocery store.

- Ask if you are unsure if a juice product is treated, especially for juices sold in refrigerated cases in grocery or health food stores, cider mills, or farmers' markets. Also, don't hesitate to ask if the labeling is unclear or if the juice or cider is sold by the glass.

When preparing juice at home:

- Wash your hands for at least 20 seconds with soap and warm water before and after preparation.

- Cut away any damaged or bruised areas on fresh fruits and vegetables. Throw away any produce that looks rotten.

- Wash all produce thoroughly under running water before cutting or cooking, including produce grown at home or bought from a grocery store or farmers' market. Washing fruits and vegetables with soap, detergent, or commercial produce wash is not recommended.

- Scrub firm produce, such as melons and cucumbers, with a clean produce brush. Even if you plan to peel the produce before juicing it, wash it first so dirt and bacteria are not transferred from the surface when peeling or cutting into it.

- After washing, dry produce with a clean cloth towel or paper towel to further reduce bacteria that may be present on the surface.

About Foodborne Illness

Know the Symptoms

Consuming dangerous foodborne bacteria will usually cause illness within 1–3 days of eating the contaminated food. However, sickness can also occur within 20 minutes or up to 6 weeks later. Although most people will recover from a foodborne illness within a short period of time, some can develop chronic, severe, or even life-threatening health problems.

Foodborne illness can sometimes be confused with other illnesses that have similar symptoms. The symptoms of foodborne illness can include:

- Vomiting, diarrhea, and abdominal pain

- Flu-like symptoms, such as fever, headache, and body ache

Take Action

If you think that you or a family member has a foodborne illness, contact your healthcare provider immediately. Also, report the suspected foodborne illness to the FDA in either of these ways:

- Contact the consumer complaint coordinator in your area

- Contact MedWatch, the FDA's Safety Information and Adverse Event Reporting Program:

  - **By Phone:** 800-FDA-1088 (800-332-1088)

  - **Online:** File a voluntary report at www.fda.gov/medwatch

Chapter 42

Technologically Altered Foods

Chapter Contents

547

Section 42.1

Food from Genetically Engineered Plants

This section includes text excerpted from "Food—Consumer Info about Food from Genetically Engineered Plants," U.S. Food and Drug Administration (FDA), January 4, 2018.

The U.S. Food and Drug Administration (FDA) regulates the safety of food for humans and animals, including foods produced from genetically engineered (GE) plants. Foods from GE plants must meet the same food safety requirements as foods derived from traditionally bred plants.

While genetic engineering is sometimes referred to as "genetic modification" producing "genetically modified organisms (GMOs)," FDA considers "genetic engineering" to be the more precise term.

Crop improvement happens all the time, and genetic engineering is just one form of it. The term "genetic engineering" is used to refer to genetic modification practices that utilize modern biotechnology. In this process, scientists make targeted changes to a plant's genetic makeup to give the plant a new desirable trait. For example, two new apple varieties have been genetically engineered to resist browning associated with cuts and bruises by reducing levels of enzymes that can cause browning.

Humans have been modifying crops for thousands of years through selective breeding. Early farmers developed cross-breeding methods to grow numerous corn varieties with a range of colors, sizes, and uses. For example, the garden strawberries that consumers buy today resulted from a cross between a strawberry species native to North America and a strawberry species native to South America.

Need for Genetically Engineered (GE) Plants

Developers breed GE plants for many of the same reasons that traditional breeding is used. They may want to create plants with better flavor, higher crop yield (output), greater resistance to insect damage, and immunity to plant diseases. Traditional breeding involves repeatedly cross-pollinating plants until the breeder identifies offspring with the desired combination of traits. The breeding process introduces a number of genes into the plant. These genes may include the gene responsible for the desired trait, as well as genes responsible for unwanted characteristics.

GE isolates the gene for the desired trait, adds it to a single plant cell in a laboratory, and generates a new plant from that cell. By narrowing the introduction to only one desired gene from the donor organism, scientists can eliminate unwanted characteristics from the donor's other genes. GE is often used in conjunction with a traditional breeding to produce the genetically engineered plant varieties on the market today.

Am I Eating Food from GE Plants?

Foods from GE plants were introduced into our food supply in the 1990s. Cotton, corn, and soybeans are the most common GE crops grown in the United States In 2012, GE soybeans accounted for 93 percent of all soybeans planted, and GE corn accounted for 88 percent of corn planted.

The majority of GE plants are used to make ingredients that are then used in other food products. Such ingredients include:

- Cornstarch in soups and sauces

- Corn syrup used as a sweetener

- Corn oil, canola oil, and soybean oil in mayonnaise, salad dressings, bread, and snack foods

- Sugar from sugar beets in various foods

Other major crops with GE varieties include potatoes, squash, apples, and papayas.

Are Foods from GE Plants Safe to Eat?

The FDA has determined that credible evidence has demonstrated that foods from the GE plant varieties marketed to date are as safe as comparable, non-GE foods.

Are Foods from GE Plants Regulated?

Yes. The FDA regulates foods from GE crops in conjunction with the U.S. Department of Agriculture (USDA) and U.S. Environmental Protection Agency (EPA).

the FDA enforces the U.S. food safety laws that prohibit unsafe food. GE plants must meet the same legal requirements that apply to all food. To help ensure that firms are meeting their obligation to market only safe and lawful foods, the FDA encourages developers of GE plants to consult with the agency before marketing their products.

The mission of the USDA's Animal and Plant Health Inspection Service (APHIS) is to safeguard the health, welfare, and value of American agriculture and natural resources, including regulating the introduction of certain genetically engineered organisms that may pose a risk to plant health.

EPA regulates pesticides, including those genetically engineered into food crops, to make sure that pesticides are safe for human and animal consumption and won't harm the environment.

How the FDA Evaluates the Safety of GE Plants

During the FDA consultation process, the food developer conducts a safety assessment. This safety assessment identifies the distinguishing attributes of the new traits in the plant and assesses whether any new material in food made from the GE plant is safe when eaten by humans or animals. As part of this assessment, the developer compares the levels of nutrients and other components in the food to those in food from traditionally bred plants or other comparable foods.

The developer submits a summary of its safety assessment to the FDA for the FDA's evaluation. When the safety assessment is received by the FDA, scientists carefully evaluate the data and information. The FDA considers the consultation to be complete only when its team of scientists is satisfied that the developer's safety assessment has adequately addressed all safety and other regulatory issues.

Section 42.2

Cloned Meat and Dairy

This section includes text excerpted from "Animal Cloning and Food Safety," U.S. Food and Drug Administration (FDA), November 29, 2017.

After years of detailed study and analysis, the U.S. Food and Drug Administration (FDA) has concluded that meat and milk from clones of cattle, swine (pigs), and goats, and the offspring of clones from any species traditionally consumed as food, are as safe to eat as food from conventionally bred animals. This conclusion stems from an extensive study of animal cloning and related food safety, culminating in the release of three FDA documents in January 2008: a risk assessment, a risk management plan, and guidance for industry.

Researchers have been cloning livestock species since 1996, starting with the famous sheep named Dolly. When it became apparent in 2001 that cloning could become a commercial venture to help improve the quality of herds, the FDA's Center for Veterinary Medicine (CVM) asked livestock producers to voluntarily keep food from clones and their offspring out of the food chain until CVM could further evaluate the issue.

FDA Studies Cloning

For more than five years, CVM scientists studied hundreds of published reports and other detailed information on clones of livestock animals to evaluate the safety of food from these animals. The resulting report, called a risk assessment, presents the FDA's conclusions that:

- cloning poses no unique risks to animal health, compared to the risks found with other reproduction methods, including natural mating

- the composition of food products from cattle, swine, and goat clones, or the offspring of any animal clones, is no different from that of conventionally bred animals

- because of the preceding two conclusions, there are no additional risks to people eating food from cattle, swine, and goat clones or the offspring of any animal clones traditionally consumed as food

The FDA issued the risk assessment, the risk management plan, and guidance for industry in draft form for public comment in December 2006. Since that time, the FDA has updated the risk assessment to reflect new scientific information that reinforces the food safety conclusions of the draft.

The FDA's concern about animal health prompted the agency to develop a risk management plan to decrease any risks to animals involved in cloning. The FDA also issued guidance to clone producers and the livestock industry on using clones and their offspring for human food and animal feed.

What Is a Clone?

"Clones are genetic copies of an animal," says Larisa Rudenko, Ph.D., a Molecular Biologist and Senior Adviser for biotechnology in CVM. "They're similar to identical twins, but born at different times." Cloning can be thought of as an extension of the assisted reproductive technologies, such as artificial insemination, and more recently, embryo transfer and in vitro fertilization, that livestock breeders have been using for centuries.

Animal cloning has been around for more than 20 years. Most cloning today uses a process called somatic cell nuclear transfer:

- Scientists take an egg from a female animal (often from ovaries at the slaughterhouse) and remove the gene-containing nucleus.

- The nucleus of a cell from an animal the breeder wishes to copy is added to the egg.

- After other steps in the laboratory take place, the egg cell begins to form into an embryo.

- The embryo is implanted in the uterus of a surrogate dam (female parent), which carries it to term and delivers it like her own offspring.

Clones may allow farmers to upgrade the quality of their herds by providing more copies of their best animals—those with naturally occurring desirable traits, such as resistance to disease, high milk production, or quality meat production. These animal clones are then used for conventional breeding, and their sexually reproduced offspring become the food-producing animals.

What Cloning Means to Consumers

- The FDA has concluded that cattle, swine, and goat clones, and the offspring of any animal clones traditionally consumed as food, are safe for human and animal consumption.

- Food labels do not have to state that food is from animal clones or their offspring. The FDA has found no science-based reason to require labels to distinguish between products from clones and products from conventionally produced animals.

- The main use of clones is to produce breeding stock, not food. These animal clones—copies of the best animals in the herd— are then used for conventional breeding, and the sexually repro- duced offspring of the animal clones become the food-producing animals.

- Due to the lack of information on clone species other than cow, goat, and pig (for example, sheep), the FDA recommends that other clone species do not enter the human food supply.

Part Six

Consumer Products and Medical Hazards

Chapter 43

Teflon (Perfluorochemicals, or PFCs)

Many of us have probably seen news stories about something commonly referred to as PFCs or perfluorochemicals. You may not know exactly what they are, but can probably guess that they have something to do with the environment and your health.

About Perfluorinated Chemicals (PFCs)

Perfluorinated chemicals (PFCs) are a large group of manufactured compounds that are widely used to make everyday products more resistant to stains, grease, and water. For example, PFCs may be used to keep food from sticking to cookware, to make sofas and carpets resistant to stains, to make clothes and mattresses more waterproof, and may also be used in some food packaging, as well as in some fire fighting materials. Because they help reduce friction, they are also used in a variety of other industries, including aerospace, automotive, building and construction, and electronics. PFCs break down very slowly in the environment and are often characterized as persistent. There is widespread wildlife and human exposure to several PFCs, including perfluorooctanoic acid (PFOA) and perfluorooctane sulfonate (PFOS). Both PFOA and PFOS are by-products of other commercial

This chapter includes text excerpted from "Perfluorinated Chemicals (PFCs)," National Institute of Environmental Health Sciences (NIEHS), July 2016.

products, meaning they are released into the environment when other products are made, used, or discarded. PFOS is no longer manufactured in the United States, and PFOA production has been reduced and will be eliminated. More research is needed to fully understand all sources of human exposure, but people are most likely exposed to these compounds by consuming PFC contaminated water or food, or by using products that contain PFCs.

Unlike many other persistent chemicals, PFCs are not stored in body fat. However, PFCs are similar to other persistent chemicals, because the half-life, or the amount of time it takes for 50 percent of the chemical to leave the human body, for some of these chemicals, is several years. This slow elimination time makes it difficult to determine how changes in lifestyle, diet, or other exposure related factors influence blood levels.

In animal studies, some PFCs disrupt normal endocrine activity; reduce immune function; cause adverse effects on multiple organs, including the liver and pancreas; and cause developmental problems in rodent offspring exposed in the womb. Data from some human studies suggests that PFCs may also have effects on human health, while other studies have failed to find conclusive links. Additional research in animals and in humans is needed to better understand the potential adverse effects of PFCs for human health. Researchers continue to study the adverse effects of PFCs in animal models.

National Toxicology Program (NTP) Studies

The U.S. Environmental Protection Agency (EPA) nominated the PFC class to the National Toxicology Program (NTP) for study, due to concerns of:

- Widespread exposure to humans

- Persistence in the environment

- Observed toxicity in animal models

- Insufficient information to properly assess human health risk across the entire structural class

One thing that differentiates each PFC is the size of what scientists refer to as chain length, or the number of carbon atoms in its chemical makeup. For example, PFOA has 8 carbons, which is why it is sometimes referred to as C8. The NTP is studying PFCs as a class, due to potential similarities in chemical properties and toxicity.

The scientists will be able to compare one PFC chemical to another, determine the relationship between chain length and toxicity, and work toward understanding a common basis for toxicity. The NTP research involves a variety of short- and long-term rodent toxicology studies, using internal dose, such as plasma levels, to relate exposure to effects. The entire research program is multifaceted.

Additional Research on PFCs

In addition to the NTP's effort, the National Institute of Environmental Health Sciences (NIEHS)-funded grantees across the country are researching PFCs. For example, some are exploring a potential link between PFCs and behavioral disorders, including attention deficit hyperactivity disorder (ADHD), while others are evaluating the potential adverse health risks of PFCs and other chemicals on neurobehavioral development and immune function.

Reducing Exposure

Some progress has been made in reducing PFCs. The EPA has been working with companies since 2000 to phase out PFOA and PFOS, and to reduce the environmental and human health impacts of other PFCs. Also, some state agencies are reviewing PFC research findings from the NIEHS and others, to help assess and evaluate the impact of these chemicals on human health in their communities.

Chapter 44

Perfluorooctanoic Acid (PFOA)

Perfluorooctanoic acid (PFOA) has been a manufactured perfluorochemical and a by-product in producing fluoropolymers. Perfluorochemicals (PFCs) are a group of chemicals used to make fluoropolymer coatings and products that resist heat, oil, stains, grease, and water. PFOA was used particularly for manufacturing polytetrafluoroethylene (PTFE). PFOA persists in the environment and does not break down. PFOA has been identified in bodies of water and in a variety of land and water animals.

In the *Fourth National Report on Human Exposure to Environmental Chemicals,* The Centers for Disease Control and Prevention (CDC) scientists found PFOA in the serum of nearly all the people tested, indicating that PFOA exposure is widespread in the United States population.

Finding measurable amounts of PFOA in serum does not imply that the levels of PFOA cause an adverse health effect. Biomonitoring studies on levels of PFOA provide physicians and public health officials with reference values so that they can determine whether people have

This chapter contains text excerpted from the following sources: Text in this chapter begins with excerpts from "Perfluorooctanoic Acid (PFOA) Factsheet," Centers for Disease Control and Prevention (CDC), April 7, 2017; Text beginning with the heading "About Perfluorooctanoic Acid (PFOA)" is excerpted from "Perfluorooctanoic Acid (PFOA)," Tox Town, National Library of Medicine (NLM), April 20, 2017.

been exposed to higher levels of PFOA than are found in the general population. Biomonitoring data can also help scientists plan and conduct research on exposure and health effects.

About Perfluorooctanoic Acid (PFOA)

PFOA is part of a larger group of chemicals called perfluoroalkyls, which are used in products to resist heat and to repel oil, grease, stains, and water. PFOA is a synthetic chemical that had many manufacturing and industrial uses. It is sometimes called C8 and is a white to off-white powder with a strong odor. The chemical formula for PFOA is C8HF15O2. The two perfluoroalkyls that were made in the largest amounts were PFOA and perfluorooctane sulfonic acid (PFOS).

Historically, PFOA was used in the United States in stain resistant carpets and fabrics, nonstick cookware, water repellent clothing, paper plates, paper and cardboard packaging, and in fire-fighting foams. Another use has been in ski wax.

Aside from industrial uses, consumer products such as those using the trademarked Teflon may have PFOA as impurities. PFOA can also be produced by the breakdown of other substances.

PFOA by itself does not break down under typical environmental conditions. It can be found in air, soil, and water. PFOA is extremely persistent in the environment and can be carried over great distances.

Companies have stopped production or have begun changing manufacturing practices to reduce releases and the amounts of PFOA and perfluoroalkyls in their products. In 2006, the U.S. Environmental Protection Agency (EPA) asked eight major companies to commit to work toward the elimination of their production and use of PFOA and chemicals that break down to PFOA from emissions and products by 2015. All companies have met the PFOA Stewardship Program goals.

How I Might Be Exposed to PFOA

At work, you can be exposed by breathing, eating, or having skin contact with PFOA if you work in a facility that makes or uses PFOA or perfluoroalkyls. You can also be exposed if you live near an industrial facility that uses PFOA. You may have a higher exposure to PFOA if you install or treat carpeting.

You can be exposed to PFOA by drinking contaminated water, breathing contaminated air or contaminated dust, or eating contaminated food. The EPA has established health advisory levels for PFOA in drinking water at 70 parts per trillion (ppt). PFOA has been detected in breast milk and this may contribute to the exposure of infants. The general population, especially children, may be exposed if they are in contact with carpets treated with PFOA.

How PFOA Can Affect My Health

Many studies have looked at exposures to PFOA and possible adverse effects. CDC has stated that finding low amounts of PFOA in blood serum does not mean that adverse effects will occur. It states that there is no conclusive evidence that PFOA can cause cancer in humans. However, some studies have reported increases in prostate, kidney, and testicular cancers in humans exposed to high levels of PFOA.

PFOA is found at very low levels in the blood of the general U.S. population, although it is not fully understood how everyone is exposed to the chemical. It can remain in the human body for many years.

The American Cancer Society (ACS) states that "Other than the possible risk of flu-like symptoms from breathing in fumes from an overheated Teflon-coated pan, there are no known risks to humans from using Teflon-coated cookware. While PFOA is used in making Teflon, it is not present (or is present in extremely small amounts) in Teflon-coated products."

EPA has not officially classified PFOA as a carcinogen. Under EPA's Guidelines for Carcinogen Risk Assessment, there is suggestive evidence of carcinogenic potential for PFOA.

If you think your health has been affected by exposure to PFOA or other perfluoroalkyls, contact your healthcare professional.

For poison emergencies or questions about possible poisons, contact your local poison control center.

Chapter 45

Insect Repellent

Did you know that insect repellents are pesticides? According to pesticide law, a pesticide is any substance or mixture of substances intended for:

- preventing
- destroying
- repelling
- mitigating any pest

People often think of the term "pesticide" as referring only to something that kills insects, but "pesticide" is a broad term and includes products that don't kill anything, such as insect repellents. Products labeled as repellents are not designed to eliminate pests. For example, in the case of the skin-applied repellents, the product makes people less attractive to the pest.

Types of Insect Repellents

Insect repellents applied to the skin are often what we think of when we want to avoid insect bites. These are the most broadly useful,

---

This chapter contains text excerpted from the following sources: Text in this chapter begins with excerpts from "What Is an Insect Repellent?" U.S. Environmental Protection Agency (EPA), August 30, 2017; Text under the heading "Ensuring Safety" is excerpted from "Using Insect Repellents Safely and Effectively," U.S. Environmental Protection Agency (EPA), May 24, 2017.

since they stay with you regardless of your movements. Other types of repellents that the U.S. Environmental Protection Agency (EPA) registers include:

- Clip on products that have a pad with the repellent and a fan or other mechanism that disperses the repellent near your body

- Spatial repellents use a heating mechanism to disperse repellent in an outdoor area. Examples of dispersal mechanisms for spatial repellents include:

  - Lanterns

  - Torches

  - Table-top diffusers

  - Candles

  - Coils

Note that both stationary and wearable spatial repellents are for outdoor use only, unless the label specifically states they can be used indoors. Read the label to understand any limitations such as:

- The area they cover

- The effect of wind on their use

- Whether or not the repellent needs to build up in an area before mosquitoes will be repelled effectively

To be registered by the EPA, these products must have safety and effectiveness data, which the EPA evaluates before allowing them on the market.

Ensuring Safety

Remember these important points to use repellents safely:

Applying the Product

- Read and follow the label directions to ensure proper use; be sure you understand how much to apply

- Apply repellents only to exposed skin and/or clothing. Do not use under clothing.

- Do not apply near eyes and mouth, and apply sparingly around ears.

* When using sprays, do not spray directly into the face; spray on hands first and then apply to face.

* Never use repellents over cuts, wounds, or irritated skin.

* Do not spray in enclosed areas.

* Avoid breathing a spray product.

* Do not use it near food.

Other Safety Tips

* Check the label to see if there are warnings about flammability. If so, do not use around open flames or lit cigarettes.

* After returning indoors, wash treated skin and clothes with soap and water.

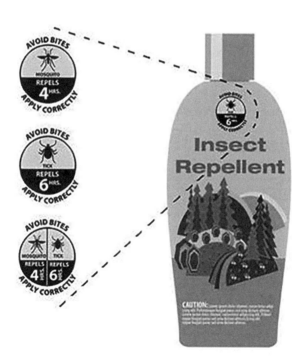

Figure 45.1. *Sample of How the Graphics Look* (Source: "Repellency Awareness Graphic," U.S. Environmental Protection Agency (EPA).)

You may see one of three versions of the graphic on a product label showing mosquitoes, ticks, or mosquitoes and ticks are repelled.

- Do not use any product on pets or other animals unless the label clearly states it is for animals.

- Most insect repellents do not work against lice or fleas.

- Store insect repellents safely out of the reach of children, in a locked utility cabinet or garden shed.

- Use other preventive actions to avoid getting bitten by:

  - Mosquitoes

  - Ticks

Chapter 46

Soaps and Triclosan

Chapter Contents

Section 46.1

Soap

This section contains text excerpted from the following
sources: Text beginning with the heading "Regulatory
Definition of the Term "Soap" is excerpted from "Cosmetics—Soap:
FAQs," U.S. Food and Drug Administration (FDA), November 15,
2017; Text under the heading "What Makes Soap 'Antibacterial'" is
excerpted from "For Consumers—Antibacterial Soap? You Can Skip
It, Use Plain Soap and Water," U.S. Food and Drug
Administration (FDA), November 6, 2017.

Regulatory Definition of the Term "Soap"

Whether a product is a "soap" in the traditional sense, or is really
a synthetic detergent, helps determine how the product is regulated.
So, let's take a look at how "soap" is defined in the U.S. Food and Drug
Administration's (FDA) regulations.

To meet the definition of soap in the FDA's regulations, a product
has to meet three conditions:

1. **What it is made of.** To be regulated as "soap," the product
    must be composed mainly of the "alkali salts of fatty acids,"
    that is, the material you get when you combine fats or oils
    with an alkali, such as lye.

2. **What ingredients cause its cleaning action.** To be regu-
    lated as "soap," those "alkali salts of fatty acids" must be the
    only material that results in the product's cleaning action. If
    the product contains synthetic detergents, it's a cosmetic, not a
    soap. You still can use the word "soap" on the label.

3. **How it is intended to be used.** To be regulated as soap,
    it must be labeled and marketed only for use as soap. If it is
    intended for purposes such as moisturizing the skin, mak-
    ing the user smell nice, or deodorizing the user's body, it's a
    cosmetic. Or, if the product is intended to treat or prevent
    disease, such as by killing germs, or treating skin conditions,

such as acne or eczema, it's a drug. You still can use the word "soap" on the label.

What the Soap Contains

Ordinary soap is made by combining fats or oils and an alkali, such as lye. The fats and oils, which may be from animal, vegetable, or mineral sources, are degraded into free fatty acids, which then combine with the alkali to form crude soap. The lye reacts with the oils, turning what starts out as liquid into blocks of soap. When made properly, no lye remains in the finished product. In the past, people commonly made their own soap using animal fats and lye that had been extracted from wood ashes.

At present, there are very few true soaps on the market. Most body cleansers—both liquid, and solid—are actually synthetic detergent products. Detergent cleansers are popular because they make suds easily in water and don't form gummy deposits. Some of these detergent products are actually marketed as "soap" but are not true soap according to the regulatory definition of the word.

What Makes Soap 'Antibacterial'

Antibacterial soaps (sometimes called antimicrobial or antiseptic soaps) contain certain chemicals not found in plain soaps. Those ingredients are added to many consumer products with the intent of reducing or preventing bacterial infection.

Many liquid soaps labeled antibacterial contain triclosan, an ingredient of concern to many environmental, academic and regulatory groups. Animal studies have shown that triclosan alters the way some hormones work in the body and raises potential concerns for the effects of use in humans.

"There's no data demonstrating that these drugs provide additional protection from diseases and infections. Using these products might give people a false sense of security," Michele says. "If you use these products because you think they protect you more than soap and water, that's not correct. If you use them because of how they feel, there are many other products that have similar formulations but won't expose your family to unnecessary chemicals. And some manufacturers have begun to revise these products to remove these ingredients."

How do you tell if a product is antibacterial? For OTC drugs, antibacterial products generally have the word "antibacterial" on the label.

Also, a drug facts label on a soap or body wash is a sign a product contains antibacterial ingredients.

Section 46.2

Triclosan

This section includes text excerpted from documents published by two public domain sources. Text under headings marked 1 are excerpted from "5 Things to Know about Triclosan—For Consumers," U.S. Food and Drug Administration (FDA), December 19, 2017; Text under heading marked 2 is excerpted from "For Consumers— Antibacterial Soap? You Can Skip It, Use Plain Soap and Water," U.S. Food and Drug Administration (FDA), November 6, 2017.

What Is Triclosan?[1]

Triclosan is an ingredient that is added to many consumer products to reduce or prevent bacterial contamination. It is added to some antibacterial soaps and body washes, toothpastes, and some cosmetics—products regulated by the U.S. Food and Drug Administration (FDA). It also can be found in clothing, kitchenware, furniture, and toys—products not regulated by the FDA.

Triclosan and Health Concerns[2]

Triclosan can be found in many places today. It has been added to many consumer products—including clothing, kitchenware, furniture, and toys—to prevent bacterial contamination. Because of that, people's long-term exposure to triclosan is higher than previously thought, raising concerns about the potential risks associated with the use of this ingredient over a lifetime.

In addition, laboratory studies have raised the possibility that triclosan contributes to making bacteria resistant to antibiotics. Some data shows this resistance may have a significant impact on the effectiveness of medical treatments, such as antibiotics.

The FDA and U.S. Environmental Protection Agency (EPA) have been closely collaborating on scientific and regulatory issues related to triclosan. This joint effort will help to ensure government wide consistency in the regulation of this chemical. The two agencies are reviewing the effects of triclosan from two different perspectives. The EPA regulates the use of triclosan as a pesticide, and is in the process of updating its assessment of the effects of triclosan when it is used in pesticides. The FDA's focus is on the effects of triclosan when it is used by consumers on a regular basis in hand soaps and body washes. By sharing information, the two agencies will be better able to measure the exposure and effects of triclosan and how these differing uses of triclosan may affect human health.

Benefits of Triclosan[1]

For some consumer products, there is evidence that triclosan provides a benefit. The FDA reviewed extensive effectiveness data on triclosan in a popular toothpaste brand. The evidence showed that triclosan in that product was effective in preventing gingivitis.

For other products, such as over-the-counter (OTC) consumer antiseptic products, the FDA has not received evidence that triclosan provides a benefit to human health. At this time, the FDA doesn't have evidence that triclosan in OTC consumer antibacterial soaps and body washes provides any benefit over washing with regular soap and water.

In December 2017, the FDA issued a final rule regarding certain OTC healthcare antiseptic products. As a result, companies will not be able to use triclosan or 23 other active ingredients in these products without premarket review due to insufficient data regarding their safety and effectiveness.

Determining the Presence of Triclosan in a Product[1]

Antibacterial soaps and body washes and fluoride toothpastes are considered OTC drugs. If an OTC drug contains triclosan, it should be listed as an ingredient on the label, in the drug facts box. If a cosmetic contains triclosan, it should be included in the ingredient list on the product label.

The FDA's Role in Evaluating the Safety of Triclosan[1]

FDA has been reviewing safety and effectiveness data on triclosan in the agency's OTC antiseptic rulemakings. It continues to monitor and follow the scientific literature available for the safety and effectiveness of triclosan.

Chapter 47

Plastics

Chapter Contents

Section 47.1

Bisphenol A

This section contains text excerpted from the following
sources: Text in this section begins with excerpts from
"Bisphenol A (BPA)," National Institute of Environmental Health
Sciences (NIEHS), May 24, 2017; Text beginning with the heading
"Use of BPA in Food Contact Application" is excerpted from
"Bisphenol A (BPA): Use in Food Contact Application," U.S. Food
and Drug Administration (FDA), February 6, 2018.

Bisphenol A (BPA) is a chemical produced in large quantities for
use primarily in the production of polycarbonate (PC) plastics and
epoxy resins.

Applications of Bisphenol A (BPA)

Polycarbonate plastics have many applications including use in
some food and drink packaging, e.g., water and infant bottles, com-
pact discs, impact-resistant safety equipment, and medical devices.
Epoxy resins are used as lacquers to coat metal products such as food
cans, bottle tops, and water supply pipes. Some dental sealants and
composites may also contribute to BPA exposure.

How BPA Gets into the Body

The primary source of exposure to BPA for most people is through
the diet. While air, dust, and water are other possible sources of exposure, BPA in food and beverages accounts for the majority of daily
human exposure.

BPA can leach into food from the protective internal epoxy resin
coatings of canned foods and from consumer products such as polycarbonate tableware, food storage containers, water bottles, and
baby bottles. The degree to which BPA leaches from polycarbonate
bottles into liquid may depend more on the temperature of the liquid
or bottle than on the age of the container. BPA can also be found in
breast milk.

Why People Are Concerned about BPA

One reason people may be concerned about BPA is because human exposure to BPA is widespread. The National Health and Nutrition Examination Survey (NHANES III) conducted by the Centers for Disease Control and Prevention (CDC) found detectable levels of BPA in 93 percent of 2,517 urine samples from people six years older and older. The CDC-NHANES data are considered representative of exposures in the United States. Another reason for concern, especially for parents, maybe because some animal studies report effects in fetuses and newborns exposed to BPA.

Steps to Prevent Exposure to BPA

Some animal studies suggest that infants and children may be the most vulnerable to the effects of BPA. Parents and caregivers can make the personal choice to reduce exposures of their infants and children to BPA:

• Don't microwave polycarbonate plastic food containers. Polycarbonate is strong and durable, but over time it may break down from overuse at high temperatures.

• Plastic containers have recycle codes on the bottom. Some, but not all, plastics that are marked with recycle codes 3 or 7 may be made with BPA.

• Reduce your use of canned foods

• When possible, opt for glass, porcelain, or stainless steel containers, particularly for hot food or liquids

• Use baby bottles that are BPA free

Use of BPA in Food Contact Application

BPA is a structural component in polycarbonate beverage bottles. It is also a component in metal can coatings, which protect the food from directly contacting metal surfaces. BPA has been used in food packaging since the 1960s.

As is the case when foods are in direct contact with any packaging material, small, measurable amounts of the packaging materials may migrate into food and can be consumed with it. As part of its premarket review of food packaging materials, U.S. Food and Drug Administration (FDA) food contact regulations and food contact notification program assesses the likely migration from the packaging material to assure that any migration to food occurs at safe levels.

Heightened interest in the safe use of BPA in food packaging has resulted in increased public awareness as well as scientific interest. As a result, many exploratory scientific studies have appeared in the public literature. Some of these studies have raised questions about the safety of ingesting the low levels of BPA that can migrate into food from food contact materials. To address these questions the U.S. National Toxicology Program (NTP), partnering with FDA's National Center for Toxicological Research (NCTR) is carrying out in-depth studies to answer key questions and clarify uncertainties about BPA.

On the regulatory front, FDA's regulations authorize FDA to amend its food additive regulations to reflect when certain uses of an additive have been abandoned. FDA can take this action on its own initiative or in response to a food additive petition that demonstrates that a use of a food additive has been permanently and completely abandoned. FDA granted two petitions requesting that FDA amend its food additive regulations to no longer provide for the use of certain BPA-based materials in baby bottles, sippy cups, and infant formula packaging because these uses have been abandoned. As a result, FDA amended its food additive regulations to no longer provide for these uses of BPA.

Background Studies Conducted for Bisphenol A

BPA is an industrial chemical used to make polycarbonate, a hard, clear plastic, which is used in many consumer products. BPA is also found in epoxy resins, which act as a protective lining on the inside of some metal-based food and beverage cans. Uses of all substances that migrate from packaging into food, including BPA, are subject to premarket approval by FDA as indirect food additives or food contact substances. FDA can make regulatory changes based on new safety or usage information. The original approvals for BPA were issued under FDA's food additive regulations and date from the 1960s.

In the fall of 2014, FDA experts from across the agency, who specialize in toxicology, analytical chemistry, endocrinology, epidemiology, and other fields completed a four-year review of more than 300 scientific studies. The FDA review has not found any information in the evaluated studies to prompt a revision of FDA's safety assessment of BPA in food packaging at this time.

Increasing Our Understanding about the Biology and Metabolism of BPA

Strong consumer and scientific interest in the safety of BPA has prompted FDA to support additional studies to provide further information and address apparent inconsistencies in the scientific literature about BPA. Many of these studies addressed how the body disposes of or metabolizes BPA. These studies also addressed questions about how long it takes for the body to dispose of BPA.

FDA Studies. FDA's regulatory Centers and FDA's National Center for Toxicological Research (NCTR) continue to pursue a set of studies on the fate of BPA in the body from various routes of exposure and the safety of low doses of BPA, including assessing novel endpoints where questions have been raised.

Research studies pursued by FDA's NCTR have:

- Found evidence in rodent studies that the level of the active form of BPA passed from expectant mothers to their unborn offspring, following oral exposure, was so low it could not be measured. The study orally dosed pregnant rodents with 100–1,000 times more BPA than people are exposed to through food, and could not detect the active form of BPA in the fetus 8 hours after the mother's exposure.

- Demonstrated that oral BPA administration results in rapid metabolism of BPA to an inactive form. This results in much lower internal exposure of BPA (i.e., the active form) than what occurs from other routes of exposure such as injection.

- Found that primates (including humans) of all ages effectively metabolize and excrete BPA much more rapidly and efficiently than rodents

- Developed physiologically based pharmacokinetic models that can be used to predict the level of internal exposure to the active and inactive forms of BPA. Based on the effects of metabolism, internal exposures to the active form of BPA following oral administration are predicted to be below 1 percent or less of the total BPA level administered.

- Completed a rodent subchronic study intended to provide information that would help in designing a long-term study that is now underway. The subchronic study was designed to characterize potential effects of BPA in a wide range of endpoints, including prostate and mammary glands, metabolic changes, and cardiovascular endpoints. The study included an in utero phase, direct dosing to pups to mimic bottle feeding in neonates, and employed a dose range covering the low doses where effects have been previously reported in some animal studies, as well as higher doses where estrogenic effects have been measured in guideline oral studies. The results of this study showed no effects of BPA at any dose in the low-dose range.

The FDA's NCTR is continuing with an additional study:

- **Rodent chronic toxicity study**, which is currently underway. Using the data and design from the rodent subchronic study, the U.S. National Toxicology Program (NTP)/U.S. Food and Drug Administration (FDA) is conducting a long-term toxicity study of BPA in rodents to assess a variety of endpoints, including novel endpoints where questions have been raised. As an addition to this core study, FDA is providing extra animals and tissues to a consortium of grantees selected and funded by the National Institute of Environmental Health Sciences (NIEHS) to address other critical questions.

Amendments in Food Additive Regulations

Food additive regulations amended to no longer provide for the use of BPA-based materials in baby bottles, sippy cups, and infant formula packaging.

- **FDA has amended its regulations to no longer provide for the use of BPA-based polycarbonate resins in baby bottles and sippy cups.** In July 2012, FDA took this action in response to a food additive petition filed by the American Chemistry Council (ACC). The ACC petition demonstrated, from publicly available information and information collected from industry sources, that the use of polycarbonate resins in baby bottles and sippy cups had been abandoned.

- **FDA has amended its regulations to no longer provide for the use of BPA-based epoxy resins as coatings in packaging for infant formula.** In July 2013, FDA took this action in response to a food additive petition filed by Congressman Edward Markey of Massachusetts. This petition demonstrated, from publicly available information and information collected from industry sources, that the use of BPA-based epoxy resins as coatings in packaging for infant formula had been abandoned.

An amendment of the food additive regulations based on abandonment is not based on safety, but is based on the fact that the regulatory authorization is no longer necessary for the specific use of the food additive because that use has been permanently and completely abandoned. The safety of a food additive is not relevant to FDA's determination regarding whether a certain use of that food additive has been abandoned.

Section 47.2

Phthalates and Polyvinyl Chloride (PVC)

This section contains text excerpted from the following sources: Text beginning with the heading "What Are Phthalates?" is excerpted from "Phthalates," U.S. Food and Drug Administration (FDA), February 22, 2018; Text under the heading "What Is Polyvinyl Chloride (PVC)?" is excerpted from "Polyvinyl Chloride (PVC)," Tox Town, National Library of Medicine (NLM), August 23, 2017.

What Are Phthalates?

Phthalates are a group of chemicals used in hundreds of products, such as toys, vinyl flooring and wall covering, detergents, lubricating oils, food packaging, pharmaceuticals, blood bags and tubing, and personal care products, such as nail polish, hair sprays, aftershave lotions, soaps, shampoos, perfumes, and other fragrance preparations.

How Phthalates Have Been Used in Cosmetics

Historically, the primary phthalates used in cosmetic products have been dibutyl phthalate (DBP), used as a plasticizer in products such as nail polishes (to reduce cracking by making them less brittle); dimethyl phthalate (DMP), used in hair sprays (to help avoid stiffness by allowing them to form a flexible film on the hair); and diethylphthalate

(DEP), used as a solvent and fixative in fragrances. According to FDA's survey of cosmetics, DBP and DMP are now used rarely. DEP is the only phthalate still commonly used in cosmetics.

Phthalates and Human Health

It's not clear what effect, if any, phthalates have on human health. An expert panel convened by the U.S. National Toxicology Program (NTP), part of the National Institute for Environmental Safety and Health (NIEHS), concluded that reproductive risks from exposure to phthalates were minimal to negligible in most cases.

The Centers for Disease Control and Prevention (CDC) released a report titled *National Report on Human Exposure to Environmental Chemicals*. The report described a survey of a small segment of the U.S. population for environmental chemicals in urine. One group of chemicals surveyed was phthalates. However, the CDC survey was not intended to make an association between the presence of environmental chemicals in human urine and disease, but rather to learn more about the extent of human exposure to industrial chemicals.

The Cosmetic Ingredient Review (CIR) expert panel reaffirmed its original conclusion, finding that DBP, DMP, and DEP were safe as used in cosmetic products. Looking at maximum known concentrations of these ingredients in cosmetics, the panel evaluated phthalate exposure and toxicity data, and conducted a safety assessment for dibutyl phthalate in cosmetic products. The panel found that exposures to phthalates from cosmetics were low compared to levels that would cause adverse effects in animals.

FDA reviewed the safety and toxicity data for phthalates, including the CDC data as well as the CIR conclusions based on reviews. While the CDC report noted elevated levels of phthalates excreted by women of child-bearing age, neither this report nor the other data reviewed by FDA established an association between the use of phthalates in cosmetic products and a health risk. Based on this information, FDA determined that there wasn't a sound, scientific basis to support taking regulatory action against cosmetics containing phthalates.

What We Know about Infant Exposure to Phthalates

Infants, like all consumers, are exposed daily to phthalates from a number of sources, including air, drugs, food, plastics, water, and cosmetics.

The American Academy of Pediatrics (AAP) has published an article stating that infants exposed to infant care products, specifically baby shampoos, baby lotions, and baby powder, showed increased levels of phthalate metabolites in their urine.

Like the CDC report, this study did not establish an association between these findings and any health effects. In addition, levels of phthalates, if any, in the infant care products were not determined.

How to Know If There Are Phthalates in the Cosmetics You Use

Under the authority of the Fair Packaging and Labeling Act (FPLA), FDA requires an ingredient declaration on cosmetic products sold at the retail level to consumers. Consumers can tell whether some products contain phthalates by reading the ingredient declaration on the labels of such products.

However, the regulations do not require the listing of the individual fragrance ingredients; therefore, the consumer will not be able to determine from the ingredient declaration if phthalates are present in a fragrance. Also, because the FPLA does not apply to products used exclusively by professionals—for example, in salons—the requirement for an ingredient declaration does not apply to these products. Based on available safety information, DEP does not pose known risks for human health as it is currently used in cosmetics and fragrances. Consumers who nevertheless do not want to purchase cosmetics containing DEP may wish to choose products that do not include "Fragrance" in the ingredient listing.

What Is Polyvinyl Chloride (PVC)?

Polyvinyl chloride (PVC) is an odorless and solid plastic. It is most commonly white but can also be colorless or amber. It can also come in the form of white powder or pellets. PVC is made from vinyl chloride. The chemical formula for vinyl chloride is C_2H_3Cl. PVC is made up of many vinyl chloride molecules that, linked together, form a polymer $(C_2H_3Cl)n$.

PVC is made softer and more flexible by the addition of phthalates. Bisphenol A (BPA) is also used to make PVC plastics. PVC contains high levels of chlorine.

PVC is used to make pipes, pipe fittings, pipe conduits, vinyl flooring, and vinyl siding. It is used to make wire and cable coatings, packaging materials, wrapping film, gutters, downspouts, door and window frames, gaskets, electrical insulation, hoses, sealant liners, paper and textile finishes, thin sheeting, roof membranes, swimming pool liners, weatherstripping, flashing, molding, irrigation systems, containers and automotive parts, tops, and floor mats.

When softened with phthalates, PVC is used to make some medical devices, including intravenous (IV) bags, blood bags, blood and respiratory tubing, feeding tubes, catheters, parts of dialysis devices, and heart bypass tubing. Phthalates are used in PVC plastics such as garden hoses, inflatable recreational toys, and other toys.

Consumer products made with PVC include raincoats, toys, shoe soles, shades and blinds, upholstery and seat covers, shower curtains, furniture, carpet backing, plastic bags, videodiscs, and credit cards. Most vinyl chloride produced in the United States is used to make PVC.

How You Might Be Exposed to PVC

You can be exposed to PVC by eating food or drinking water contaminated with it. At home, you can be exposed to PVC if you have PVC pipes, vinyl flooring, or other consumer products made with PVC. You can be exposed if your home has vinyl siding or if you are building or renovating your home. Exposure may occur through food packaging and containers or "shrink-wrapped" packages.

You can be exposed to PVC outdoors if you have a plastic swimming pool or plastic furniture. You can be exposed if you live or work on a farm that has an irrigation system containing PVC.

You can be exposed to PVC if you are a patient in a hospital and use medical devices made with PVC.

At work, you can be exposed to PVC if you work in a facility that manufactures PVC pipes and pipe fittings, tubing, and other building and construction products. You can be exposed if you work in a facility that manufactures vinyl chloride, BPA, or phthalates. You can be exposed if you are a plumber, home builder, construction worker, healthcare professional, farmer, or worker in an auto manufacturing facility or repair shop.

How Can PVC Affect My Health?

Exposure to PVC often includes exposure to phthalates, which are used to soften PVC and may have adverse health effects. Because of PVC's heavy chlorine content, dioxins are released during the manufacturing, burning, or landfilling of PVC. Exposure to dioxins can cause reproductive, developmental, and other health problems, and at least one dioxin is classified as a carcinogen.

PVC is made from vinyl chloride, which is listed as a human carcinogen in the Fourteenth Report on Carcinogens published by the NTP. Dioxins, phthalates, and BPA are suspected to be endocrine disruptors, which are chemicals that may interfere with the production or activity of hormones in the human endocrine system. Tetrachlorodibenzodioxin (TCDD) dioxin is listed as a human carcinogen, and di(2-ethylhexyl) phthalate (DEHP) is listed as "reasonably anticipated to be a human carcinogen" in the Fourteenth Report on Carcinogens published by the NTP. Exposure to PVC dust may cause asthma and affect the lungs.

If you think your health has been affected by exposure to PVC, contact your healthcare professional.

Chapter 48

Contaminants in Consumer Products

Chapter Contents

Section 48.1

Overview: Importation of Food and Cosmetics

This section includes text excerpted from "Food—Overview: Importation of Food and Cosmetics," U.S. Food and Drug Administration (FDA), December 7, 2017.

The U.S. Food and Drug Administration's (FDA) Import Program

The U.S. Food and Drug Administration (FDA) is responsible for enforcing the Federal Food, Drug, and Cosmetic Act (FD&C Act) and other laws which are designed to protect consumers' health, safety, and pocketbook. These laws apply equally to domestic and imported products.

With the exception of most meat and poultry, all food and cosmetics as defined in the FD&C Act, are subject to examination by the FDA when imported or offered for import into the United States. Most meat and poultry products are regulated by the U.S. Department of Agriculture (USDA).

All color additives used in foods and cosmetics in the United States must be approved by the FDA; many cannot be used unless certified in the FDA's own laboratories.

Food

Food imported into the United States must meet the same laws and regulations as food produced in the United States. It must be safe and contain no prohibited ingredients, and all labeling and packaging must be informative and truthful, with the labeling information in English (or Spanish in Puerto Rico).

Imported food products are subject to the FDA review when the food is offered for import at the U.S. ports of entry. The FDA does not certify, license, or otherwise approve individual food importers, products, labels, or shipments prior to importation. Importers can import food into the United States as long as the facilities that produce, pack, store, or otherwise handle the products are registered with the FDA and meet other the FDA requirements, such as sanitation.

During the entry process, firms must provide to the FDA information related to the specific products and the manufacturers of the products. Based on the entry information provided and other information FDA has, FDA will decide whether the product meets the U.S. requirements and can be released into the U.S. commerce.

In the wake of various acts of terrorism, the FDA exercises heightened vigilance in assessing food defense risk and maintaining the safety of the nation's food supply.

Prior Notice

Under the prior notice requirements, the FDA must receive notice before food is imported or offered for import into the United States. The purpose of prior notice is to enable the FDA to target inspections or examinations of the imported food at U.S. ports of entry more effectively and to determine whether there is any credible information that the imported food shipment presents a threat or serious risk to public health. Food imported or offered for import into the United States without adequate prior notice may be refused admission into the United States.

The prior notice requirement applies to all foods unless excluded, for humans or animals, including:

- Dietary supplements and dietary ingredients

- Infant formula

- Beverages (including alcoholic beverages and bottled water)

- Fruits and vegetables

- Fish and seafood

- Dairy products and eggs

- Raw agricultural commodities for use as food or as components of food

- Animal feed (including pet food)

- Food and feed additives

- Live food animals

Exclusions from the prior notice requirements include:

- Food carried by or accompanying an individual arriving in the United States for his or her personal use (i.e., for consumption

589

by themselves, family, or friends, and not for sale or other distribution)

- Food that is imported is then exported without leaving the port of arrival until export

- Meat food products, poultry products, and egg products that are subject to the exclusive jurisdiction of the USDA

- Food made by an individual in his or her personal residence and sent by that individual as a personal gift to an individual in the United States

- Food shipped as baggage or cargo constituting the diplomatic bag (e.g., from one nation's government office to its embassy in the United States)

Generally, the FDA's' prior notice regulations apply to all food for humans and other animals imported or offered for import into the United States, for use, storage, or distribution in the United States, including food for gifts. The FDA's website contains information about the FDAs' prior notice policy regarding sending gifts to your friends and family and regarding importing gift packs.

Cosmetics

Cosmetic products imported into the United States must meet the same laws and regulations as those produced in the United States. They must be safe for their intended uses and cannot contain prohibited ingredients. All labeling and packaging must be informative and truthful, with the labeling information in English (or Spanish in Puerto Rico). Certain cosmetic products must be labeled with warning statements.

FDA encourages cosmetic firms to register their establishments and file Cosmetic Product Ingredient Statements with the FDA's Voluntary Cosmetic Registration Program (VCRP). However, firms importing products considered to be cosmetics in the United States are not required to register with the FDA. The VCRP can only accept Cosmetic Product Ingredient Statements (CPIS) for cosmetics that are already on the market in the United States. A registration number is not required for importing cosmetics into the United States.

Section 48.2

Melamine

This section includes text excerpted from "Food—Melamine
in Tableware: Questions and Answers," U.S. Food and Drug
Administration (FDA), December 12, 2017.

Melamine is a chemical that has many industrial uses. In the
United States, it is approved for use in the manufacturing of some
cooking utensils, plates, plastic products, paper, paperboard, and
industrial coatings, among other things. In addition, although it is
not registered as a fertilizer in the United States, melamine has been
used as a fertilizer in some parts of the world.

Melamine may be used in the manufacturing of packaging for food
products, but is not the U.S. Food and Drug Administration (FDA)
approved for direct addition to human food or animal feeds marketed
in the United States.

Frequently Asked Questions on Melamine

*I Recently Read That Plastic Tableware from China
Contained High Levels of Melamine. Can the Melamine from
These Products Get into Foods and Drinks?*

The Taiwan Consumers' Foundation tested plastic tableware made
in China and found that it contained melamine at a level of 20,000
parts per billion (ppb). This type of tableware is manufactured with
a substance called melamine formaldehyde resin. It forms molecular
structures that are molded, with heat, to form the shape of the tableware. A small amount of the melamine used to make the tableware is
"left over" from this chemical reaction and remains in the plastic. This
left over melamine can migrate very slowly out of the plastic into food
that comes into contact with the tableware.

If Melamine from Plastic Tableware Can Get into Foods and Drinks, Does It Make the Foods or Drinks Harmful to Health?

It has been found that melamine does not migrate from melamine formaldehyde tableware into most foods. The only measured migration, in tests, was from some samples (three out of 19 commercially available plates and cups) into acidic foods, under exaggerated conditions (that is, the food was held in the tableware at 160°F for two hours). When adjusted for actual use conditions (cold orange juice held in the tableware for about 15 minutes), the migration would be less than 10 parts of melamine per billion parts of juice.

This is 250 times lower than the level of melamine (alone or even in combination with related compounds analogs known to increase its toxicity) that the FDA has concluded is acceptable in foods other than infant formula (2,500 ppb); in other words, well below the risk level. In addition, such highly acidic foods make up only about 10 percent of the total diet, so the dietary level of melamine in these scenarios would be less than one part per billion.

However, when highly acidic foods are heated to extreme temperatures (e.g., 160°F or higher), the amount of melamine that migrates out of the plastic can increase. Foods and drinks should not be heated on melamine-based dinnerware in microwave ovens. Only ceramic or other cookware which specifies that the cookware is microwave safe should be used. The food may then be served on melamine-based tableware.

Should I Stop Using Plastic Tableware?

Foods and drinks may be served on plastic tableware. Plastic tableware that does not specify that it's microwave safe should not be used to heat foods and drinks.

How Did the U.S. Food and Drug Administration (FDA) Decide What Level of Melamine in Food Doesn't Pose a Risk to Health?

A safety and risk assessment estimates the risk that specific substances have on human health, based on the best scientific data available at the time. The FDA has done this type of assessment to identify the risk posed by melamine and its analogues in foods.

The risk assessment was conducted by scientists from the FDA's Center for Food Safety and Applied Nutrition (CFSAN) and the FDA's Center for Veterinary Medicine (CVM) and included a review of the scientific literature on melamine toxicity. Animal studies also provided valuable information for this work. The assessment underwent peer review by a group of experts identified by an independent contractor.

What Problems Can Melamine Cause If People Eat or Drink Food Contaminated with It?

Products with melamine contamination above the levels noted in the FDA's risk assessment may put people at risk of conditions such as kidney stones, and kidney failure, and of death. Signs of melamine poisoning may include irritability, blood in urine, little or no urine, signs of kidney infection, and/or high blood pressure.

Chapter 49

Fragrance Additives

Many products we use every day contain fragrances. Some of these products are regulated as cosmetics by the U.S. Food and Drug Administration (FDA). Some belong to other product categories and are regulated differently, depending on how the product is intended to be used. This chapter offers information about fragrances that people often ask about.

How to Know If a Fragrance Product Is Regulated as a Cosmetic

If a product is intended to be applied to a person's body to make the person more attractive, it's a cosmetic under the law. Here are some examples of fragrance products that are regulated as cosmetics:

- Perfume

- Cologne

- Aftershave

Fragrance ingredients are also commonly used in other products, such as shampoos, shower gels, shaving creams, and body lotions. Even some products labeled "unscented" may contain fragrance ingredients. This is because the manufacturer may add just enough fragrance to

---

This chapter includes text excerpted from "Cosmetics—Fragrances in Cosmetics," U.S. Food and Drug Administration (FDA), November 25, 2017.

mask the unpleasant smell of other ingredients, without giving the product a noticeable scent.

Some fragrance products that are applied to the body are intended for therapeutic uses, such as treating or preventing disease, or affecting the structure or function of the body. Products intended for this type of use are treated as drugs under the law, or sometimes as both cosmetics and drugs. Here are some examples of labeling statements that will cause a product containing fragrances to be treated as a drug:

- Easing muscle aches

- Soothing headaches

- Helping people sleep

- Treating colic

Many other products that may contain fragrance ingredients, but are not applied to the body, are regulated by the Consumer Product Safety Commission (CPSC). Here are some examples:

- Laundry detergents

- Fabric softeners

- Dryer sheets

- Room fresheners

- Carpet fresheners

Statements on labels, marketing claims, consumer expectations, and even some ingredients may determine a product's intended use.

"Essential Oils" and "Aromatherapy"

There is no regulatory definition for "essential oils," although people commonly use the term to refer to certain oils extracted from plants. The law treats Ingredients from plants the same as those from any other source. For example, "essential oils" are commonly used in so called "aromatherapy" products. If an "aromatherapy" product is intended to treat or prevent disease, or to affect the structure or function of the body, it's a drug.

Similarly, a massage oil intended to lubricate the skin is a cosmetic. But if claims are made that a massage oil relieves aches or relaxes muscles, apart from the action of the massage itself, it's a drug, or possibly both a cosmetic and a drug.

Safety Requirements

Fragrance ingredients in cosmetics must meet the same require-ment for safety as other cosmetic ingredients. The law does not require FDA approval before they go on the market, but they must be safe for consumers when they are used according to labeled directions, or as people customarily use them. Companies and individuals who man-ufacture or market cosmetics have a legal responsibility for ensuring that their products are safe and properly labeled.

Labeling of Fragrance Ingredients

If a cosmetic is marketed on a retail basis to consumers, such as in stores, on the Internet, or person to person, it must have a list of ingredients. In most cases, each ingredient must be listed individually. But under U.S. regulations, fragrance and flavor ingredients can be listed simply as "fragrance" or "flavor."

Here's why: FDA requires the list of ingredients under the Fair Packaging and Labeling Act (FPLA). This law is not allowed to be used to force a company to tell "trade secrets." Fragrance and flavor formulas are complex mixtures of many different natural and synthetic chemical ingredients, and they are the kinds of cosmetic components that are most likely to be "trade secrets."

Fragrance Allergies and Sensitivities

Some individuals may be allergic or sensitive to certain ingredients in cosmetics, food, or other products, even if those ingredients are safe for most people. Some components of fragrance formulas may have a potential to cause allergic reactions or sensitivities for some people.

FDA does not have the same legal authority to require allergen labeling for cosmetics as for food. So, if you are concerned about fra-grance sensitivities, you may want to choose products that are fra-grance free, and check the ingredient list carefully. If consumers have questions, they may choose to contact the manufacturer directly.

Phthalates as Fragrance Ingredients

Phthalates are a group of chemicals used in hundreds of products. The phthalate commonly used in fragrance products is diethyl phthal-ate, or DEP. DEP does not pose known risks for human health as it is currently used in cosmetics and fragrances.

Chapter 50

Beauty Products

Chapter Contents

Section 50.1

1,4-Dioxane in Cosmetics

This section includes text excerpted from "Cosmetics—1,4-Dioxane in Cosmetics: A Manufacturing Byproduct," U.S. Food and Drug Administration (FDA), December 31, 2017.

The U.S. Food and Drug Administration (FDA) has received questions about 1,4-dioxane, a contaminant that may occur in trace amounts in certain cosmetics. The following information is from responses to those questions, scientific literature, and other public sources.

What Is 1,4-Dioxane?

The compound 1,4-dioxane is a trace contaminant in some cosmetic products. It is not used as an ingredient in cosmetics, but may be present in extremely small amounts in some cosmetics. 1,4-dioxane forms as a by-product during the manufacturing process of certain cosmetic ingredients. These ingredients include certain detergents, foaming agents, emulsifiers, and solvents identifiable by the prefix, word, or syllables "PEG," "polyethylene," "polyethylene glycol," "polyoxyethylene," "-eth-," or "-oxynol-."

Is 1,4-Dioxane in Cosmetic Products Harmful?

1,4-dioxane is a potential human carcinogen. A 2016 report by the U.S. Department of Health and Human Services (HHS) National Toxicology Program (NTP) found that 1,4-dioxane is "reasonably anticipated to be a human carcinogen-based on sufficient evidence of carcinogenicity from studies in experimental animals," although the data available from human epidemiological studies are not adequate to evaluate the relationship between human cancer and exposure to 1,4-dioxane. The U.S. Environmental Protection Agency (EPA) has classified 1,4-dioxane as "likely to be carcinogenic to humans," based on a finding of sufficient evidence of carcinogenicity in animals intentionally exposed to 1,4-dioxane but inadequate evidence of carcinogenicity in humans.

The FDA has not independently conducted a hazard identification and risk assessment concerning exposure to 1,4-dioxane as a contaminant in cosmetic products. However, two international scientific studies of trace contamination levels of 1,4-dioxane in cosmetics (by the International Cooperation on Cosmetics Regulations (ICCR), an international group of regulatory authorities from the United States, the European Union, Japan, Canada, and Brazil), and by the European Commission Scientific Committee on Consumer Safety (SCCS)), have examined this issue. The ICCR workgroup determined that all of the levels reported in the recent literature are within acceptable margins of exposure based on available safety assessments from Canada, Europe, and Japan. In an independent risk assessment, SCCS concluded that 1,4-dioxane amounts in cosmetic products are considered safe for consumers at trace levels of ≤10 parts per million (ppm).

The FDA periodically monitors the levels of 1,4-dioxane in cosmetics products and we have observed that changes made in the manufacturing process have resulted in a significant decline over time in the levels of this contaminant in these products.

The FDA also conducted skin absorption studies, which showed that 1,4-dioxane can penetrate animal and human skin when applied in certain preparations, such as lotions. However, further research by the FDA determined that 1,4-dioxane evaporates readily, further diminishing the already small amount available for skin absorption, even in products that remain on the skin for hours.

How Much 1,4-Dioxane Is Present in Cosmetics?

The FDA has periodically monitored specific levels of 1,4-dioxane in cosmetic products since the late 1970s. the FDA conducted surveys on the amount of 1,4-dioxane in finished cosmetic products, which showed a decline over that period. It's survey showed that 1,4-dioxane was not detected in 80 percent of the 35 samples tested, where 1 ppm was the level of detection. About 6 percent were between 1–5 ppm, about 6 percent were between 5–10 ppm, and about 8 percent were between 10–12 ppm (the highest level detected was 11.6 ppm).

What Is the FDA Doing about of 1,4-Dioxane in Cosmetics?

Since the 1980s the FDA recommended that manufacturers use the "vacuum stripping" technique, as a way of reducing 1,4-dioxane. It continues to monitor information about 1,4-dioxane and its levels in cosmetics and plans to conduct a survey in 2018. If the FDA were to determine that a health hazard exists, it would advise the industry and the public, and would consider appropriate actions for protecting the health and welfare of consumers.

Section 50.2

Latex in Cosmetics

This section includes text excerpted from "Cosmetics—
Latex in Cosmetics," U.S. Food and Drug
Administration (FDA), March 6, 2017.

Most people use cosmetic products containing latex without adverse effects. However, some people may have had allergic reactions to latex-containing products. Because of this, the U.S. Food and Drug Administration (FDA) is concerned that consumers might not be aware that some cosmetic products contain natural rubber latex.

What We Know about Latex Allergy

Roughly 1–6 percent of the general population is allergic to natural rubber latex. Natural rubber latex is a milky fluid that contains extremely small particles of rubber that comes from plants, principally from the H. brasiliensis rubber tree. Natural rubber latex also contains a variety of naturally occurring substances, including the polymer cis-1,4-polyisoprene and various plant proteins, including what are called antigenic proteins that may trigger an immune response. Some of these antigenic proteins may also be allergenic: that is, they can cause a latex-sensitive person to have an allergic reaction. Sensitivity to latex may develop over time, especially for people who are often exposed to it.

From January 2015 to September 2017, the FDA received 30 reports of allergic reactions involving cosmetic products that typically contain natural rubber latex, including hair bonding adhesives, face and body paints, eyeliner, and eyelash adhesives. Allergic reactions can range from skin irritations or rashes to respiratory problems and even to a more severe reaction called anaphylactic shock. Four of these reports appeared to be of anaphylactic reactions. Because reporting is not required, the actual number of cases is likely to be higher than what is reported to the FDA. The only way that the FDA learns about incidents like these is when consumers, physicians or companies voluntarily report them. The current laws regulating cosmetics do not require companies to submit reports about cosmetic-related adverse events to the FDA.

How to Know If a Cosmetic Contains Natural Rubber Latex

Read the Label

Although cosmetic products are not required to include a latex allergy warning, the FDA does require that the labels of cosmetics include a list of ingredients, in order of decreasing amount. Consumers should review labeling information prior to purchase. Usually, the ingredient list is on the package, where the consumer can easily find it. If the product is sold by mail order, including online, the list may be on the package directly or consumers may be directed to a product catalog or a website, or there may be specific information about how to request a copy of the ingredient list. The FDA regulations require that mail order distributors respond promptly to your request.

Here are some ingredient names to watch for, all of which indicate the presence of latex:

- Natural rubber latex
- Natural latex rubber
- Rubber latex
- Natural latex
- Latex rubber
- Natural centrifuged latex
- Natural liquid latex
- Aqueous latex adhesive
- Latex

Manufacturers can change their products' ingredients at any time, so it's a good idea to check the ingredient list every time you buy the product even if you have used it before.

603

Consumers who are concerned about natural rubber latex allergy may want to take more precautions, such as:

- Avoiding all products that commonly contain natural rubber latex ingredients (body paints, theatrical cosmetics, hair bonding adhesives, and eyelash adhesives), even if latex isn't listed as an ingredient

- Contacting the manufacturer to learn more about the ingredients in the product

- Speaking with your healthcare professional or dermatologist about your concerns

- Telling your salon professional if you have or suspect that you have a latex allergy, to avoid possible exposure

Products marketed only to professionals may not have a list of ingredients. That's because the Fair Packaging and Labeling Act (FPLA) doesn't apply to those cosmetic products sold for professional use. Salon professionals may need to contact the manufacturer to find out what's in these products.

Having Doubts of Problem with Latex

If you are allergic to natural rubber latex and you have a reaction to a cosmetic product, stop using the product and contact your healthcare professional.

How to Report a Problem

If you are a consumer, health professional, attorney, or member of the cosmetics industry who wants to report a complaint or an adverse event (such as an allergic reaction) related to a cosmetic, you have three choices:

- Call an FDA consumer complaint coordinator if you wish to speak directly to a person about your problem

- Complete an electronic Voluntary MedWatch form online

- Complete a paper Voluntary MedWatch form that can be mailed to the FDA

When you report a reaction, be sure to include as much information as possible. It is helpful for the FDA to know the precise product name, place, and time of purchase, lot number, labeling, and ingredients, especially if you believe you have experienced a reaction to latex. It is also important to let us know if you have a latex allergy or sensitivity.

The law does not require cosmetic companies to report problems to the FDA. Therefore, your report is very important in order to help the FDA monitor the cosmetics market.

Section 50.3

Lead in Cosmetics

This section includes text excerpted from
"Cosmetics—Lead in Cosmetics," U.S. Food and Drug
Administration (FDA), November 15, 2017.

Lead: A Cause for Concern

Questions sometimes arise about the presence of lead in cosmetics. Lead is an element that occurs naturally in the earth. Trace amounts of lead may occur in the foods we eat and the water we drink. The U.S. Food and Drug Administration (FDA) works hard to limit consumers' exposure to lead in all the FDA regulated products, including cosmetics. This section provides some background on what the law says about the safety of cosmetics. It also describes some cosmetic products and ingredients that the FDA has looked at closely with regard to lead content.

Cosmetic Safety and U.S. Law

The FDA regulates cosmetics under a law passed by Congress: the Federal Food, Drug, and Cosmetic Act (FFDCA). This law does not require cosmetic products or most ingredients to have the FDA approval before they go on the market. The only exception is for the color additives used in cosmetics. But cosmetics must be safe when consumers use them following directions on the label, or in the customary or expected way.

If a cosmetic contains an ingredient or impurity that may make the product harmful to consumers when they use it according to the labeling or in the customary or expected way, that product is considered "adulterated" under the law. Misuse of color additives also makes a cosmetic adulterated. It's against the law to market an adulterated cosmetic. The FDA can take action when it finds out about a cosmetic with a safety problem. But first, we need to have reliable scientific information proving that the product is adulterated under the law.

Color Additives

The law treats color additives differently from other cosmetic ingredients. Except for coal-tar hair dyes, color additives need the FDA approval before they may be used in cosmetics, foods, drugs, or many medical devices. Each color additive that the FDA approves is listed in a regulation, called a "listing regulation." That regulation describes the color additive, tells how it is permitted to be used, and provides limits on impurities. Typically, color additives used in cosmetics are limited to 10–20 parts per million (ppm) lead as an impurity.

Kohl, Kajal, Al-Kahal, Surma, Tiro, Tozali, or Kwalli

These traditional eyeliners, popular in many parts of the world, are a serious health concern because they commonly contain large amounts of lead, as well as other heavy metals. Products containing kohl and similar ingredients have been linked to lead poisoning, especially among children, and are not allowed to be sold in the United States Nevertheless, these products sometimes make their way into specialty markets in this country.

The FDA has an Import Alert advising import inspectors to be on the lookout for shipments of these products, and they have posted information to alert consumers to the dangers of using them.

Lipstick, Other Cosmetic Lip Products, and Externally Applied Cosmetics

Over the years, there have been reports alleging dangerous levels of lead in lipstick. The FDA has analyzed hundreds of lipsticks and other cosmetic lip products, such as lip glosses, for the lead. They have found that levels of lead in these products were from below the detection limit to about 7 parts per million (ppm). They published the method developed by them for analyzing lipstick for lead disclaimer icon.

The FDA has also analyzed hundreds of externally applied cosmetics (cosmetics applied to the skin, such as eye shadows, blushes, shampoos, and body lotions) for lead and other impurities. The levels of lead they found were from below the detection limit to 14 ppm. Their data show that over 99 percent of the cosmetic lip products and externally applied cosmetics on the U.S. market contain lead at levels below 10 ppm.

The FDA has issued guidance to industry on limiting lead as an impurity in cosmetic lip products and externally applied cosmetics to a maximum of 10 ppm. This recommended maximum supports the public health goal to limit consumers' exposure to lead in the FDA-regulated products.

Progressive Hair Dyes

Under the law, coal-tar hair dyes don't need the FDA's approval, unlike color additives in general. But hair dyes from plant or mineral sources do.

Lead acetate is a color additive that is approved for use in coloring hair on the scalp. It is used in progressive hair dye products that darken the hair gradually over time, with repeated applications. But because of the dangers of lead exposure, hair dyes that contain lead acetate as an ingredient must have a special warning on the label: "Caution: Contains lead acetate. For external use only. Keep this product out of children's reach. Do not use on cut or abraded scalp. If skin irritation develops, discontinue use. Do not use to color mustaches, eyelashes, eyebrows, or hair on parts of the body other than the scalp. Do not get in eyes. Follow instructions carefully and wash hands thoroughly after each use."

Section 50.4

Hair Dyes

This section includes text excerpted from "Cosmetics—Hair Dyes," U.S. Food and Drug Administration (FDA), November 3, 2017.

The U.S. Food and Drug Administration (FDA) often receives questions about the safety and regulation of hair dyes. Most of these products belong to a category called "coal-tar" hair dyes. Color additives, with the exception of coal-tar hair dyes, need the FDA approval before they're permitted for use in cosmetics.

The FDA's ability to take action against coal-tar hair dyes associated with safety concerns is limited by law. It's important to follow the directions on the label. It is also important to be an informed consumer and understand the risks.

What Are Coal-Tar Hair Dyes?

The term "coal-tar colors" dates back to the time when these coloring materials were by-products of the coal industry. Today, most are made from petroleum, but the original name is still used. Coal-tar hair dyes—those coal-tar colors used for dyeing hair—include permanent, semi-permanent, and temporary hair dyes.

Coal-tar colors are also called "synthetic-organic" colors. That's because, to a chemist, a "synthetic" compound is one formed from simpler compounds and an "organic" compound is one that contains carbon atoms.

What the Law Says about Coal-Tar Hair Dyes

Under the Federal Food, Drug, and Cosmetic Act (FD&C Act), a law passed by Congress, color additives must be approved by the FDA for their intended use before they are used in the FDA-regulated products, including cosmetics. Other cosmetic ingredients do not need the FDA approval. The FDA can take action against a cosmetic on the market if it is harmful to consumers when used in the customary or expected way and used according to labeled directions.

How the law treats coal-tar hair dyes:

- The FDA cannot take action against a coal-tar hair dye, as long as the label includes a special caution statement and the product comes with adequate directions for consumers to do a skin test before they dye their hair. This is the caution statement:

Caution: This product contains ingredients which may cause skin irritation on certain individuals and a preliminary test according to accompanying directions should first be made. This product must not be used for dyeing the eyelashes or eyebrows; to do so may cause blindness. (FD&C Act, 601(a))

- Coal-tar hair dyes, unlike color additives in general, do not need the FDA's approval. (FD&C Act, 601(e)).

But there are limits to this exception:

- The FDA may take action if a harmful coal-tar hair dye product if:

- it does not have the caution statement on its label or come with adequate directions for a skin test, or

- an ingredient other than the coal-tar hair dye itself is harmful.

- "Coal-tar hair dyes" are not eyebrow or eyelash dyes. Color additives intended for dyeing the eyebrows or eyelashes need the FDA approval for that use. No color additives are approved for dyeing the eyebrows or eyelashes.

Safety Issues

While many people use coal-tar hair dyes, the FDA is aware of the following problems:

Eye injuries. Hair dyes have caused eye injuries, including blindness, when used in the eye area. Eyebrow and eyelash dyeing are not permitted uses of coal-tar hair dyes.

Allergic reactions. Some coal-tar hair dyes can cause allergic reactions or sensitization that may result in skin irritation and hair loss. People can develop sensitivities with repeated exposure. In addition, formulations may change over time. So, it's possible to have a reaction even if you have dyed your hair in the past, without a problem. That's why it's important to follow the instructions and do the skin

609

test before every use. Even if you don't see a reaction to the skin test, it's still possible to have a reaction when you dye your hair.

One hair dye ingredient, p-phenylenediamine, or "PPD," has been implicated more prominently in leading to allergic reactions. Some people may become allergic to PPD from other exposures, including occupational exposures. This is called "cross-sensitization." Here are some examples:

- Some temporary tattoo inks, sometimes marketed as "black henna"

- Certain textile dyes, ballpoint pen inks, some color additives used in foods and drugs, and other dyes used in semi-permanent and temporary hair dyes

- Rubber and other latex products

- Benzocaine and procaine, local anesthetics used by doctors and dentists

- Para-aminosalicylic acid, a drug used to treat tuberculosis (TB)

- Sulfonamides, sulfones, and sulfa drugs

- Para-aminobenzoic acid (PABA), a naturally occurring compound used in some sunscreens disclaimer icon and in some cosmetics

Temporary tattoo artists who use coal-tar hair dyes to color people's skin are misusing these products and ingredients, because coal tar hair dyes are not intended to be used for staining the skin. While the FDA regulates cosmetics products on the market, professional practice is generally subject to state and local authorities, not the FDA.

If you have a reaction to a hair dye or tattoo, ask your healthcare provider about treatment. If you know what ingredient caused the problem, you may be able to find a product that doesn't contain that ingredient. If you color your hair yourself, check the list of ingredients on the label for any you wish to avoid. If you have your hair colored at a salon, your stylist may be able to tell you the ingredients, or you may wish to check with the manufacturer.

Hair dyes and cancer. In the 1980s, some coal-tar hair dyes were found to cause cancer in animals. The FDA published a regulation requiring a special warning statement for all hair dye products containing these two ingredients:

1. 4-methoxy-m-phenylenediamine 2,4-diaminoanisole

2. 2, 4-methoxy-m-phenylenediamine sulfate 2,4-diaminoanisole sulfate

The cosmetic industry has since reformulated coal-tar hair dye products, and these two ingredients are no longer seen in hair dyes. The FDA continues to monitor research on hair dye safety. They do not have reliable evidence showing a link between cancer and coal-tar hair dyes on the market today. They are collecting adverse event data that helps assess the safety of this class of ingredients. If you experience an adverse event or bad reaction, please report that to the FDA.

Other Types of Hair-coloring Products

Hair-coloring materials made from plant or mineral sources are regulated the same as other color additives. They must be approved by the FDA and listed in the color additive regulations. Color additives approved for use on hair include henna (from the Lawsonia plant) as well as lead acetate, and bismuth citrate, both of which are used in "progressive" hair dyes that darken hair gradually with repeated applications. Of note, temporary tattoos marketed as "black henna" contain p-phenylenediamine (PPD) and may increase your risk of allergy to hair dyes. Hair dyes are not meant to be used for staining your skin.

Unusual Colors

People sometimes ask whether unusual colors such as pink, orange, blue, and green are regulated differently from other hair dyes. How a hair dye is regulated depends on whether it is a coal-tar hair dye or is made from plant or mineral materials, not on the shade.

Coal-Tar Hair Dye Safety Checklist:

• Follow all directions on the label and in the package

• Do a patch test on your skin every time before dyeing your hair

• Keep hair dyes away from your eyes, and do not dye your eyebrows or eyelashes. This can hurt your eyes and may even cause blindness.

• Wear gloves when applying hair dye

• Do not leave the product on longer than the directions say you should. Keep track of time using a clock or a timer.

- Rinse your scalp well with water after using hair dye

- Do not scratch or brush your scalp three days before using hair dyes

- Do not dye or relax your hair if your scalp is irritated, sunburned, or damaged

- Wait at least 14 days after bleaching, relaxing, or perming your hair before using dye

- Read the ingredient statement to make certain that ingredients that may have caused a problem for you in the past, such as p-phenylenediamine (PPD) are not present

- If you have a problem, tell your healthcare provider

- Keep hair dyes out of the reach of children

How to Report a Problem

If you have a reaction to a hair dye—or any other cosmetic—first contact your healthcare provider for any necessary medical help.

Then, please tell the FDA. The law doesn't require cosmetic companies, including hair dye manufacturers, to share their safety data or consumer complaints with the FDA. So, the information you report is very important to help the FDA monitor the safety of cosmetics on the market.

You can report a problem with a cosmetic to the FDA in either of these ways:

- Contact MedWatch, the FDA's problem-reporting program, at 800-332-1088, or file a MedWatch Voluntary report online

- Contact the consumer complaint coordinator in your area

Section 50.5

Microbiological Safety and Cosmetics

This section includes text excerpted from "Cosmetics —
Microbiological Safety and Cosmetics," U.S. Food and Drug
Administration (FDA), March 6, 2018.

Cosmetics can become harmful to consumers if they're contaminated with harmful microorganisms, such as certain bacteria and fungi. The U.S. Food and Drug Administration (FDA) is looking closely at the microbiological safety of cosmetics.

What the Law Says about Cosmetic Safety

Under the law, cosmetic products and ingredients, except for color additives, do not need the FDA approval before they go on the market. However, they must not be "adulterated" or "misbranded." This means they must be safe for consumers when used according to directions on the label, or in the customary or expected way, and they must be properly labeled. It also means they must not be prepared, packed, or stored in a way in which they may have become contaminated or harmful to health.

Companies and individuals who manufacture or distribute cosmetics are legally responsible for the safety of their products. This includes, for example, making sure cosmetics are free of harmful microorganisms. While the law doesn't require cosmetics to have the FDA's approval before they go on the market, they do monitor the safety of cosmetics, including their microbiological safety. The FDA can take action against cosmetics on the market that don't comply with the law.

How Microorganisms Get into Cosmetics

Remember, cosmetic firms are legally responsible for making sure their products are safe. Some of the ways cosmetics may become contaminated with bacteria or fungi are:

- Contaminated raw materials, water or other ingredients

- Poor manufacturing conditions

613

- Ingredients that encourage the growth of microorganisms, without an effective preservative system

- Packaging that doesn't protect a product adequately

- Poor shipping or storage conditions

- Consumer use, such as the need to dip fingers into the product

Questions the FDA Is Asking, and Why

The FDA bases its actions on reliable information. It makes sure its knowledge and actions reflect the current state of science, industry practice, and products on the market. Even if injuries from contaminated cosmetics are not common, they can be serious. For example, contaminated tattoo inks, eye-area cosmetics, and lotions and mouthwashes used in hospitals all have caused serious infections.

Here are some of the questions the FDA microbiologists are exploring:

- What's the best way to test cosmetics for microbiological safety?

- What types of preservative systems are cosmetic companies using, and how effective are they?

- What kinds of microorganisms pose health risks in cosmetics?

- How are people exposed to microorganisms in cosmetics?

- Which contaminated cosmetics pose the greatest risk to consumers?

For example, in November 2011, the FDA held a public meeting, requesting information on the microbiological safety of cosmetics from industry and consumer advocacy organizations.

How Consumers Can Help Protect against Microbial Contamination

Don't share cosmetics with anyone. You may be sharing germs.

- Don't add water or saliva to cosmetics, such as mascara. You may be adding bacteria or other microorganisms. You'll also be watering down a preservative that's intended to keep bacteria from growing.

- Store cosmetics carefully. If cosmetics get too warm, some microorganisms may grow faster and preservatives may break down.

- Keep containers clean.

- Wash your hands before applying cosmetics, especially if you need to dip your fingers into the container.

- Pay attention to recalls and safety alerts. Microbial contamination is a common reason for recalls of cosmetics.

How to Report a Problem

If you've experienced a problem with a cosmetic, from a minor rash or a headache to an illness that put you in the hospital, please tell the FDA. You can even report something that didn't cause a reaction, but alerted you to a problem with the product, such as a bad smell or other sign of contamination.

You can report a problem with a cosmetic to the FDA in either of these ways:

- Contact MedWatch, the FDA's problem reporting-program, at 800-332-1088, or file a MedWatch voluntary report online

- Contact the consumer complaint coordinator in your area.

Section 50.6

Parabens in Cosmetics

This section includes text excerpted from "Cosmetics—
Parabens in Cosmetics," U.S. Food and Drug
Administration (FDA), February 22, 2018.

Parabens are commonly used as preservatives in cosmetics. Here are answers to questions that consumers often ask about the safety and use of these ingredients.

What Are Frequently Asked Questions on Parabens

What Are Parabens, and Why Are They Used in Cosmetics?

Parabens are a family of related chemicals that are commonly used as preservatives in cosmetic products. Preservatives may be used in cosmetics to prevent the growth of harmful bacteria and mold, in order to protect both the products and consumers. The parabens used most commonly in cosmetics are methylparaben, propylparaben, Butylparaben, and ethylparaben.

Product ingredient labels typically list more than one paraben in a product, and parabens are often used in combination with other types of preservatives to better protect against a broad range of microorganisms.

What Kinds of Products Contain Parabens?

Parabens are used in a wide variety of cosmetics, as well as in foods and drugs. Cosmetics that may contain parabens include makeup, moisturizers, hair care products, and shaving products, among others. Many major brands of deodorants do not currently contain parabens, although some may.

Cosmetics sold to consumers in stores or online must have a list of ingredients, each listed by its common or usual name. This is important information for consumers who want to find out whether a product contains an ingredient they wish to avoid. Parabens are usually easy to identify by their names, such as methylparaben, propylparaben, butylparaben, or ethylparaben.

Does the U.S. Food and Drug Administration (FDA) Regulate the Use of Preservatives in Cosmetics?

The FDA doesn't have special rules that apply only to preservatives in cosmetics. The law treats preservatives in cosmetics the same as other cosmetic ingredients. Under the Federal Food, Drug, and Cosmetic Act (FD&C Act), cosmetic products and ingredients, other than color additives, do not need the FDA's approval before they go on the market.

However, it is against the law to market a cosmetic in interstate commerce if it is adulterated or misbranded. This means, for example, that cosmetics must be safe for consumers when used according to directions on the label or in a customary way, and they must be properly labeled.

The FDA can take action against a cosmetic on the market that does not comply with the laws enforced by them. However, to take action against a cosmetic for safety reasons, they must have reliable scientific information showing that the product is harmful when consumers use it according to directions on the label or in a customary way.

Are Parabens Safe as They're Used in Cosmetics? Are They Linked to Breast Cancer or Other Health Problems?

The FDA scientists continue to review published studies on the safety of parabens. At this time, they do not have information showing that parabens, as they are used in cosmetics, have an effect on human health. Here are some of the questions they are considering:

• What do published studies show about the possible hazards of parabens, and on the effects of parabens on human health? For example, do experimental findings with various parabens also happen in real life?

• What are the hazards and risks of not using parabens? If we stop using parabens to protect cosmetics and consumers from harmful bacteria, are there safer alternatives to preservatives?

• If there are paraben-related health effects that are scientifically supported and documented, how do these effects relate to the use of parabens in cosmetics?

• Do the different kinds of parabens act the same or different in our bodies?

The FDA continues to evaluate new data in this area. If they determine that a health hazard exists, they will advise the industry and the public, and will consider the agency's legal options under the authority of the FD&C Act to protect the health and welfare of consumers.

Section 50.7

Phthalates in Cosmetics

This section includes text excerpted from "Cosmetics—Phthalates," U.S. Food and Drug Administration (FDA), February 22, 2018.

The U.S. Food and Drug Administration (FDA) has received a number of inquiries on the safety of phthalates, which are used in a variety of cosmetics as well as other consumer products. Here are answers to questions consumers often ask about these ingredients.

Frequently Asked Questions on Phthalates

What Are Phthalates?

Phthalates are a group of chemicals used in hundreds of products, such as toys, vinyl flooring and wall covering, detergents, lubricating oils, food packaging, pharmaceuticals, blood bags and tubing, and personal care products, such as nail polish, hair sprays, aftershave lotions, soaps, shampoos, perfumes, and other fragrance preparations.

How Phthalates Have Been Used in Cosmetics

Historically, the primary phthalates used in cosmetic products have been dibutyl phthalate (DBP), used as a plasticizer in products such as nail polishes (to reduce cracking by making them less brittle); dimethyl phthalate (DMP), used in hair sprays (to help avoid stiffness by allowing them to form a flexible film on the hair); and diethylphthalate (DEP), used as a solvent and fixative in fragrances.

Phthalates and Human Health

It's not clear what effect, if any, phthalates have on human health. An expert panel convened by the National Toxicology Program (NTP), part of the National Institute for Environmental Safety and Health (NIEHS), concluded that reproductive risks from exposure to phthalates were minimal to negligible in most cases.

The Centers for Disease Control and Prevention (CDC) released a report titled National Report on Human Exposure to Environmental Chemicals. The report described a survey of a small segment of the U.S. population for environmental chemicals in urine. One group of chemicals surveyed was phthalates. However, the CDC survey was not intended to make an association between the presence of environmental chemicals in human urine and disease, but rather to learn more about the extent of human exposure to industrial chemicals.

The Cosmetic Ingredient Review (CIR) expert panel reaffirmed its original conclusion (reached in 1985), finding that DBP, DMP, and DEP were safe as used in cosmetic products. Looking at maximum known concentrations of these ingredients in cosmetics, the panel evaluated phthalate exposure and toxicity data, and conducted a safety assessment for dibutyl phthalate in cosmetic products. The panel found that exposures to phthalates from cosmetics were low compared to levels that would cause adverse effects in animals.

The FDA reviewed the safety and toxicity data for phthalates, including the CDC data, as well as the CIR conclusions. While the CDC report noted elevated levels of phthalates excreted by women of child-bearing age, neither this report nor the other data reviewed by the FDA established an association between the use of phthalates in cosmetic products and a health risk. Based on this information, the FDA determined that there wasn't a sound, scientific basis to support taking regulatory action against cosmetics containing phthalates.

How the FDA Has Followed Up

The FDA continues to monitor levels of phthalates in cosmetic products. They have developed an analytical method for determining the levels of phthalates in cosmetic products and conducted surveys of products to determine these levels in cosmetics on the market. Their survey revealed that use of phthalates in cosmetics decreased considerably from 2004–2010.

Infant Exposure to Phthalates

Infants, like all consumers, are exposed daily to phthalates from a number of sources, including air, drugs, food, plastics, water, and cosmetics. The American Academy of Pediatrics (AAP) has published an article stating that infants exposed to infant care products, specifically baby shampoos, baby lotions, and baby powder, showed increased levels of phthalate metabolites in their urine.

Like the CDC report, this study did not establish an association between these findings and any health effects. In addition, levels of phthalates, if any, in the infant care products were not determined.

How to Know If There Are Phthalates in the Cosmetics You Use

Under the authority of the Fair Packaging and Labeling Act (FPLA), the FDA requires an ingredient declaration on cosmetic products sold at the retail level to consumers. Consumers can tell whether some products contain phthalates by reading the ingredient declaration on the labels of such products.

However, the regulations do not require the listing of the individual fragrance ingredients; therefore, the consumer will not be able to determine from the ingredient declaration if phthalates are present in a fragrance. Also, because the FPLA does not apply to products used exclusively by professionals—for example, in salons—the requirement for an ingredient declaration does not apply to these products. Based on available safety information, DEP does not pose known risks to human health as it is currently used in cosmetics and fragrances. Consumers who nevertheless do not want to purchase cosmetics containing DEP may wish to choose products that do not include "Fragrance" in the ingredient listing.

The FDA's Role

Under the law, cosmetic products and ingredients, with the exception of color additives, are not subject to the FDA approval before they go on the market. The FDA can take action against unsafe cosmetics that are on the market, but only if they have dependable scientific evidence showing that a product or ingredient is unsafe for consumers under labeled or customary conditions of use.

At the present time, the FDA does not have evidence that phthalates, as used in cosmetics, pose a safety risk. If it is determined that a health hazard exists, it will advise the industry and the public, and will take action within the scope of its authority under the Federal Food, Drug, and Cosmetic Act (FFDCA) in protecting the health and welfare of consumers.

Section 50.8

Sunscreen

This section includes text excerpted from "Understanding Over-the-Counter Medicines—Sunscreen: How to Help Protect Your Skin from the Sun," U.S. Food and Drug Administration (FDA), July 14, 2017.

As the U.S. Food and Drug Administration (FDA) regulated product, sunscreens must pass certain tests before they are sold. But how you use this product, and what other protective measures you take, make a difference in how well you are able to protect yourself and your family from sunburn, skin cancer, early skin aging, and other risks of overexposure to the sun. Some key sun safety tips include:

- Limit time in the sun, especially between the hours of 10am and 2pm, when the sun's rays are most intense

- Wear clothing to cover skin exposed to the sun, such as long-sleeved shirts, pants, sunglasses, and broad-brimmed hats

- Use broad-spectrum sunscreens with sun protection factor (SPF) values of 15 or higher regularly and as directed

- Reapply sunscreen at least every two hours, and more often if you're sweating or jumping in and out of the water

How to Apply and Store Sunscreen

- Apply 30 minutes before you go outside. This allows the sunscreen (of SPF 15 or higher) to have enough time to provide the maximum benefit.

- Use enough to cover your entire face and body (avoiding the eyes and mouth). An average sized adult or child needs at least one ounce of sunscreen (about the amount it takes to fill a shot glass) to evenly cover the body from head to toe.

- Know your skin. Fair-skinned people are likely to absorb more solar energy than dark-skinned people under the same conditions.

- Re-apply at least every two hours, and more often if you're swimming or sweating.

Frequently Forgotten Spots

- Ears
- Nose
- Lips
- Back of neck

- Hands
- Tops of feet
- Along the hairline
- Areas of the head exposed by the balding or thinning hair

Storing Your Sunscreen

To keep your sunscreen in good condition, the FDA recommends that sunscreen containers should not be exposed to direct sun. Protect the sunscreen by wrapping the containers in towels or keeping them in the shade. Sunscreen containers can also be kept in coolers while outside in the heat for long periods of time. This is why all sunscreen labels must say: "Protect the product in this container from excessive heat and direct sun."

Sunscreens for Infants and Children

Sunscreens are not recommended for infants. The FDA recommends that infants be kept out of the sun during the hours of 10am and 2pm, and to use protective clothing if they have to be in the sun. Infants are at greater risk than adults of sunscreen side effects, such as a rash. The best protection for infants is to keep them out of the sun entirely. Ask a doctor before applying sunscreen to children under six months of age.

Types of Sunscreen

Sunscreen comes in many forms, including:

• Lotions

• Creams

• Sticks

• Gels

• Oils

• Butters

• Pastes

• Sprays

The directions for using sunscreen products can vary according to their forms. For example, spray sunscreens should never be applied directly to your face. This is just one reason why you should always read the label before using a sunscreen product.

Understanding the Sunscreen Label

Broad Spectrum

Not all sunscreens are broad spectrum, so it is important to look for it on the label. Broad spectrum sunscreen provides protection from the sun's ultraviolet (UV) radiation. There are two types of UV radiation that you need to protect yourself from—UVA and UVB. Broad spectrum provides protection against both by providing a chemical barrier that absorbs or reflects UV radiation before it can damage the skin.

Sunscreens that are not broad spectrum or that lack an SPF of at least 15 must carry the warning:

Sun Protection Factor (SPF)

Sunscreens are made in a wide range of SPFs. The SPF value indicates the level of sunburn protection provided by the sunscreen product. All sunscreens are tested to measure the amount of UV radiation exposure it takes to cause sunburn when using a sunscreen compared to how much UV exposure it takes to cause a sunburn when not using a sunscreen. The product is then labeled with the appropriate SPF value. Higher SPF values (up to 50) provide greater sunburn protection. Because SPF values are determined from a test that measures protection against sunburn caused by UVB radiation, SPF values only indicate a sunscreen's UVB protection.

Sunscreens that pass the broad spectrum test can demonstrate that they also provide UVA protection. Therefore, under the label requirements, for sunscreens labeled "Broad Spectrum SPF [value]," they will indicate protection from both UVA and UVB radiation.

To get the most protection out of sunscreen, choose one with an SPF of at least 15.

If your skin is fair, you may want a higher SPF of 30–50.

There is a popular misconception that SPF relates to the time of solar exposure. For example, many people believe that, if they normally get sunburned in one hour, then an SPF 15 sunscreen allows them to stay in the sun for 15 hours (e.g., 15 times longer) without getting sunburn. This is not true because SPF is not directly related to the time of solar exposure but to amount of solar exposure.

The sun is stronger in the middle of the day compared to early morning and early evening hours. That means your risk of sunburn is higher at mid-day. Solar intensity is also related to geographic location, with greater solar intensity occurring at lower latitudes.

Sunscreen Ingredients

Every drug has active ingredients and inactive ingredients. In the case of sunscreen, active ingredients are the ones that are protecting your skin from the sun's harmful UV rays. Inactive ingredients are all other ingredients that are not active ingredients, such as water or oil that may be used in formulating sunscreens. Below is a list of acceptable active ingredients in products that are labeled as the sunscreen:

• Aminobenzoic acid

- Avobenzone

- Cinoxate

- Dioxybenzone

- Homosalate

- Menthyl anthranilate

- Octocrylene

- Octyl methoxycinnamate

- Octyl salicylate

- Oxybenzone

- Padimate O

- Phenylbenzimidazole sulfonic acid

- Sulisobenzone

- Titanium dioxide

- Trolamine salicylate

- Zinc oxide

Although the protective action of sunscreen products takes place on the surface of the skin, there is evidence that at least some sunscreen active ingredients may be absorbed through the skin and enter the body. This makes it important to perform studies to determine whether, and to what extent, use of sunscreen products as directed may result in unintended, chronic, systemic exposure to sunscreen active ingredients.

Sunscreen Expiration Dates

The FDA regulations require all sunscreens and other nonprescription drugs to have an expiration date unless stability testing conducted by the manufacturer has shown that the product will remain stable for at least three years. That means, a sunscreen product that doesn't have an expiration date should be considered expired three years after purchase.

To make sure that your sunscreen is providing the sun protection promised in its labeling, the FDA recommends that you do not use sunscreen products that have passed their expiration date (if there is one), or that have no expiration date and were not purchased within the last three years. Expired sunscreens should be discarded because there is no assurance that they remain safe and fully effective.

Sunscreens from Other Countries

In Europe and in some other countries, sunscreens are regulated as cosmetics, not as drugs, and are subject to different marketing requirements. Any sunscreen sold in the United States is regulated as a drug because it makes a drug claim—to help prevent sunburn or to decrease the risks of skin cancer and early skin aging caused by the sun.

If you purchase a sunscreen outside the United States, it is important to read the label to understand the instructions for use and any potential differences between the product and U.S. products.

Section 50.9

Talc

This section includes text excerpted from "Cosmetics—
Talc," U.S. Food and Drug Administration (FDA), March 12, 2018.

Talc is an ingredient used in many cosmetics, from baby powder to blush. From time to time, the U.S. Food and Drug Administration (FDA) has received questions about its safety and whether talc contains harmful contaminants, such as asbestos.

The FDA's Authority over Cosmetic Safety

Under the Federal Food, Drug and Cosmetic Act (FD&C Act), cosmetic products and ingredients, with the exception of color additives, do not have to undergo the FDA review or approval before they go on the market. Cosmetics must be properly labeled, and they must be safe for use by consumers under labeled or customary conditions of use. Cosmetic companies have a legal responsibility for the safety and labeling of their products and ingredients, but the law does not require them to share their safety information with the FDA.

The FDA monitors for potential safety problems with cosmetic products on the market and takes action when needed to protect public health. Before they can take such action against a cosmetic, they need sound scientific data to show that it is harmful under its intended use.

Talc: What It Is and How It Is Used in Cosmetics

Talc is a naturally occurring mineral, mined from the earth, composed of magnesium, silicon, oxygen, and hydrogen. Chemically, talc is a hydrous magnesium silicate with a chemical formula of $Mg_3Si_4O_{10}(OH)_2$.

Talc has many uses in cosmetics and other personal care products; in food, such as rice and chewing gum; and in the manufacture of tablets. For example, it may be used to absorb moisture, to prevent caking, to make facial makeup opaque, or to improve the feel of a product.

Asbestos: Concern and Need for Prevention of Its Occurrence in Cosmetics

Asbestos is also a naturally occurring silicate mineral, but with a different crystal structure. Both talc and asbestos are naturally occurring minerals that may be found in close proximity to the earth. Unlike talc, however, asbestos is a known carcinogen. To prevent contamination of talc with asbestos, it is essential to select talc mining sites carefully and take steps to purify the ore sufficiently.

How the FDA Followed Up on the Latest Reports

Because safety questions about the possible presence of asbestos in talc are raised periodically, the FDA decided to conduct an exploratory survey of currently marketed cosmetic grade raw material talc, as well as some cosmetic products containing talc.

The Results of the FDA's Survey and What They Mean

The survey found no asbestos fibers or structures in any of the samples of cosmetic grade raw material talc or cosmetic products containing talc. The results were limited, however, by the fact that only four talc suppliers submitted samples and by the number of products tested. For these reasons, while the FDA finds these results informative, they do not prove that most or all talc or talc containing cosmetic products currently marketed in the United States are likely to be free of asbestos contamination. As always, when potential public health concerns are raised, the FDA will continue to monitor for new information and take appropriate actions to protect the public health.

Chapter 51

X-Rays

Medical imaging has led to improvements in the diagnosis and treatment of numerous medical conditions in children and adults. There are many types or modalities of medical imaging procedures, each of which uses different technologies and techniques. Computed tomography (CT), fluoroscopy, and radiography (conventional X-ray including mammography) all use ionizing radiation to generate images of the body. Ionizing radiation is a form of radiation that has enough energy to potentially cause damage to deoxyribonucleic acid (DNA) and may elevate a person's lifetime risk of developing cancer.

CT, radiography, and fluoroscopy all work on the same basic principle: an X-ray beam is passed through the body where a portion of the X-rays are either absorbed or scattered by the internal structures, and the remaining X-ray pattern is transmitted to a detector (e.g., film or a computer screen) for recording or further processing by a computer. These exams differ in their purpose:

- **Radiography.** A single image is recorded for later evaluation. Mammography is a special type of radiography to image the internal structures of breasts.

- **Fluoroscopy.** A continuous X-ray image is displayed on a monitor, allowing for real-time monitoring of a procedure or passage of a contrast agent (dye) through the body. Fluoroscopy

This chapter includes text excerpted from "Radiation-Emitting Products—Medical X-ray Imaging," U.S. Food and Drug Administration (FDA), March 15, 2018.

can result in relatively high radiation doses, especially for complex interventional procedures (such as placing stents or other devices inside the body) which require fluoroscopy be administered for a long period of time.

- **CT.** Many X-ray images are recorded as the detector moves around the patient's body. A computer reconstructs all the individual images into cross-sectional images or "slices" of internal organs and tissues. A CT exam involves a higher radiation dose than conventional radiography because the CT image is reconstructed from many individual X-ray projections.

Benefits and Risks

Benefits

The discovery of X-rays and the invention of CT represented major advances in medicine. X-ray imaging exams are recognized as a valuable medical tool for a wide variety of examinations and procedures. They are used to:

- noninvasively and painlessly help to diagnosis disease and monitor therapy

- support medical and surgical treatment planning

- guide medical personnel as they insert catheters, stents, or other devices inside the body, treat tumors, or remove blood clots or other blockages

Risks

As in many aspects of medicine, there are risks associated with the use of X-ray imaging, which uses ionizing radiation to generate images of the body. Ionizing radiation is a form of radiation that has enough energy to potentially cause damage to DNA. Risks from exposure to ionizing radiation include:

- a small increase in the possibility that a person exposed to X-rays will develop cancer later in life

- tissue effects such as cataracts, skin reddening, and hair loss, which occur at relatively high levels of radiation exposure and are rare for many types of imaging exams. For example, the typical use of a CT scanner or conventional radiography equipment should not result in tissue effects, but the dose to the skin from some long, complex interventional fluoroscopy procedures might, in some circumstances, be high enough to result in such effects.

Another risk of X-ray imaging is possible reactions associated with an intravenously injected contrast agent, or "dye," that is sometimes used to improve visualization.

The risk of developing cancer from medical imaging radiation exposure is generally very small, and it depends on:

- **Radiation dose.** The lifetime risk of cancer increases the larger the dose and the more X-ray exams a patient undergoes.

- **Patient's age.** The lifetime risk of cancer is larger for a patient who receives X-rays at a younger age than for one who receives them at an older age.

- **Patient's sex.** Women are at a somewhat higher lifetime risk than men for developing radiation associated cancer after receiving the same exposures at the same ages.

- **Body region.** Some organs are more radiosensitive than others.

The above statements are generalizations based on scientific analyses of large population data sets, such as survivors exposed to radiation from the atomic bomb. While specific individuals or cases may not fit into such generalizations, they are still useful in developing an overall approach to medical imaging radiation safety by identifying at risk populations or higher-risk procedures.

Because radiation risks are dependent on exposure to radiation, an awareness of the typical radiation exposures involved in different imaging exams is useful for communication between the physician and patient.

The medical community has emphasized radiation dose reduction in CT because of the relatively high radiation dose for CT exams (as compared to radiography) and their increased use, as reported in the National Council on Radiation Protection and Measurements (NCRP) Report No. 160. Because tissue effects are extremely rare for typical use of many X-ray imaging devices (including CT), the primary radiation risk concern for most imaging studies is cancer; however, the long exposure times needed for complex interventional fluoroscopy exams and resulting high skin doses may result in tissue effects, even when the equipment is used appropriately.

Balancing Benefits and Risks

While the benefit of a clinically appropriate X-ray imaging exam generally far outweighs the risk, efforts should be made to minimize this risk by reducing unnecessary exposure to ionizing radiation. To help reduce risk to the patient, all exams using ionizing radiation should be performed only when necessary to answer a medical question, treat a disease, or guide a procedure. If there is a medical need for a particular imaging procedure and other exams using no or less radiation are less appropriate, then the benefits exceed the risks, and radiation risk considerations should not influence the physician's decision to perform the study or the patient's decision to have the procedure. However, the "As Low as Reasonably Achievable" (ALARA) principle should always be followed when choosing equipment settings to minimize radiation exposure to the patient.

Patient factors are important to consider in this balance of benefits and risks. For example:

- Because younger patients are more sensitive to radiation, special care should be taken in reducing radiation exposure to pediatric patients for all types of X-ray imaging exams.

- Special care should also be taken in imaging pregnant patients due to possible effects of radiation exposure to the developing fetus.

- The benefit of possible disease detection should be carefully balanced against the risks of an imaging screening study on healthy, asymptomatic patients.

Information for Patients

X-ray imaging (CT, fluoroscopy, and radiography) exams should be performed only after careful consideration of the patient's health needs. They should be performed only when the referring physician judges them to be necessary to answer a clinical question or to guide treatment of a disease. The clinical benefit of a medically appropriate X-ray imaging exam outweighs the small radiation risk. However, efforts should be made to help minimize this risk.

Questions to Ask Your Healthcare Provider

Patients and parents of children undergoing X-ray imaging exams should be well informed and prepared by:

- Keeping track of medical-imaging histories as part of a discussion with the referring physician when a new exam is recommended

- Informing their physician if they are pregnant or think they might be pregnant

- Asking the referring physician about the benefits and risks of imaging procedures, such as:

  - How will the results of the exam be used to evaluate my condition or guide my treatment (or that of my child)?

  - Are there alternative exams that do not use ionizing radiation that are equally useful?

- Asking the imaging facility:

  - If it uses techniques to reduce radiation dose, especially to sensitive populations such as children

  - About any additional steps that may be necessary to perform the imaging study (e.g., administration of oral or intravenous contrast agent to improve visualization, sedation, or advanced preparation)

  - If the facility is accredited (accreditation may only be available for specific types of X-ray imaging such as CT)

Part Seven

Additional Help and Information

Chapter 52

Glossary of Terms Related to Mental Health Disorders

acid deposition: Acidic materials that falls from the atmosphere to the Earth in either wet (rain, sleet, snow, fog) or dry (gases, particles) forms. More commonly referred to as acid rain, acid deposition has two components: wet and dry deposition.

acid rain: The result of sulfur dioxide (SO_2) and nitrogen oxides (NO_x) reacting in the atmosphere with water and returning to earth as rain, fog, or snow. Broadly used to include both wet and dry deposition. The acid rain page provides a great deal of information about this issue.

aerosol: A small droplet or particle suspended in the atmosphere, typically containing sulfur. Aerosols are emitted naturally (e.g., in volcanic eruptions) and as the result of human activities (e.g., by burning fossil fuels).

aflatoxins: A group of closely related toxic metabolites that are designated mycotoxins. They are produced by *Aspergillus flavus* and A. parasiticus. Members of the group include AFLATOXIN B1, aflatoxin B2, aflatoxin G1, aflatoxin G2, AFLATOXIN M1, and aflatoxin M2.

air quality index (AQI): A numerical index used for reporting severity of air pollution levels to the public. The AQI incorporates five criteria pollutants—ozone, particulate matter, carbon monoxide, sulfur dioxide and nitrogen dioxide—into a single index.

This glossary contains terms excerpted from documents produced by several sources deemed reliable.

637

algal blooms: Sudden spurts of algal growth, which can affect water quality adversely and indicate potentially hazardous changes in local water chemistry.

allergen: A material that, as a result of coming into contact with appropriate tissues of an animal body, induces a state of allergy or hypersensitivity; generally associated with idiosyncratic hypersensitivities.

ambient air: The portion of the atmosphere external to buildings and breathed by the general public.

anaerobic: Able to live, grow, or take place where free oxygen is not present.

anaphylaxis: An immediate and severe allergic reaction to a substance (e.g., food or drugs). Symptoms include breathing difficulties, loss of consciousness, and a drop in blood pressure.

animal dander: Tiny scales of animal skin.

antimicrobial: Agent that kills microbial growth.

antitoxin: Antibodies capable of destroying toxins generated by microorganisms including viruses and bacteria.

antiviral: Literally "against-virus"—any medicine capable of destroying or weakening a virus.

benchmark dose (BMD): A dose that produces a predetermined change in response rate of an adverse effect (called the benchmark response or BMR) compared to background.

bioaccumulation: The process in which a substance is taken up by an aquatic organism through any route, including respiration, ingestion, or direct contact with water or sediment.

bioassay: A method used to determine the toxicity of specific chemical contaminants.

biological contaminants: Debris from or pieces of dead organisms.

biological pesticides: Certain microorganism, including bacteria, fungi, viruses, and protozoa, that are effective in controlling pests.

biomagnification: The increased accumulation and concentration of a contaminant at higher levels of the food chain.

body burden: The concentration of a substance which has accumulated in the body.

cancer cluster: The occurrence of a larger-than-expected number of cases of cancer within a group of people in a geographic area over a period of time.

carcinogen: Any substance that causes cancer.

carcinogenicity: The complex process whereby normal body cells are transformed to cancer cells.

chronic exposure: An exposure to a chemical or hazardous substance that occurs over a period of time usually more than 3 months.

cloning: Asexual reproduction of animals using somatic cell nuclear transfer (SCNT).

coronavirus: One of a group of viruses that have a halo or crown-like (corona) appearance when viewed under a microscope.

detection limit: The minimum concentration of an analyte in a sample, that with a high level of confidence is not zero.

dichlorodiphenyltrichloroethane (DDT): A group of colorless chemicals, no longer made today, that was used to kill insects

differentiation: The process whereby relatively unspecialized cells, e.g., embryonic or regenerative cells, acquire specialized structural and/or functional features that characterize the cells, tissues, or organs of the mature organism.

disinfectants: One of three groups of antimicrobials registered by EPA for public health uses. EPA considers an antimicrobial to be a disinfectant when it destroys or irreversibly inactivates infectious or other undesirable organisms.

dose: The amount of a substance to which a person is exposed (air, soil, dust, or water) over some time period.

dose-response assessment: The relation between dose levels and associated effects.

dry deposition: The falling of small particles and gases to the Earth without rain or snow. Dry deposition is a component of acid deposition, more commonly referred to as acid rain.

effluent: Something that flows out, especially a liquid or gaseous waste stream.

electromagnetic radiation: A traveling wave motion that results from changing electric and magnetic fields.

emulsifier: Substance added to products, such as meat spreads, to prevent separation of product components to ensure consistency.

environmental agents: Conditions other than indoor air contaminants that cause stress, comfort, and/or health problems (e.g., humidity extremes, drafts, noise, and over-crowding).

epidemiology: The study of the distribution and determinants of health-related states or events in specified populations; and the application of this study to the control of health problems.

exacerbation: Any worsening of asthma. Onset can be acute and sudden, or gradual over several days.

exposure assessment: The analysis or estimation of the intensity, frequency, and duration of human exposures to an agent.

exposure pathway: A route by which a radionuclide or other toxic material can enter the body.

flashing: Material for allowing proper drainage around the joints and angles of the roof and penetrations through the roof and walls.

fossil fuels: Oil, natural gas, and coal. Fossil fuels were made in nature from ancient plants and animals, and today we burn them to make energy.

free chlorine: The chlorine in water not combined with other constituents; therefore, it is able to serve as an effective disinfectant.

fungicide: A substance or chemical that kills fungi.

genetic engineering: A process of inserting new genetic information into existing cells in order to modify a specific organism for the purpose of changing one of its characteristics.

genome: The full set of genes in an individual, either haploid (the set derived from one parent) or diploid (the set derived from both parents).

greenhouse gases: Gases that occur naturally in the Earth's atmosphere and trap heat to keep the planet warm.

Haemophilus influenzae type B (Hib): Haemophilus influenzae type b. A bacterial infection that may result in severe respiratory infections, including pneumonia, and other diseases such as meningitis.

half-life: The time any substance takes to decay by half of its original amount.

high-efficiency particulate air (HEPA) filter: Type of air filter that removes >99.97 percent of particles 0.3 um or larger at a specified flow rate of air.

house dust mite: Either of two widely distributed mites of the genus Dermatophagoides (D. farinae and D. pteronyssinus) that commonly occur in house dust and often induce allergic responses, especially in children.

humectant: Substance added to foods to help retain moisture and soft texture. An example is glycerine, which may be used in dried meat snacks.

humidifier fever: A respiratory illness caused by exposure to toxins from microorganisms found in wet or moist areas in humidifiers and air conditioners.

hypersensitivity pneumonitis: A group of respiratory diseases that cause inflammation of the lung (specifically granulomatous cells).

immune globulin: A protein found in the blood that fights infection. Also known as gamma globulin.

*in vitro***:** Outside the organism, or in an artificial environment. This term applies, for example, to cells, tissues or organs cultured in glass or plastic containers.

incubation period: Time interval between infection (i.e., introduction of the infectious agent into the susceptible host) and the onset of the first symptom of illness known to be caused by the infectious agent.

infiltration: The downward movement of water through a soil in response to gravity and capillary suction.

irradiation: Exposure to radiation.

landfills: 1) Sanitary landfills are disposal sites for nonhazardous solid wastes, 2) Secure chemical landfills are disposal sites for hazardous waste.

leaching: Process by which water removes chemicals from soil through chemical reactions and the downward movement of water.

lesion: An abnormal change in the structure of an organ, due to injury or disease.

lifetime exposure: Total amount of exposure to a substance that a human would receive in a lifetime (usually assumed to be 70 years).

lowest observed adverse effect level (LOAEL): The lowest dose in a study in which there was an observed toxic or adverse effect.

magnetron: The physical component of a microwave system that generates the microwaves.

maximum ventilation: The volume of air breathed in one minute during repetitive maximal respiratory effort. Synonymous with maximum ventilatory minute volume.

microwaves: Electromagnetic waves at frequencies 915, 2450, 5800, and 24225 MHz.

monosodium glutamate (MSG): Describes a climate pattern with a wind system that changes direction with the seasons; this pattern is dominant over the Arabian Sea and Southeast Asia.

mucus: The clear, viscid secretion of mucous membranes, consisting of mucin, epithelial cells, leukocytes, and various inorganic salts suspended in water.

municipal solid waste (MSW): Residential solid waste and some nonhazardous commercial, institutional, and industrial wastes. This material is generally sent to municipal landfills for disposal.

neurotoxin: A toxic agent or substance that inhibits, damages or destroys the tissues of the nervous system, especially neurons, the conducting cells of your body's central nervous system.

nonionizing radiation: Radiation that has lower energy levels and longer wavelengths than ionizing radiation. Examples include radio waves, microwaves, visible light, and infrared from a heat lamp.

ozone: Ozone, the triatomic form of oxygen ($O3$), is a gaseous atmospheric constituent. In the troposphere, it is created by photochemical reactions. In high concentrations, tropospheric ozone can be harmful to a wide range of living organisms.

papain: An enzyme that can dissolve or degrade the proteins collagen and elastin to soften meat and poultry tissue. It is derived from the tropical papaya tree and is used as a meat tenderizer.

particulates: 1) Fine liquid or solid particles such as dust, smoke, mist, fumes, or smog found in air or emissions. 2) Very small solids suspended in water; they can vary in size, shape, density, and electrical charge and can be gathered together by coagulation and flocculation.

Perfluorinated chemicals (PFCs): Perfluorinated chemicals have all carbon-hydrogen bonds in a chain replaced by carbon-fluorine bonds. Examples include perfluorooctanoic acid (PFOA) and perfluorooctane sulfonate (PFOS).

Perfluorooctane sulfonic acid (PFOS): Perfluorooctane sulfonic acid is a fully fluorinated, eight chain sulfonic acid (CAS RN 1763-23-1) sometimes used to refer to the anionic salt form.

Perfluorooctanoic acid (PFOA): Perfluorooctanoic acid is a fully fluorinated, eight-carbon chain carboxylic acid (C8) (CAS RN 335-67-1) sometimes used to refer to the anionic salt form.

PM2.5: Tiny particles with an aerodynamic diameter less than or equal to 2.5 microns. This fraction of particulate matter penetrates most deeply into the lungs.

point source: Pollutant loads discharged at a specific location from pipes, outfalls, and conveyance channels from either municipal wastewater treatment plants or industrial waste treatment facilities.

polycyclic aromatic hydrocarbons (PAHS): A group of organic chemicals that includes several petroleum products and their derivatives.

precursor: A chemical that can be transformed to produce another chemical. For example, some residual monomer chemicals from the telomer manufacturing process, such as telomer alcohols and telomer iodides.

rancid/rancidity: Oxidation/breakdown of fat that occurs naturally causing undesirable smell and taste. BHA/BHT and tocopherols are used to keep fats from becoming rancid.

reflectivity: The ability of a surface material to reflect sunlight including the visible, infrared, and ultraviolet wavelengths.

relative humidity: Partial pressure of water vapor at the atmospheric temperature divided by the vapor pressure of water at that temperature, expressed as a percentage.

residual: Amount of a pollutant remaining in the environment after a natural or technological process has taken place; e.g., the sludge remaining after initial wastewater treatment.

resilience: A capability to anticipate, prepare for, respond to, and recover from significant multi-hazard threats with minimum damage to social well-being, the economy, and the environment.

respirator: A personal protective device that is worn over the nose and mouth to reduce the risk of inhaling hazardous airborne particles, gases, or vapors.

route of exposure: The way people come into contact with a hazardous substance. Three routes of exposure are breathing (inhalation], eating or drinking (ingestion], or contact with the skin (dermal contact].

shielding: The material between a radiation source and a potentially exposed person that reduces exposure.

sink: Any process, activity or mechanism which removes a greenhouse gas, an aerosol or a precursor of a greenhouse gas or aerosol from the atmosphere.

spirometry: A medical test that measures how well the lungs exhale.

stressor: Any physical, chemical, or biological entity that can induce an adverse response.

surface runoff: Precipitation, snowmelt, or irrigation water in excess of what can infiltrate the soil surface and be stored in small surface depressions; a major transporter of nonpoint source pollutants.

thimerosal: Thimerosal is a mercury-containing preservative used in some vaccines and other products since the 1930's.

toxicity: The degree to which a substance or mixture of substances can harm humans or animals.

toxicodynamics: The study of the cellular and molecular mechanisms of the action of a poison.

tremolite: A mineral in the amphibole group, that occurs as a series in which magnesium and iron can freely substitute for each other. Tremolite is the mineral when magnesium is predominant.

ultraviolet A (UVA): A band of ultraviolet radiation with wavelengths from 320–400 nanometers produced by the sun: UVA is not absorbed by ozone. This band of radiation has wavelengths just shorter than visible violet light.

ultraviolet B (UVB): A band of ultraviolet radiation with wavelengths from 280–320 nanometers produced by the sun: UVB is a kind of ultraviolet light from the sun (and sun lamps) that has several harmful effects.

ultraviolet C (UVC): A band of ultraviolet radiation with wavelengths shorter than 280 nanometers: UVC is extremcly dangerous, but it is completely absorbed by ozone and normal oxygen (O2).

uncertainty factors: Factors used in the adjustment of toxicity data to account for unknown variations. An uncertainty factor would adjust measured toxicity upward and downward to cover the sensitivity range of potentially more or less sensitive species.

vermiculite: A chemically inert, lightweight, fire resistant, and odorless magnesium silicate material that is generally used in construction and horticultural applications.

volatile organic compound (VOC): Any organic compound that participates in atmospheric photochemical reactions except those designated by EPA as having negligible photochemical reactivity.

wet deposition: The process by which chemicals are removed from the atmosphere and deposited on the Earth's surface via rain, sleet, snow, cloudwater, and fog.

X-ray: Electromagnetic radiation caused by deflection of electrons from their original paths, or inner orbital electrons that change their orbital levels around the atomic nucleus.

Chapter 53

Directory of Environmental Health Organizations and Resources

Agency for Toxic Substances and Disease Registry (ATSDR)
Centers for Disease Control and Prevention (CDC)
4770 Buford Hwy N.E.
Atlanta, GA 30341
Toll-Free: 800-CDC-INFO
(800-232-4636)
Toll-Free TTY: 888-232-6348
Website: www.atsdr.cdc.gov
E-mail: cdcinfo@cdc.gov

Asthma and Allergy Foundation of America (AAFA)
8201 Corporate Dr.
Ste. 1000
Landover, MD 20785
Toll-Free: 800-7-ASTHMA
(800-727-8462)
Website: www.aafa.org

Resources in this chapter were compiled from several sources deemed reliable; all contact information was verified and updated in April 2018.

Beyond Pesticides
701 E. St. S.E.
Ste. 200
Washington, DC 20003
Phone: 202-543-5450
Fax: 202-543-4791
Website: www.beyondpesticides.
org
E-mail: info@beyondpesticides.
org

Birth Defect Research for Children, Inc.
976 Lake Baldwin Ln.
Ste. 104
Orlando, FL 32814
Phone: 407-895-0802
Website: www.birthdefects.org
E-mail: staff@birthdefects.org

Campaign for Tobacco-Free Kids
1400 I St. N.W.
Ste. 1200
Washington, DC 20005
Phone: 202-296-5469
Fax: 202-296-5427
Website: www.tobaccofreekids.
org
E-mail: info@tobaccofreekids.org

Center for Environmental Health (CEH)
2201 Bdway.
Ste. 302
Oakland, CA 94612
Phone: 510-655-3900
Fax: 510-655-9100
Website: www.ceh.org

Center for Food Safety and Applied Nutrition (CFSAN)
5001 Campus Dr. HFS-009
College Park, MD 20740-3835
Toll-Free: 888-723-3366
Toll-Free TTY: 800-877-8339
Website: www.fda.gov/
AboutFDA/CentersOffices/
OfficeofFoods/CFSAN/
ContactCFSAN/default.htm
E-mail: consumer@fda.gov

Center for Health, Environment, and Justice (CHEJ)
7139 Shreve Rd.
Falls Church, VA 22046
Phone: 703-237-2249
Wesite: www.chej.org
E-mail: info@chej.org

Center for Science in the Public Interest (CSPI)
1220 L St. N.W.
Ste. 300
Washington, DC 20005
Phone: 202-332-9110
Fax: 202-265-4954
Website: www.cspinet.org
E-mail: cspi@cspinet.org

Chemical Injury Information Network (CIIN)
P.O. Box 301
White Sulphur Springs, MT 59645
Phone: 406-547-2255
Website: www.ciin.org
E-mail: chemicalinjury@ciin.org

Children's Environmental Health Network (CEHN)
110 Maryland Ave. N.E.
Ste. 404
Washington, DC 20002
Phone: 202-543-4033
Fax: 202-543-8797
Website: www.cehn.org
E-mail: cehn@cehn.org

Clean Air Task Force (CATF)
114 State St.
Fl. 6
Boston, MA 02108
Phone: 617-624-0234
Fax: 617-624-0230
Website: www.catf.us

Clean Water Fund (CWF)
1444 St. N.W.
Ste. 400
Washington, DC 20005
Phone: 202-895-0420
Fax: 202-895-0438
Website: www.cleanwaterfund.
org

Collaborative on Health and the Environment (CHE)
P.O. Box 316
Bolinas, CA 94924
Phone: 415-868-0970
Fax: 415-868-2230
Website: www.
healthandenvironment.org
E-mail: info@
healthandenvironment.org

Environment & Human Health, Inc. (EHHI)
1191 Ridge Rd.
North Haven, CT 06473
Phone: 203-248-6582
Fax: 203-288-7571
Website: www.ehhi.org
E-mail: info@ehhi.org

Environmental Defense Fund (EDF)
1875 Connecticut Ave.
Ste. 600
Washington, DC 20009
Toll-Free: 800-684-3322
Phone: 212-505-2100
Fax: 212-505-2375
Website: www.edf.org

Environmental Health Strategy Center
565 Congress St.
Portland, ME 04101
Phone: 207-699-5795
Website: www.ourhealthyfuture.
org
E-mail: info@preventharm.org

Environmental Working Group (EWG)
1436 U St. N.W.
Ste. 100
Washington, DC 20009
Phone: 202-667-6982
Website: www.ewg.org

Federal Emergency Management Agency (FEMA)
500 C St. S.W.
Washington, DC 20472
Phone: 202-646-2500
Website: www.fema.gov

Food and Water Watch
1616 P St. N.W.
Washington, DC 20036
Toll-free: 855-340-8083
Phone: 202-683-2500
Fax: 202-683-2501
Website: www.
foodandwaterwatch.org
E-mail: info@fwwatch.org

Food Safety and Inspection Service (FSIS)
U.S. Department of Agriculture (USDA)
1400 Independence Ave. S.W.
Washington, DC 20250-3700
Toll-Free: 800-877-8339
Phone: 202-720-9113
Website: www.fsis.usda.gov

Food Safety Research Information Office (FSRIO)
National Agricultural Library (NAL)
10301 Baltimore Ave.
Beltsville, MD 20705-2351
Phone: 301-504-5755
Fax: 301-504-7042
Website: www.nal.usda.gov

Friends of the Earth
1100 15th St. N.W.
Fl. 11
Washington, DC 20005
Phone: 202-783-7400
Fax: 202-783-0444
Website: www.foe.org

Greenpeace USA
702 H St. N.W.
Ste. 300
Washington, DC 20001
Toll-Free: 800-722-6995
Phone: 202-462-1177
Fax: 202-462-4507
Website: www.greenpeace.org
E-mail: info@wdc.greenpeace.org

Healthy Building Network (HBN)
1710 Connecticut Ave.
Fl. 4
Washington, DC 20009
Toll-Free: 877-974-2767
Phone: 202-741-5717
Website: www.healthybuilding.
net

Inform, Inc.
Toll-Free: 800-987-654
Website: www.informinc.org
E-mail: contact@informinc.org

KidsHealth
Nemours Foundation
Website: www.kidshealth.org

March of Dimes
1275 Mamaroneck Ave.
White Plains, NY 10605
Website: www.marchofdimes.
com

National Cancer Institute (NCI)
NCI Public Inquiries Office
BG 9609 MSC 9760
9609 Medical Center Dr.
Bethesda, MD 20892-9760
Toll-Free: 800-422-6237
Website: www.cancer.gov

National Center for Environmental Health (NCEH)
4770 Buford Hwy N.E.
Atlanta, GA 30341-3717
Toll-Free: 800-232-4636
Toll-Free TTY: 888-232-6348
Website: www.cdc.gov/nceh

National Council for Science and the Environment (NCSE)
740 15th St. NW
Ste. 900
Washington, DC 20005
Phone: 202-530-5810
Fax: 202-628-4311
Website: www.ncseonline.org
E-mail: NCSE@NCSEGlobal.org

National Environmental Health Association (NEHA)
720 S. Colorado Blvd.
Ste. 1000-N
Denver, CO 80246-1926
Phone: 303-756-9090
Fax: 303-691-9490
Website: www.neha.org
E-mail: staff@neha.org

National Institute for Occupational Safety and Health (NIOSH)
1600 Clifton Rd.
Atlanta, GA 30329-4027
Toll-Free: 800-232-4636
Toll-Free TTY: 888-232-6348
Website: www.cdc.gov/niosh

National Institute of Allergy and Infectious Diseases (NIAID)
Office of Communications and
Government Relations (OCGR)
5601 Fishers Ln.
MSC 9806
Bethesda, MD 20892-9806
Toll-Free: 866-284-4107
Phone: 301-496-5717
Fax: 301-402-3573
Website: www.niaid.nih.gov
E-mail: ocpostoffice@niaid.nih.gov

National Institute of Environmental Health Sciences (NIEHS)
P.O. Box 12233
MD K3-16
Research Triangle Park, NC 27709-2233
Phone: 919-541-3345
Fax: 301-480-2978
Website: www.niehs.nih.gov
E-mail: webcenter@niehs.nih.gov

National Institute on Aging (NIA)
31 Center Dr. MSC 2292
Bldg. 31, Rm. 5C27
Bethesda, MD 20892
Toll-Free: 800-222-2225
Toll-Free TTY: 800-222-4225
Website: www.nia.nih.gov
E-mail: niaic@nia.nih.gov

National Institutes of Health (NIH)
9000 Rockville Pike
Bethesda, MD 20892
Phone: 301-496-4000
TTY: 301-402-9612
Website: www.nih.gov
E-mail: NIHinfo@od.nih.gov

National Resources Defense Council (NRDC)
40 W. 20th St.
Fl. 11
New York, NY 10011
Phone: 212-727-2700
Website: www.nrdc.org
E-mail: nrdcinfo@nrdc.org

National Safety Council (NSC)
1121 Spring Lake Dr.
Itasca, IL 60143-3201
Toll-Free: 800-621-7615
Phone: 630-285-1121
Fax: 630-285-1434
Website: www.nsc.org
E-mail: customerservice@nsc.org

National Service Center for Environmental Publications (NSCEP)
P.O. Box 42419
Cincinnati, OH 45242-0419
Toll-Free: 800-490-9198
Fax: 301-604-3408
Website: www.epa.gov/ncepihom
E-mail: nscep@lmsolas.com

Occupational Safety and Health Administration (OSHA)
200 Constitution Ave. N.W.
Washington, DC 20210
Toll-Free: 800-321-6742
Toll-Free Fax: 877-889-5627
Website: www.osha.gov

Office of Children's Health Protection (OCHP)
U.S. Environmental Protection Agency (EPA)
1200 Pennsylvania Ave. N.W.
MC 1107-T
Washington, DC 20460
Phone: 202-564-2188
Fax: 202-564-2733
Website: www.epa.gov/aboutepa/
about-office-childrens-health-
protection-ochp

Office of Disease Prevention and Health Promotion (ODPHP)
1101 Wootton Pkwy
LL-100
Rockville, MD 20852
Website: www.healthypeople.gov
E-mail: healthypeople@hhs.gov

*Office of Environmental
Health Hazard Assessment
(OEHHA)*
California Environmental
Protection Agency (CalEPA)
1001 I St.
Sacramento, CA 95814
Phone: 916-323-2514
Website: www.oehha.ca.gov
E-mail: cepacomm@calepa.ca.gov

*Office on Women's Health
(OWH)*
U.S. Department of Health and
Human Services (HHS)
200 Independence Ave. S.W.
Rm. 712E
Washington, DC 20201
Toll-Free: 800-994-9662
Website: www.womenshealth.
gov

*Organic Consumers
Association (OCA)*
6771 S. Silver Hill Dr.
Finland, MN 55603
Phone: 218-226-4164
Fax: 218-353-7652
Website: www.
organicconsumers.org

*Pesticide Action Network
North America (PANNA)*
2029 University Ave.
Ste. 200
Berkeley, CA 94704
Phone: 510-788-9020
Website: www.panna.org

*Physicians for Social
Responsibility (PSR)*
1111 14th St. N.W.
Ste. 700
Washington, DC 20005
Phone: 202-667-4260
Website: www.
envirohealthaction.org
E-mail: psrnatl@psr.org

Right-to-Know Network
2040 S. St. N.W.
Fl. 2
Washington, DC 20009
Website: www.rtk.net
E-mail: matt.dempsey@chron.
com

*Science and Environmental
Health Network (SCHN)*
P.O Box 50733
Eugene, OR 97405
Website: www.sehn.org
E-mail: moreinfo@sehn.org

Toxic-Free Future
4649 Sunnyside Ave. N.
Ste. 540
Seattle, WA 98103
Phone: 206-632-1545
Website: www.toxicfreefuture.
org
E-mail: admin@toxicfreefuture.
org

*Union of Concerned
Scientists (UCS)*
Two Brattle Sq.
Cambridge, MA 02138-3780
Phone: 617-547-5552
Fax: 617-864-9405
Website: www.ucsusa.org

U.S. Access Board
1331 F St. N.W.
Ste. 1000
Washington, DC 20004-1111
Toll-Free: 800-872-2253
Phone: 202-272-0080
Toll-Free TTY: 800-993-2822
TTY: 202-272-0082
Fax: 202-272-0081
Website: www.access-board.gov
E-mail: info@access-board.gov

U.S. Consumer Product Safety Commission (CPSC)
4330 E. W. Hwy
Bethesda, MD 20814
Toll-Free: 800-638-2772
Phone: 301-504-7923
TTY: 301-595-7054
Fax: 301-504-0124; 301-504-0025
Website: www.cpsc.gov

U.S. Department of Agriculture (USDA)
1400 Independence Ave. S.W.
Washington, DC 20250
Toll-Free: 888-674-6854
Phone: 202-720-2791
Toll-Free TTY: 800-256-7072
Website: www.usda.gov

U.S. Environmental Protection Agency (EPA)
1200 Pennsylvania Ave. N.W.
Washington, DC 20005
Phone: 202-895-0420
Fax: 202-895-0438
Website: www.epa.gov

U.S. Food and Drug Administration (FDA)
10903 New Hampshire Ave.
Silver Spring, MD 20993
Toll-Free: 888-INFO-FDA
(888-463-6332)
Website: www.fda.gov

U.S. National Library of Medicine (NLM)
8600 Rockville Pike
Bethesda, MD 20894
Toll-Free: 888-346-3656
Fax: 301-402-1384
Website: www.nlm.nih.gov

Washington State Department of Health (DOH)
20425 72nd Ave. S.
Bldg. 2, Ste. 310
Kent, WA 98032
Toll-Free: 800-525-0127
Website: www.doh.wa.gov

World Resources Institute (WRI)
10 G St. N.E.
Ste. 800
Washington, DC 20002
Phone: 202-729-7600
Fax: 202-729-7610
Website: www.wri.org

Index

Index